THE ESSENTIALS OF HERBAL DRUGS

THE ESSENTIALS OF HERBAL DRUGS

Varsha Tiwari, PhD
Abhishek Tiwari, PhD
Ajay Sharma, PhD
Editors

APPLE ACADEMIC PRESS

First edition published 2026

Apple Academic Press Inc.
1265 Goldenrod Circle, NE,
Palm Bay, FL 32905 USA

760 Laurentian Drive, Unit 19,
Burlington, ON L7N 0A4, Canada

CRC Press
2385 NW Executive Center Drive,
Suite 320, Boca Raton FL 33431

4 Park Square, Milton Park,
Abingdon, Oxon, OX14 4RN, UK

Library and Archives Canada Cataloguing in Publication

CIP data on file with Canada Library and Archives

Library of Congress Cataloging-in-Publication Data

CIP data on file with US Library of Congress

ISBN: 978-1-99851-176-1 (hbk)
ISBN: 978-1-99851-177-8 (ebk)
DOI: 10.1201/9781998511778

About the Editors

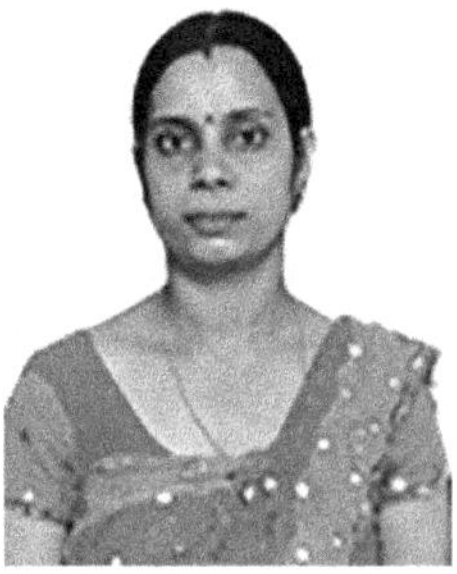

Varsha Tiwari, PhD
Professor, Amity Institute of Pharmacy, Amity University Uttar Pradesh, Lucknow Campus, India

Varsha Tiwari, PhD, is a Professor at the Amity Institute of Pharmacy, Amity University Uttar Pradesh, Lucknow Campus, India. Dr Tiwari has received more than nearly the equivalent of $1 million USD in grants from the Central Council for Research in Unani Medicine, New Delhi, India. She has been granted 18 Indian, three South African, and three Australian patents. In addition, she has submitted a number of patents for approval. She has published 10 books and 28 book chapters with Elsevier, Springer, Bentham, Wiley, and Astral International. She has published more than 65 research papers and has guided several doctoral, postgraduate, and graduate students. She has organized many conferences and also delivered many invited lectures at conferences. Dr. Varsha received a young scientist award, young author award, and pharmacy recognition award at the national level. She completed her doctorate at Uttarakhand Technical University in 2016 and her MPharm at M. S. Ramaiah University, Bengaluru, India.

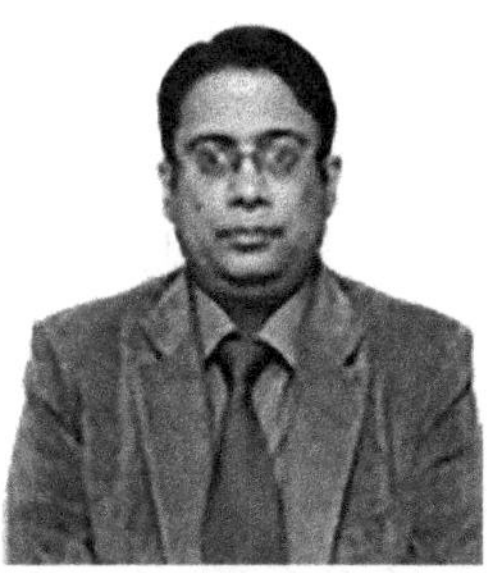

Abhishek Tiwari, PhD
Professor, Amity Institute of Pharmacy, Amity University Uttar Pradesh, Lucknow Campus, India

Abhishek Tiwari, PhD, is a Professor at the Amity Institute of Pharmacy, Amity University Uttar Pradesh, Lucknow Campus, India. Dr. Tiwari has received grants totaling more than $108,000 USD from various funding agencies, including the Central Council for

Research in Unani Medicine, New Delhi, India. He has been granted 32 patents and has filed nine patents for approval. Dr. Tiwari has published 76 papers in national and international journals and has authored more than 22 Indian and international books, along with 40 book chapters with Elsevier, Springer, Bentham, Wiley, and Astral International. He has supervised two PhD students and is currently guiding seven PhD students. Dr. Tiwari serves as an editorial board member for various national and international journals. He received the "Best Author Award" in 2019, the "Best Teacher Award" in 2019, and the "Outstanding Teacher Award" in 2014 and 2015. Dr. Tiwari completed his Bachelor of Pharmacy (BPharm) at Jiwaji University, Gwalior, India, his Master of Pharmacy (MPharm) at M. S. Ramaiah College of Pharmacy, Bangalore, and his PhD at Uttarakhand Technical University, Dehradun, India.

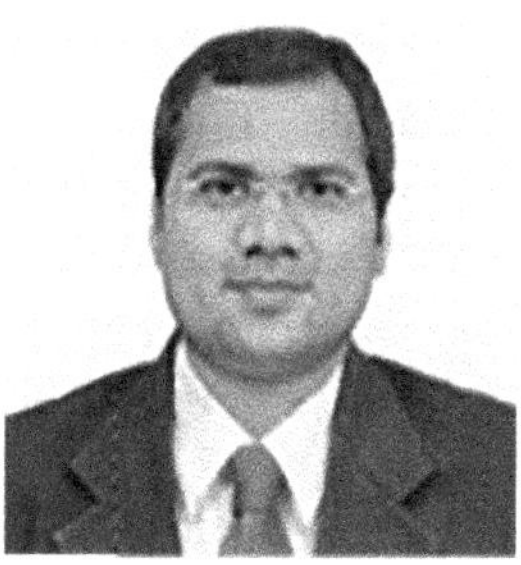

Ajay Sharma, PhD
Professor and Head, Department of Pharmacognosy, School of Pharmaceutical Sciences, Delhi Pharmaceutical Sciences and Research University, New Delhi, India

Ajay Sharma, PhD, is currently working as Professor and Head of the Department of Pharmacognosy, School of Pharmaceutical Sciences, Delhi Pharmaceutical Sciences and Research University, New Delhi, India. He has more than 15 years of teaching and research experience. His research areas include drug discovery and development from natural sources, ethnopharmacology, natural product chemistry, metabolomics, plant biotechnology, bioactivity-guided fractionation, and bioconversions. He has published more than 90 research articles in peer-reviewed journals of national and international repute. He has presented more than 150 papers at national and international conferences. Additionally, he has contributed four books and six book chapters and has published 10 Indian patents. He has received research grants from the Central Council for Research in Unani Medicine (CCRUM), the Ministry of AYUSH, the Department of Biotechnology (DBT), the All India Council for Technical Education (AICTE), and the Madhya Pradesh Council of Science and Technology (MPCST).

Dr. Sharma has been the recipient of several prestigious awards, including the Claude Leon Foundation Scholarship (2013), University of KwaZulu-Natal, Pietermaritzburg, Research Center for Plant Growth and Development, South Africa; the Postdoctoral Research Scholarship, College of Pharmacy, International Islamic University, Pahang, Malaysia; the Best Teacher Award during the Eminent Teachers Award-2019 Program, organized by Amity University Madhya Pradesh in conjunction with Dainik Bhaskar, Gwalior; the APP Young Achiever Award during the Two-Day International Conference on "Current Trends in Pharmaceutical Education and Research," Edinburgh International College, Biratnagar, Nepal; the Innovation Award for Scientific Research (2018); and the AYUSH Award of the Central Council for Research in Ayurvedic Sciences (CCRAS) 2017 under the category "Best Research Paper Award." He is a member of various national and international scientific bodies. He has also been listed among the top 2% of scientists as per the Stanford University rankings for the past two years. He obtained his PhD from Poona College of Pharmacy, Bharati Vidyapeeth University, Pune. During his studies, he was awarded a Postdoctoral Research Fellowship from Yeungnam University, Republic of Korea; a Senior Research Fellowship from the Department of Biotechnology (DBT), New Delhi, India; and a Junior Research Fellowship from the University Grants Commission (UGC), New Delhi, India.

Contents

Contributors

Suneetha Achanti
Department of Pharmaceutical Analysis, KVSR Siddhartha College of Pharmaceutical Sciences, Vijayawada, Andhra Pradesh, India

Muhammad Arif
Department of Pharmaceutical Chemistry, Faculty of Pharmacy, Integral University, Lucknow, Uttar Pradesh, India

Tejaswini T. Asawe
Department of Pharmaceutical Chemistry, Siddhi's Institute of Pharmacy, Thane, Maharashtra, India

M. S. Ashawat
Laureate Institute of Pharmacy, Kathog, Kangra, Himachal Pradesh, India

Ashish Baldi
Pharma Innovation Lab, Department of Pharmaceutical Sciences and Technology, Maharaja Ranjit Singh Punjab Technical University, Bathinda, Punjab, India

Deshraj Chumbale
Amrutwahini College of Pharmacy, Sangamner, Ahmednagar, Maharashtra, India

Savita S. Deokar
Department of Pharmaceutics, School of Pharmacy, Pimpri Chinchwad University, Vadgaon, Sate Maval, Pune, Maharashtra, India

Syed Kaynat Fatima
Department of Molecular Biology, Staffordshire University, Stoke-on-Trent, UK

Neeraj Kumar Fuloria
Faculty of Pharmacy, AIMST University, Kedah, Malaysia

Shivkanya Fuloria
Faculty of Pharmacy, AIMST University, Kedah, Malaysia

Mansour Ghorbanpour
Department of Medicinal Plants, Faculty of Agriculture and Natural Resources, Arak University, Iran

Sahil Hussain
Department of Pharmaceutical Chemistry, Faculty of Pharmacy, Integral University, Lucknow, Uttar Pradesh, India

Tomy M. Joseph
Department of Polymer Technology, Faculty of Chemistry, Gdańsk University of Technology, Gdańsk, Poland

Archita Katrolia
Department of Pharmaceutics, College of Pharmacy, JSS Academy of Technical Education, Noida, Uttar Pradesh, India

Krishna G. Khamkar
Department of Pharmaceutics, Siddhi's Institute of Pharmacy, Thane, Maharashtra, India

Mohemmed Faraz Khan
Department of Pharmaceutical Chemistry, Faculty of Pharmacy, Integral University, Lucknow, Uttar Pradesh, India

Ajay Kumar
Department of Pharmacology, Sardar Patel College of Pharmacy, Gorakhpur, Uttar Pradesh, India

Anoop Kumar
Department of Pharmacology, Delhi Pharmaceutical Sciences and Research University (DPSRU), New Delhi, India

Arun Kumar
Department of Pharmaceutical Chemistry, Faculty of Pharmacy, Integral University, Lucknow, Uttar Pradesh, India

Deepak Kumar
Faculty of Pharmaceutical Sciences, Mahayogi Gorakhnath University Gorakhpur, Uttar Pradesh, India

Jayant Kumar
Department of Pharmaceutical Sciences,
Hemwati Nandan Bahuguna Garhwal University (A Central University), Srinagar, Jammu and Kashmir, India

Jitendra Kumar
Department of Pharmacy, MJP Rohilkhand University, Bareilly, Uttar Pradesh, India

Jitender Madan
Department of Pharmaceutics, National Institute of Pharmaceutical Education and Research, Hyderabad, Telangana, India

Debarshi Kar Mahapatra
Associate Professor, Chitkara College of Pharmacy, Chitkara University, Rajpura, Punjab, India

Arya Lakshmi Marisetti
Department of Pharmacognosy and Phytochemistry, School of Pharmaceutical Sciences,
Delhi Pharmaceutical Sciences and Research University, New Delhi, India

Popat Mohite
AET's St. John Institute of Pharmacy and Research, Palghar, Maharashtra, India

Mohd. Mujeeb
Department of Pharmacognosy and Phytochemistry, School of Pharmaceutical Education and Research, Jamia Hamdard, New Delhi, India

Shubham Munde
AET's St. John Institute of Pharmacy and Research, Palghar, Maharashtra, India

Mohd. Mursal
Department of Pharmaceutical Chemistry, Faculty of Pharmacy, Integral University, Lucknow, Uttar Pradesh, India

Subh Naman
Pharma Innovation Lab, Department of Pharmaceutical Sciences and Technology,
Maharaja Ranjit Singh Punjab Technical University, Bathinda, Punjab, India; Faculty of Pharmaceutical Sciences, ICFAI University, Himachal Pradesh, India

Ved Pal
Department of Pharmacognosy, College of Pharmacy, JSS Academy of Technical Education, Noida, Uttar Pradesh, India

Ramdas Pandhare
MES's College of Pharmacy, Sonai, Ahmednagar, Maharashtra, India

Vijender Kumar Pareekh
Department of Pharmacognosy and Phytochemistry, School of Pharmaceutical Sciences, Delhi Pharmaceutical Sciences and Research University, New Delhi, India

Praveen Kumar Pasala
Department of Pharmacology, Raghavendra Institute of Pharmaceutical Education and Research, Anantapuramu, Andhra Pradesh, India

D. S. N. B. K. Prasanth
School of Pharmacy and Technology Management, SVKM's Narsee Monjee Institute of Management Studies (NMIMS), Polepally SEZ, TSIIC, Jadcherla, Mahbubnagar, Hyderabad, India

Abhijeet Puri
AET's St. John Institute of Pharmacy and Research, Palghar, Maharashtra, India

Vilas Shivaji Sawale
Pathrikar Institute of Pharmacy, Aurangabad, Maharashtra, India

Prerna Saxena
Department of Pharmacognosy and Phytochemistry, School of Pharmaceutical Education and Research, Jamia Hamdard, New Delhi, India

Shoheb S. Shaikh
NN Sattha College of Pharmacy, Ahilyanager, Maharashtra, India

Surabhi Shakya
Department of Pharmacy, MJP Rohilkhand University, Bareilly, Uttar Pradesh, India

Sanyam Sharma
Pharma Innovation Lab, Department of Pharmaceutical Sciences and Technology, Maharaja Ranjit Singh Punjab Technical University, Bathinda, Punjab, India

Jyoti Shrivastava
Department of Pharmaceutical Chemistry, The Oxford College of Pharmacy, Hongasandra, Bangalore, India

Kuldeep Singh
Department of Pharmaceutical Chemistry, Faculty of Pharmacy, Integral University, Lucknow, Uttar Pradesh, India

Pradeep Singh
Department of Pharmacy, College of Health Sciences, Debre Tabor University, Ethiopia

Rohit Singh
Department of Pharmaceutical Chemistry, College of Pharmacy, JSS Academy of Technical Education, Noida, Uttar Pradesh, India

Sudarshan Singh
Office of Research Administration, Chiang Mai University, Chiang Mai, Thailand; Faculty of Pharmacy, Chiang Mai University, Chiang Mai, Thailand

Varinder Singh
Pharma Innovation Lab, Department of Pharmaceutical Sciences and Technology, Maharaja Ranjit Singh Punjab Technical University, Bathinda, Punjab, India

Anuj K. Srivastava
Department of Pharmacognosy, Sardar Patel College of Pharmacy, Gorakhpur, Uttar Pradesh, India

Ashima Thakur
Faculty of Pharmaceutical Sciences, ICFAI University, Baddi, Himachal Pradesh, India

Prashant Upadhyay
School of Pharmaceutical Sciences, Faculty of Pharmacy, IFTM University, Moradabad, Uttar Pradesh, India

Sukirti Upadhyay
School of Pharmaceutical Sciences, Faculty of Pharmacy, IFTM University, Moradabad, Uttar Pradesh, India

Amit Kumar Verma
Department of Pharmacy, MJP Rohilkhand University, Bareilly, Uttar Pradesh, India

Harshal A. Vishe
Department of Pharmaceutical Quality Assurance, Siddhi's Institute of Pharmacy, Thane, Maharashtra, India

Preface

The book *The Essentials of Herbal Drugs* is a comprehensive guide to understanding the fundamental aspects of herbal drugs and their significance in modern healthcare. Comprising eleven insightful chapters, this book serves as a valuable resource for exploring the rich history, quality control measures, cultivation practices, metabolic pathways, extraction techniques, regulatory considerations, and future trends of herbal medicines.

- **Chapter 1: Introduction to Herbal Drugs**

  Throughout history, herbal drugs have played a crucial role in traditional healing practices across cultures. From ancient civilizations to modern times, the use of plants and plant extracts for medicinal purposes has been deeply ingrained in human society. This chapter introduces herbal drugs, highlighting their diverse forms and therapeutic benefits.

- **Chapter 2: Quality Control of Herbal Drugs**

  Quality control is essential for ensuring the safety and efficacy of herbal medicines. This chapter focuses on the methods and parameters used to evaluate the quality of natural products, addressing concerns such as adulteration and standardization.

- **Chapter 3: Cultivation, Collection and Processing of Drugs of Natural Origin: The Quality Perceptions**

  Cultivation, collection, processing, and storage practices significantly impact the potency of medicinal plants. This chapter discusses the factors influencing the quality of herbal drugs at every stage, emphasizing the importance of proper cultivation techniques and environmental conditions.

- **Chapter 4: Metabolic Pathways in Higher Plants and Their Determination**

  Understanding metabolic pathways in plants is key to unlocking the potential of herbal medicines. This chapter reviews the intricate biochemical processes that lead to the production of secondary metabolites, which are essential for therapeutic purposes.

- **Chapter 5: Evolving Approaches in the Extraction and Assessment of Herbal Medicines: Progress in Methodologies and Utilization of Analytical Instruments**

  The extraction and assessment of herbal medicines require advanced methodologies and analytical instruments. This chapter discusses evolving approaches in extraction techniques and the utilization of spectroscopy, chromatography, and electrophoresis for analyzing herbal constituents.

- **Chapter 6: Isolation, Identification and Analysis of Phytoconstituents**

  The isolation, identification, and analysis of phytoconstituents provide valuable insights into the bioactive compounds present in plants. This chapter discusses classical and modern separation methods as well as analytical techniques for characterizing phytochemicals.

- **Chapter 7: Advancements in Plant Tissue Culture: A Historical Perspective**

  Plant tissue culture offers innovative opportunities for propagating plants and studying their medicinal properties. This chapter explores the principles of tissue culture and its applications in pharmacognosy.

- **Chapter 8: Nutraceuticals**

  Nutraceuticals, derived from food sources with added health benefits, represent a growing segment of the herbal medicine market. This chapter examines the regulatory requirements and challenges associated with nutraceuticals.

- **Chapter 9: Biological Screening, Toxicity and Regulations of Herbal Drugs**

  Biological screening, toxicity assessment, and regulatory guidelines are crucial for ensuring the safety and efficacy of herbal drugs. This chapter provides an overview of these aspects, emphasizing the importance of evidence-based practices.

- **Chapter 10: Pharmacovigilance of Natural Products**

  Pharmacovigilance plays a vital role in monitoring the safety of natural products. This chapter discusses the challenges and future perspectives of pharmacovigilance for herbal medicines.

- **Chapter 11: Conclusion and Future Trends in Phyto-Pharmaceutical Research**

  In conclusion, this chapter explores future trends in phyto-pharmaceutical research, highlighting emerging opportunities for drug discovery and the potential of natural compounds in healthcare.

The Essentials of Herbal Medicine aims to serve as a comprehensive resource for students, researchers, and practitioners interested in herbal drugs and their therapeutic applications. We hope that this book will inspire further exploration and innovation in the field of herbal medicine, ultimately contributing to the advancement of healthcare worldwide.

We extend our heartfelt gratitude to the contributing authors whose chapters were instrumental in completing this book. Our indebtedness extends to all who supported its completion, particularly Apple Academic Press (CRC Press), whose role has been indispensable.

Special thanks go to Ms. Sheetal Kumar, Assistant Publishing Manager, for helpful demeanor and encouragement. Furthermore, we express our gratitude to Prof. M. P. Pandey, Vice-Chancellor, and Prof. Navneet Verma of IFTM University, Moradabad, India, for their generous support. Lastly, we offer profound thanks to our parents, whose unwavering encouragement has played a pivotal role in bringing this book to fruition.

—Editors

Introduction

The Essentials of Herbal Drugs provides a thorough exploration of the complex world of herbal medicines, emphasizing their significance in modern healthcare systems. Herbal drugs have been an integral part of traditional healing practices across various cultures for centuries. From ancient civilizations to contemporary society, the use of plants and plant extracts for medicinal purposes has been deeply embedded in human history. This book aims to bridge the gap between traditional knowledge and modern scientific advancements, offering a comprehensive guide to understanding the fundamental aspects of herbal drugs and their increasing relevance in today's healthcare landscape.

The journey begins with an overview of herbal drugs, examining their diverse forms and therapeutic benefits. The first chapter sets the stage by tracing the historical significance of herbal medicines, highlighting their role in traditional healing practices and their evolution into modern therapeutic agents. It underscores the broad spectrum of herbal drugs, ranging from crude plant materials to highly refined plant extracts, each offering distinct health benefits. This foundational understanding paves the way for more in-depth discussions in the subsequent chapters.

Quality control is paramount in ensuring the safety and efficacy of herbal medicines. This book focuses on various methods and parameters used to evaluate the quality of natural products, addressing critical concerns such as adulteration, contamination, and standardization of herbal drugs. By emphasizing rigorous quality control measures, it highlights the importance of maintaining high standards to ensure that herbal medicines are both safe and effective for consumer use.

The potency and therapeutic efficacy of medicinal plants are significantly influenced by their cultivation, collection, processing, and storage practices. This book discusses the various factors that impact the quality of herbal drugs at every stage of their production, emphasizing the importance of proper cultivation techniques, environmental conditions, and sustainable harvesting practices. By providing insights into the entire lifecycle of herbal drugs, it underscores the need for meticulous handling to preserve the integrity and potency of medicinal plants.

Understanding the metabolic pathways in plants is essential for unlocking their full therapeutic potential. This book reviews the complex biochemical processes that lead to the production of secondary metabolites, which are crucial for the medicinal properties of plants. It explores the intricate networks of metabolic pathways and the techniques used to study these processes, offering a deeper understanding of how plants synthesize bioactive compounds.

Advancements in extraction techniques and analytical instruments have revolutionized the field of herbal medicine. This book discusses evolving methodologies for extracting herbal constituents and the use of sophisticated instruments such as spectroscopy, chromatography, and electrophoresis for their analysis. It highlights progress in these areas and how they contribute to the accurate assessment of the efficacy and safety of herbal medicines.

The isolation, identification, and analysis of phytoconstituents provide critical insights into the bioactive compounds present in plants. This book delves into both classical and modern methods for separating and characterizing phytochemicals, emphasizing the importance of understanding the chemical composition of herbal drugs to fully harness their therapeutic potential.

Plant tissue culture offers innovative opportunities for the propagation of medicinal plants and the study of their properties. This book traces the historical development of plant tissue culture techniques and their applications in pharmacognosy, discussing the principles and benefits of tissue culture and highlighting its role in producing high-quality plant material for medicinal use.

Nutraceuticals, derived from food sources with additional health benefits, represent a growing segment of the herbal medicine market. This book explores the concept of nutraceuticals, their regulatory requirements, and the challenges associated with their development and marketing, offering an overview of how nutraceuticals bridge the gap between nutrition and pharmacology while presenting new opportunities for preventive healthcare.

Ensuring the safety and efficacy of herbal drugs involves rigorous biological screening and toxicity assessment. This book provides an overview of the methods used to evaluate the pharmacological activity and safety profiles of herbal medicines, discusses the regulatory frameworks governing their approval and marketing, and emphasizes the importance of evidence-based practices in their development.

Pharmacovigilance plays a crucial role in monitoring the safety of natural products. This book examines the challenges and future perspectives of pharmacovigilance in the context of herbal medicines, highlighting the need for robust surveillance systems to detect and manage adverse effects, ensuring that herbal drugs remain safe for widespread use.

In its final chapter, this book explores emerging trends and future directions in phyto-pharmaceutical research. It highlights the potential of natural compounds in drug discovery and the innovative approaches being developed to harness their therapeutic benefits. Emphasizing ongoing research efforts aimed at integrating herbal medicines into mainstream healthcare, it presents a promising future for phyto-pharmaceuticals.

Designed to be a comprehensive resource for students, researchers, and practitioners interested in herbal medicine, *The Essentials of Herbal Drugs* combines traditional knowledge with modern scientific insights. This book aims to inspire further exploration and innovation, ultimately contributing to the advancement of healthcare worldwide.

CHAPTER 1

Introduction to Herbal Drugs

SUKIRTI UPADHYAY,[1,*] PRASHANT UPADHYAY,[2]
NEERAJ KUMAR FULORIA,[3] and SHIVKANYA FULORIA[3]

[1]*School of Pharmaceutical Sciences, Faculty of Pharmacy, IFTM University, Moradabad, Uttar Pradesh, India*

[2]*School of Pharmaceutical Sciences, IFTM University, Moradabad, Uttar Pradesh, India*

[2]*Faculty of Pharmacy, AIMST University, Kedah, Malaysia*

*Corresponding author

ABSTRACT

Herbal drugs, also known as herbal medicines or phytotherapeutics, involve the utilization of plants and plant extracts for medicinal purposes. These remedies have been integral to traditional healing practices across cultures for centuries. The active compounds in herbs can offer therapeutic benefits, and herbal medicine encompasses a wide range of forms, including teas, powders, fermented formulations, tinctures, tablets, capsules, and topical applications. While herbal remedies are often considered natural, it is crucial to approach their use with awareness, considering potential interactions and consulting healthcare professionals for guidance. The history of herbal drugs dates back thousands of years, with various cultures incorporating plant-based remedies into their traditional medicine. Ancient Chinese, Egyptian, Indian, and Greco-Roman civilizations extensively used herbs for therapeutic purposes. In the Middle Ages, herbal knowledge was preserved and expanded upon by Islamic scholars. The Renaissance saw a restoration of interest in herbalism, and by the 19th century, herbal medicine was widely practiced.

The Essentials of Herbal Drugs. Varsha Tiwari, Abhishek Tiwari, and Ajay Sharma (Eds.)

DOI: 10.1201/9781998511778-1

In the 20th century, the rise of modern medicine led to a decline in herbal remedies in Western societies, but interest persisted and experienced a resurgence in recent decades. Today, herbal drugs are studied for their potential medicinal benefits, and some traditional remedies have been integrated into mainstream healthcare. The sources of herbal drugs vary from organized parts of plants to unorganized parts of plants. Therefore, there is a need for proper identification of herbs. These herbal drugs are classified on the basis of various parameters.

1.1 INTRODUCTION TO HERBAL DRUGS

1.1.1 SOURCES OF DRUGS

1.1.1.1 PLANTS

For centuries, plants have been a major source of medicinal compounds. Plant extracts are the source of many medications, such as analgesics, anti-inflammatory agents, and anticancer medications. Aspirin, derived from willow bark, and the cancer treatment Paclitaxel, derived from Pacific yew trees, are two prominent examples. Pharmacognosy is the study of pharmaceuticals originating from plants. German botanist Seydler is credited with coining the term "Pharmacognosy" [1].

The earliest source of drugs is plants. The two main categories of plants are food and drugs. The majority of medicines used to be made from plants. Nearly each part of the plant is utilized, including the stem, roots, fruits, and leaves [2] (Figure 1.1).

1. **Leaves:** *Digitalis purpurea* leaves are the source of the cardiac glycoside's digoxin and digitoxin. The essential ingredient in cough syrup is eucalyptus oil, which is extracted from eucalyptus leaves. Cigarette leaves contain nicotine. The leaves of *Atropa belladonna* contain atropine.

2. **Flowers:** *Vincarosea* yields vincristine and vinblastine, while clove yields eugenol. Rose provides the tonic rose water.

3. **Fruits:** Senna pods contain the purgative anthracene, which is used to treat constipation. The cholinomimetic agent physostigmine is produced by Calabar beans.

4. **Seeds:** Nux vomica seeds contain strychnine, a stimulant of the central nervous system. Castor oil comes from castor seeds.

5. **Roots:** Ipecacuanha root yields emetin, which is used to cause vomiting in cases of unintentional poisoning. It possesses amoebicidal qualities as well. Reserpine, a hypotensive drug, is produced by *Rauwolfia serpentina*. The medication reserpine was used to treat hypertension.
6. **Bark:** Cinchona bark contains the antimalarial medications quinine and quinidine. Quinidine possesses antiarrhythmic qualities as well.
7. **Stem:** The well-established hepatoprotective Kalmegh [3].

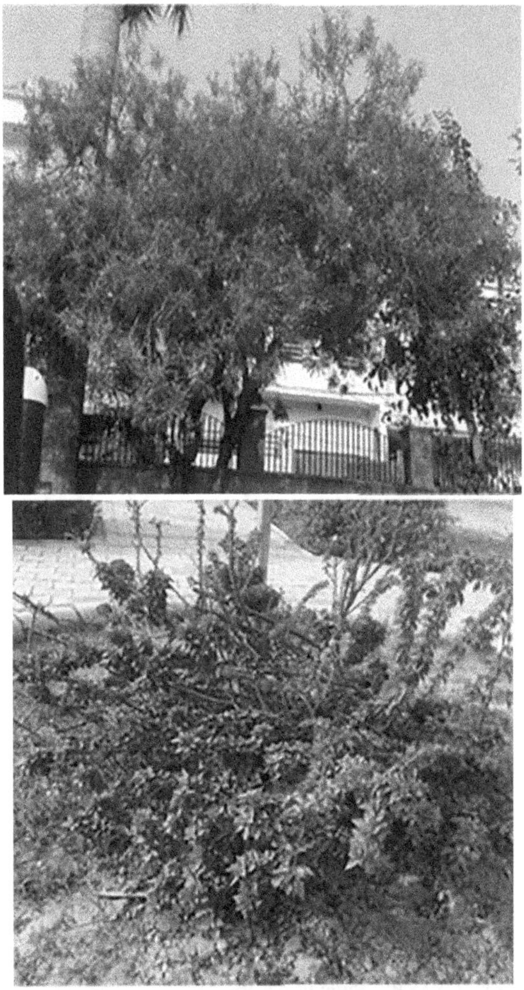

FIGURE 1.1 *(Continued)*

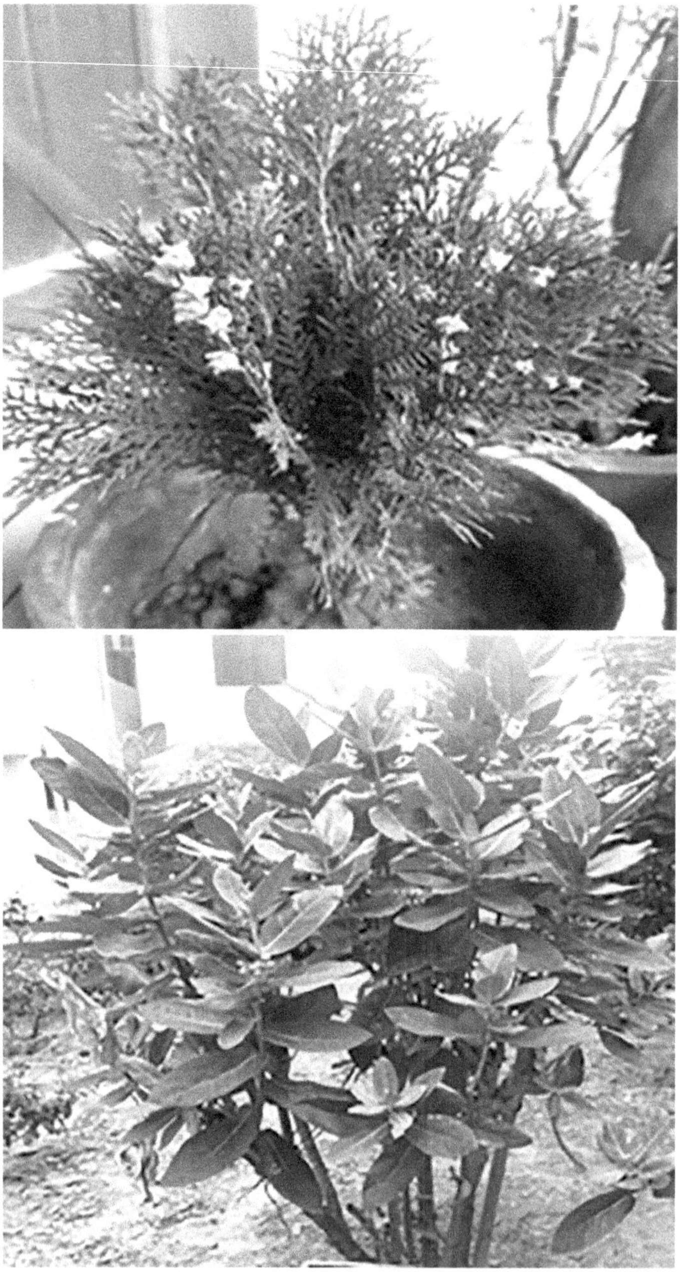

FIGURE 1.1 Some medicinal plants – (a) *Nerium oleander*; (b) *Bougainvillea glabra*; (c) *Thuja orientalis*; and (d) *Calotropis procera*.

1.1.1.2 ANIMALS

Some medications come from animals or animal byproducts. For example, pancreas tissue from animals such as pigs and cows were originally used to produce insulin, which is used to treat diabetes. The medicinal potential of snake venom has been investigated, and the pharmaceutical potential of materials derived from marine organisms is also being explored. Animals and the natural world are still great sources of information for drug research. Hormones, enzymes, and animal organs used in extractives, as well as bile acids, comprise the main category of animal products used in medicine. Pancreatin, pepsin, fibrinolysin, trypsin, chymotrypsin, and bile are examples of enzymes. Thyroid hormones, conjugated estrogens, insulin, gonadotropins, vasopressin, and oxytocin are among the hormones. Insulin is obtained from the pancreas and is used to treat diabetes. Thyroxin, which is needed for growth, differentiation, and metabolism, can be obtained from sheep thyroid. Vitamins A and D are found in cod liver. Vaccines are made with the blood of animals. Dried, fully grown female cochineal insects are used to make cosmetics, medications, and food coloring. Cochineal also contains carminic acid [4].

1.1.1.3 MARINES

Over 5000 species of marine life can be found in the seas and oceans that cover the majority of the planet's surface. Numerous substances have demonstrated strong biological activity. The recognized marine medicinal products in Western medicine include agar, alginic acid, carrageenan, protamine sulfate, spermaceti, cod, and halibut liver oils [5]. Seaweeds, or macroalgae, have long been utilized as unrefined medications to treat iodine deficiency conditions like goiter. Certain seaweeds have also been used to treat anemia in pregnant women and as sources of extra vitamins. Many novel compounds with biological activities, including antiviral, antibacterial, antitumor, antiparasitic, anticoagulant, anti-inflammatory, antimicrobial, and cardiovascular products, have been isolated from marine organisms over the past 30 to 40 years. Bio-indol derivatives (anti-inflammatory), octopamine (cardiovascular agent), bryostatin (anticancer agent), and ara-A (semisynthetic antiviral agent) have been identified.

Marine drugs, or bioactive compounds with potential medicinal uses, are abundant in marine organisms. These include compounds derived from different invertebrates, algae, and marine sponges. Marine-derived compounds have demonstrated potential for use in antiviral drugs, pain relief, and cancer treatment. Searches for novel medicinal compounds in the diverse marine ecosystem are ongoing. Miscellaneous marine compounds include Kainic acid (anti-convulsant), Domoic acid (anti-ascariatic), Flustramine (muscle relaxant), and Aplysinopin (antidepressant) [6].

1.1.1.4 TISSUE CULTURE

Tissue culture is a biological research technique whereby tissue fragments from plants or animals are cultivated in artificial environments to maintain their viability and functionality. A solitary cell, a population of cells, or an entire or partial organ may make up the cultured tissue [7]. In culture, cells can divide, vary in shape, size, or function, show specialized behavior (muscle cells, for instance, can contract), or engage in cellular interactions [8].

1.1.1.4.1 Ancient expansions

German zoologist Wilhelm Roux experimented with tissue culture in 1885, growing material from a chick embryo in a warm saline solution. But in 1907, American zoologist Ross G. Harrison made a significant breakthrough when he showed how frog nerve cell methods could grow in a clotted lymph medium. Harrison's method was later improved upon by French surgeon Alexis Carrel and his subordinate Montrose Burrows, who documented their preliminary findings in a sequence of papers published in 1910–1911. Tissue culture was first described, and the term was coined by Carrel and Burrows. Subsequently, several researchers were able to successfully cultivate animal cells by employing a range of biological fluids as culture media, including tissue extracts, blood serum, lymph, and plasma. Mammalian embryonic stem cells could be successfully grown *in vitro* thanks to techniques developed in the 1980s and 1990s. These discoveries eventually made it possible to create and maintain human embryonic stem cell lines, which improved knowledge of human biology and aided in the development of new treatments and regenerative drug techniques [9].

1.1.1.4.2 Culture atmospheres

Cells can be cultured in a chemically defined synthetic medium, a biological culture medium like blood serum or tissue extract, or a combination of the two. The right amounts of the nutrients needed for the cells being studied must be present in a medium that is either suitably alkaline or acidic. Cultures are frequently developed as single cell layers on glass or plastic surfaces, or as suspensions in liquid or semisolid media [8]. To begin a culture, a small model of tissue is placed on top of or within the medium. The culture is then incubated in the flask, tube, or plate, usually at a temperature that is comparable to the natural environment of the tissue. Sterile environments are maintained to avoid microbial contamination. Occasionally, cultures are initiated from single cells, resulting in constant biological populations referred to as replicas. After being placed in culture conditions, single cells usually form colonies in 10–14 days [7].

1.1.1.4.3 Primary cultures and well-known cell lines

The two key varieties of cultures are primary (mortal) cultures and cultures of reputable (immortal) cell lines [9]. Primary cultures are composed of normal cells, tissues, or organs that are taken straight from tissue obtained through biopsy from a living organism [10]. One of the advantages of primary cultures is that they are essentially models of the typical purpose of the cell, tissue, or organ under study. However, samples that are cultured for longer periods of time typically accumulate more mutations, which can change the function of cells and the structure of chromosomes. Primitive societies are also usually mortal. Cells age by multiplying for a mere 50 to 100 generations, after which their rate of multiplication sharply declines. The term “Hayflick limit” refers to the point in primary cultures where cells undergo replicative senescence, or stop growing. It was discovered by American microbiologist Leonard Hayflick [11]. Well-known cell lines, on the other hand, have an endless lifespan. These cell lines are typically obtained from patient biopsies of their tumors, or they may be produced from primary cells that have experienced alterations that allow them to pass the Hayflick limit and multiply indefinitely. Like cells in primary cultures, established line cells also undergo character-changing mutations over time. Therefore, in order for researchers from various laboratories to match the outcomes of their experiments conducted with the same cell lines, they first need to verify which cell line they are working with. The process of authentication verifies the identity of cells by comparing their DNA profile to a standard or known profile specific to that cell line. Treatment of cultured cells and tissues [12].

A microscope can be used to directly examine live cultures, or it can be used to view them through still and moving images captured through the lens. For additional examination, it is also possible to kill, fix (preserve), and stain cells, tissues, and organs. Samples can also be thinly sectioned and embedded (in resin, for example) after they have been fixed, which will expose additional information when examined under a light or electron microscope. Tissue-cultured cells undergo a multitude of different experimental protocols. For example, viruses, drugs, vitamins, hormones, bacteria that cause disease, or substances that could cause cancer could be added to the culture. Next, following the observation of the cells, researchers look for both general alterations in the actions or roles of the cells and specific molecular changes, such as adjustments in the aspect of a specific protein or gene [13].

1.1.1.4.4 Biotic visions

Numerous biological science discoveries have been made possible by tissue culture. For instance, it has disclosed fundamental details about the makeup and structure of cells; their biochemical, inherited, and generative activities; their nourishment, metabolism, particular roles, and aging and healing methods; the impact of physical, chemical, and biological agents (like viruses as well as drugs) on cells; and the distinctions between normal and aberrant cells, such as tumor cells [14]. Tissue culture research has aided in the classification of tumors, the discovery of infections, chromosomal abnormalities, and enzyme deficits, as well as the development and testing of medications and vaccines. Since it was discovered that some viruses can also grow in tissue culture, vaccines against poliomyelitis, influenza, mumps, measles, and other transmissible diseases have been created using this technique. Interferon is one of the viral inhibitors that have been produced by cell cultures. Cultures of cells or organs can also produce hormones. Tissue transplant recipients and potential donors can be matched using cultured white blood cells from two different people.

It is possible to determine whether a pregnant woman's fetus has specific chromosomal faults, such as those linked to Down syndrome and others, by removing and culturing her cells [15].

The field of somatic cell genetics has made significant progress in the detection and analysis of chromosome abnormalities and congenital disorders. Through the use of tissue culture techniques, a variety of hybrid cells containing chromosomes from different species have been cultured, enabling the distinct definition of the functions of individual chromosomes. Techniques for identifying environmental substances that may cause gene damage have been developed, and tissue culture studies have shed light on the hereditary sources of some genetic illnesses [9]. The identification of certain genes and chromosomal abnormalities linked to the disease has illuminated the nature of some cancers. Somatic cell heredity techniques have also been applied to plant cells; for instance, new strains of cereal crops with enhanced nutritional qualities have been developed through the use of these techniques.

The process of aseptically growing cells, tissues, or organs in a synthetic medium is known as tissue culture. The typical steps in the process are as follows: culture is the *in vitro* gardening of plant cells or tissue in a liquid or semisolid well-defined nutrient medium, under aseptic and controlled environmental conditions, with the goal of producing primary and secondary metabolites or regenerating plants. This method offers an alternative approach to issues brought about by the current rate of extinction and the devastation of the ecosystem and flora. A nutrient medium and a well-equipped culture laboratory are necessary for the entire process. This procedure includes a number of steps, including sterilizing the explant (a plant tissue source), inoculating and incubating glassware and extra accessories, and preparing nutrient medium with inorganic and organic salts, along with vitamins, amino acids, and plant growth hormones [16].

1. **Tissue Selection:** Usually from plants or animals, a tiny piece of tissue is chosen as the starting sample.
2. **Surface Sterilization:** To get rid of impurities, the tissue is surface sterilized.
3. **Culture Medium:** The tissue is submerged in a rich culture medium that is fortified with growth regulators, vitamins, and other necessary nutrients.

4. **Incubation:** To promote cell growth, the culture is kept under carefully regulated lighting, humidity, and temperature levels.
5. **Subculturing:** To ensure continuous growth as the cells multiply, they are periodically moved to new medium [17].

The production of therapeutic proteins and vaccines, as well as biological research, heavily relies on tissue culture techniques.

Drugs can be made from different sections of plants:

1. **Leaves:** Marijuana (cannabis), coca (used to make cocaine), and tea leaves (for caffeine) are a few examples.
2. **Roots:** The opium poppy, which yields opioids like morphine, is one example of a plant whose roots are used to make certain drugs.
3. **Flowers:** Certain plants, such as cannabis, opium poppies, and some types of mushrooms, release psychoactive compounds in their blossoms.
4. **Seeds:** Two types of seeds that may contain psychoactive substances are morning glory and poppy seeds.

It is noteworthy that there are significant variations in the usage and legality of these substances, with certain ones being subject to stringent guidelines or outright bans.

1.1.1.4.5 Phytopharmaceutical in plant tissue culture

Due to young, dispersed, rapidly dividing cells that mature slowly and divide into meristem tissue, there is a poor yield of phytoconstituents. Sluggish-growing cells in a massed arrangement vary in product production over time in tissue culture [8].

These days, tissue culture technology is thought to be an extremely effective method for producing these phytochemicals under carefully monitored circumstances. Plants are widely used in the treatment of human ailments and are a rich source of many secondary metabolites, including flavonoids, alkaloids, terpenoids, polyphenols, and saponins [18].

Due to the repression and dormancy of the desired biosynthetic pathway, as well as the non-excretion of the product from tissue culture, two types of tissue culture are used to avoid these problems: hairy root culture and immobilized cell systems [19].

The following phytoconstituents are obtained in large amounts from tissue culture:

- Anthraquinone: 18%
- Ajmalicine: 1.8%
- Benzylisoquinoline: 15%
- Berberine alkaloid: 10%
- Diosgenin: 7.8%
- Acetoside: 5%
- Nicotine: 5%
- Rosmarinic acid: 21.4%
- Serpentine: 2.2%
- Shikmic Acid: 10%
- Shikonin: 12.4%

The productivity for economic consideration is defined as grams of product per liter of culture per day. The overall production of secondary metabolites in culture is proportional to the rate of accumulation. Generally, cultures produce 1 gram per liter. The hairy root culture of *Catharanthus roseus* is capable of producing ajmalicine and serpentine [20].

1.1.1.4.6 Applications

Biochemical conversions, clonal propagation (micro-propagation), immobilized plant cell production, and phytopharmaceutical production are all necessary. There is a need for highly skilled personnel. It is an intricate and challenging technique [21].

The relatively new field of biosynthetic sources (genetically engineered drugs) is being developed through the integration of findings from immunology, immune pharmacology, DNA splicing, recombinant DNA technology, molecular biology, and gene splicing. Biopharmaceuticals, biologics, bioengineered products, recombinant DNA-expressed products, or genetically engineered drugs are medications created utilizing living organisms with the aid of biotechnology or genetic engineering. Recombinant insulin and the hepatitis B vaccine are two examples.

In recombinant DNA technology, the enzyme restriction endonucleases are used to cleave DNA. When the desired gene is linked to DNA that replicates quickly (bacterial, viral, or plasmid), it can be inserted into bacterial cultures to produce large amounts of genetic material. There is a huge potential for drug production. The drug is available in its purest form and has lower antigenicity [22].

1.1.1.5 OTHER SOURCES

1. **Semi-Synthetic Sources/Synthetic Sources:**
   - i. **Synthetic Sources:** A drug is considered synthetic when both its chemical structure and nucleus are changed from a natural source. Example: Emetine Bismuth Iodide.
   - ii. **Semi-Synthetic Source:** A drug is considered semi-synthetic if its chemical structure is changed but its nucleus is still derived from a natural source. Methyl testosterone, ethyl estradiol, homatropine, ampicillin, apomorphine, and diacetylmorphine are a few examples. Nowadays, semi-synthetic versions of most medications—including anticonvulsants and anxiety medications—are in use.
2. **Mineral/Earth Sources:**
   - i. **Metallic as well as Non-Metallic Sources:** Iron is used to treat anemia due to iron deficiency. Syphilis is treated with mercurial salts. Zinc supplements are used, and zinc oxide paste is applied to wounds and eczema. The antiseptic is iodine, and supplements with iodine are also used. Rheumatoid arthritis patients are treated with gold salts. Shilajit is used for immunity modulation and sexual problems.
   - ii. **Miscellaneous Sources:** Fluorine has antiseptic qualities. Additionally, borax has antiseptic properties. Shampoos intended to treat dandruff contain selenium in the form of selenium sulfide. Liquid paraffin is prepared using petroleum.
3. **Microbiological Sources:** The source of many biological immunizations, such as different vaccines, is microorganisms. Vaccination against viruses (smallpox, rabies, influenza, poliomyelitis, measles virus, yellow fever, hepatitis virus, etc.) and bacterial vaccines (vaccines against whooping cough, pertussis, BCG,

Mycobacterium tuberculosis, plague, and cholera) are important. Penicillin is produced by the fungus *Penicillium notatum*. Streptomycin is produced by actinobacteria. Micromonospora and Streptomyces are the sources of aminoglycosides like tobramycin and gentamicin. The vaccine against rickettsia is a class of minuscule gram-negative bacteria utilized to develop active immunity to prevent typhus fever. Both diphtheria and tetanus toxoids are examples of microbiological products [23].

1.1.2 ORGANIZED DRUGS AND UNORGANIZED DRUGS

Drugs that are organized and unorganized, as the name suggests, are plant or animal organs composed of cells or specific structural elements. These medications go by names like fruits, flowers, seeds, insects, and so forth. They are obtained through various processes such as extraction, distillation, incision, expression, exudation, and secretion purification from plant or animal parts. For instance, juices, extracts, resins, and so forth, are dependable in character. Natural materials such as oils, gums, and balsams can be solid, semisolid, or liquid. Terms from botany or zoology can be used to characterize these medications. They cannot be adequately described by such terminology; instead, one must look for physical characteristics such as density, optical rotation, viscosity, refractive index, and solubility in different solvents [24].

Microscopic characters are one of the key factors in identifying drugs that are organized as T.S. and L.S. Confirmatory tests include physical standards and chemical tests.

For instance, Cinchona, Ephedra, Fennel, Clove, Digitalis, Aloe, Agar, Colophony, Opium, Castor oil, Beeswax, and Pepsin are a few examples.

Many plant-based products, including gums, mucilages, juices, extracts, and dried latex, are utilized in the nutrition, cosmetics, and medicinal industries. To concentrate their properties, these substances can be obtained through drying processes.

1.1.2.1 ORGANIZED DRUGS

Organized drugs represent the cellular body found in organized drugs. Most of these are unrefined medications derived from plants.

Nearly every morphological component of a plant, or the plant in its entirety, can be classified as an organized drug. There is a lengthy list of such illegal substances. A few examples of these groups of crude drugs are cinchona bark, digitalis leaves, quassia wood, sandalwood, senna, nux vomica seeds, rauwolfia roots, and so forth. These groups of crude drugs can also be described as organized crude drugs when they are represented by other morphological organs.

For such raw medications, microscopic and anatomical research is paramount. These can be used directly in medicine, or the active ingredient can be extracted or modified and used instead. Herbal teas, extracts, tinctures, and other simple medicines can be made from these drugs by processing them thoroughly to separate and purify the pure therapeutically active ingredient that gives the drug its final effect [25].

Examples of organized drugs:

1. **Woods:** Red Sandalwood, Quassia, and Sandalwood.
2. **Barks:** Arjuna, Ashoka, Cassia, Cascara, Cinchona, and Wild Cherry.
3. **Leaves:** Digitalis, Eucalyptus, Gymnema, Mint, Tulsi, Senna, Spearmint, Squill, Vasaka, Coca, Buchu, Belladonna, and Tea.
4. **Flowering Parts:** Chamomile, Santonica, Pyrethrum, Saffron, Clove.
5. **Seeds:** Bitter almond, Black Mustard, Colchicum, Cardamom, Nutmeg, Nux vomica, Psyllium, Physostigma, Strophanthus, and White Mustard.
6. **Fruits:** Dill, fennel, gokhru, hirda, lemon peel, senna pod, star anise, tamarind, vidang, amla, anise, bael, bahera, bitter orange peel, capsicum, caraway, cardamom, colocynth, coriander, cumin, ginger, and fennel.
7. **Roots and Rhizomes:** Podophyllum, Ipecac, Ipomoea, Jalap, Jatamansi, Rauwolfia, Rhubarb, Senega, Shatavari, Turmeric, Valerian, Squill, Dioscorea, Galanga, Garlic, Gention, Ginger, Ginseng, Glycyrrhiza, Squill, and Ashwagandha [26].
8. **Plants and Herbs:** Ergot, Ephedra, Bacopa, Andrographis, Kalmegh, Yeast, Vinca, Datura, and Centella.
9. **Hair and Fibers:** Hemp, Cotton, Jute, Flax, Silk.

1.1.2.2 UNORGANIZED DRUGS

The anatomical or morphological organization is absent from unorganized drugs. Even though these products are sold directly to customers, their main suppliers are still living things like plants, animals, and minerals. Such unrefined medications do not need to be studied under a microscope. This category includes products like agar, alginic acid, dried extracts of black and pale catechu, plant lattices like opium, and plant exudates like gums, oleogums, and oleogum resins. Direct commodities for use include essential oils, fixed oils, fats, and waxes derived from vegetable or animal sources, even though they are hydro-distilled or extracted from plants. Unorganized raw substances may include different mineral products like shilajit. With the use of analytical, chemical, and physical standards, the quality and purity of these products can be examined. They can be liquid, semisolid, or solid [5].

Examples of unorganized drugs:

1. **Mucilages:** They are glue-like substances produced by most plants; they are slimy in nature. The formation of gum is known as gummosis. Mucilages are found in agar, senna, and isapgol.

2. **Dried Latex:** It is produced from specialized tissue of a plant. Physically, it is a white aqueous suspension, and it contains proteins, sugars, and minerals, as well as starch. Under microscopic vision, it shows globules of oil, for example, opium and papain.

3. **Dried Juice:** These are obtained from the fleshy leaves of aloe, the stems of trees, or the heartwood of Acacia catechu. For example, aloe and kino.

4. **Dried Extracts:** Pectin, alginate, agar, black and pale catechu.

5. **Gums:** These are pathological products produced by the plant when it suffers unfavorable conditions or is injured. For example, acacia, tragacanth, guar gum, Indian gum, and sterculia.

6. **Waxes:** Carnauba, spermaceti, and beeswax agar.

7. **Resins:** These are often associated with volatile oils and are called oleoresins. They may be combined in a glycosidic manner with sugar, as in the Convolvulaceae family. Resins are found in

schizogenous or schizolysigenous ducts or cavities. The association of resin with gum makes it oleo gum resin. Examples include – asafoetida, benzoin, copaiba, guaiacum, colophony, coal tar, guggul, mastic, tar, tolu balsam, sandarac, and storax.

7. **Volatile Oils:** Anise, coriander, rosemary, sandalwood, peppermint, cinnamon, lemon, caraway, dill, clove, eucalyptus, nutmeg, camphor, and turpentine.
8. **Animal Products:** Beeswax, cantharides, cod-liver oil, gelatin, halibut liver oil, honey, shark liver oil, shellac, spermaceti wax, wool fat, musk, and lactose.
9. **Fossil Organisms and Minerals:** Bentonite, talc, kaolin, and kieselguhr.
10. **Fixed Oils and Fats:** Almond, arachis, castor, chalmoogra, coconut, cottonseed, halibut liver, linseed, olive, sesame, theobroma, cod-liver, and kokum butter (27).

1.1.3 CLASSIFICATION OF CRUDE DRUGS

Advanced plants, animals, microbes, and marine organisms are the most significant natural origins of pharmaceuticals. Both organic and inorganic minerals can be used to produce a number of beneficial products. A system of drug classification is the specific order of arrangement that must be followed in order to study the distinct drugs. A classification technique ought to be: (i) straightforward; (ii) user-friendly; and (iii) devoid of uncertainty and confusion [27].

Due to their widespread distribution, each classification scheme has advantages and disadvantages of its own; however, for the purposes of this learning, the medicines are categorized in the following ways [28]:

- Alphabetical classification;
- Taxonomical classification;
- Morphological classification;
- Pharmacological classification;
- Chemical classification;
- Chemotaxonomical classification; and
- Serotaxonomical classification.

1.1.3.1 ALPHABETICAL CLASSIFICATION

For any disconnected item, the easiest method of classification is alphabetical. The Latin, English, and occasionally native language names (vernacular names) of raw drugs are listed in alphabetical order. The following are a few pharmacopoeias, dictionaries, and reference books that use this system to categorize crude drugs [28]:

- Indian Pharmacopoeia;
- European Pharmacopoeia;
- British Herbal Pharmacopoeia;
- British Pharmacopoeia;
- British Pharmaceutical Codex;
- United States Pharmacopoeia and National Formulary.

Whereas these are organized in English in the British Pharmaceutical Codex (B.P.C.) and United States Pharmacopoeia (USP) [29] according to their terms, they are arranged in Latin in the European Pharmacopoeia.

- ➢ **Merits:**
  - This system's location makes it simple to trace and add drug entries.
  - It is quick and easy to use.
  - There is no confusion or redundant entry.
- ➢ **Demerits:** There is no connection between drug entries that came before and those that came after.

Examples: Benzoin, Acacia, Cinchona, Dill, Opium, Ergot, Fennel, Gentian, Hyoscyamus, Ipecacuanha, Jalap, Kurchi, Liquorice, Mints, Nux vomica, Rauwolfia, Podophyllum, Quassia, Senna, Wool fat, Vasaka, Yellow beeswax, Zeodary.

1.1.3.2 TAXONOMICAL CLASSIFICATION

Every plant has unique morphological, microscopic, chemical, embryological, serological, and genetic characteristics. The following categories are used in this classification to group crude drugs: kingdom, subkingdom, division, class, order, family, genus, and species [30].

1. **Class:** Plants classified as *Angiospermae* (Angiosperms) or Gymnospermae (Gymnosperms) do not yield flowers.
2. **Subclass:** Plants classified as Monocotyledonae (Monocotyledons, Monocots) have a single seed leaf, whereas Dicotyledonae (Dicotyledons, Dicots) have two seed leaves.
3. **Superorder:** A collection of closely associated plant families arranged according to the order in which their differences are believed to have arisen from a common predecessor. *Magnoliidae, Hamamelidae, Caryophyllidae, Dilleniidae, Rosidae,* and *Asteridae* are the six superorders in the Dicotyledonae, while *Alistimatidae, Commelinidae, Arecidae,* and *Liliidae* are the four superorders in the Monocotyledonae. The superorders' names finish in *-idae*.
4. **Order:** There are multiple orders that subdivide each superorder.

   The orders' names finish in *-ales*.
5. **Family:** Families are created within each order. These plants are the highest classification typically used, and they share many common botanical features. At this stage, the untrained eye can frequently distinguish the similarities between plants with ease. Each family is given a type of plant by modern botanical classification, which possesses the unique qualities that set this collection of plants apart from others. The family is then named after this type of plant.

Plant families vary in number depending on which botanist's classification is used. While some botanists recognize nearly 500 plant families, others recognize only about 150 families, favoring the categorization of other related plants as subfamilies. Cronquist's 1968 system, which has only undergone minor revisions since then, is a commonly used one. The titles of the families end in *-aceae*.

1. **Subfamily:** The family can be additionally subdivided into several subfamilies, which are groups of plants that share certain notable botanical characteristics. The subfamilies' titles finish in *-oideae*.
2. **Tribe:** Even after being further divided into smaller botanical divisions within a family, these divisions typically include a large number of distinct species. The tribe's names finish in *-eae*.

3. **Subtribe:** An additional classification based on minute botanical distinctions, which are frequently only apparent to botanists. The subtribe names finish in *-inae*.
4. **Genus:** The most recognizable portion of the plant name is this one; this is the common name you give a plant, such as Papaver (poppies), Aquilegia (columbines), and so forth. A genus's plants are frequently easily identified as being appropriate to the similar group.
5. **Species:** This is the level at which a particular plant is defined. The name of the plant usually refers to one or more characteristics of it, such as the color of the flowers, the size or form of the leaves, or the location where it was discovered. The combined terms "genus" and "species" designate a single plant and are used to identify it. Species can occasionally be further subdivided into subspecies, which contain plants that are not quite different enough to be considered varieties. Following the genus name, the species name should be written in lowercase letters without a capital letter.
6. **Variety:** A plant variety is characterized by minor differences from the species plant that are more pronounced than those in form. *Varietas* is the Latin term, typically shortened to var. Names of genera and species come first, followed by var., which comes before names of specific varieties.
7. **Form:** A plant that falls under a species but exhibits subtle botanical variations, like variations in flower color or leaf shape, is referred to as a form. Names of genera and species come first, with form (or f.) coming before names of specific varieties.
8. **Cultivar:** A cultivar is a type of plant that has been intentionally hybridized or has arisen naturally. It can be grown vegetatively or through seed to create additional similar plants.

   The genus and species names come first in the name:

Kingdom [31]	Plantae
Subkingdom	Tracheobionta
Division	Magnoliophyta
Class	Monocotyledons
Subclass	Zinziberidae

Kingdom [31]	Plantae
Order	Zinziberales
Family	Zinziberaceae
Genus	Curcuma
Species	longa

- **Merits:** Taxonomical classification is advantageous when researching evolutionary developments.
- **Demerits:** Additionally, there is no correlation found in this system among the drugs' chemical components and biological activity.

1.1.3.3 MORPHOLOGICAL CLASSIFICATION

The drugs in this system are arranged based on the external characteristics or morphology of the plant or animal parts, that is, the parts of the plant that are utilized as drugs, such as the leaves, stem, roots, and so forth. Medications derived from the plant's direct parts that contain cellular tissues are referred to as organized drugs; these include barks, rhizomes, leaves, fruits, whole plants, hairs, and fibers. Unorganized drugs are those that are made from plants using intermediate physical procedures like cutting, drying, or solvent extraction and do not include any plant tissues that are cells. Unorganized drugs include things like agar, aloe juice, opium latex, Gambir, gelatin, tragacanth, benzoin, beeswax, honey, lemongrass oil, and so forth [32].

- **Merits:** Morphological classification is more useful in recognizing and detecting adulteration. For practical research, this classification scheme is more effective, particularly in cases where the drug's chemical makeup is unclear.
- **Demerits:** The primary limitation of morphological classification is the lack of a relationship between the chemical components and the therapeutic effects. There is drug or plant repetition.

1.1.3.4 PHARMACOLOGICAL CLASSIFICATION

Pharmacological or therapeutic classification of drugs refers to the grouping of drugs established on their main constituent, pharmacological action, or therapeutic usage. This classification is more widely used and is a more pertinent approach. Drugs with a cardiotonic action, such as digitalis, squill, and strophanthus, are categorized according to their phylogenetic connection, the category of phytoconstituents they comprise, or the parts they use [33] (Table 1.1).

TABLE 1.1 Various Pharmacological Categories of Herbs

Sl. No.	Pharmacological Category	Herbs
1.	Drugs performing on gastrointestinal tract:	Kalmegh
	• Bitter	Coriander, cumin
	• Carminative	Ipecac
	• Emetic	Kurchi
	• Antiamoebic	Senna
	• Laxative	
2.	Drugs performing on respiratory system:	Honey
	• Antitussive	Mint
	• Expectorant	Glycyrrhiza
	• Branchodilators	
3.	Drugs performing on cardiovascular system:	Terminalia arjuna
	• Cardiotonic	Motherwort
	• Cardiac depressant	Beetroot
	• Vasodilator	*Rauwolfia serpentina*
	• Antihypertensive	
4.	Drug performing on autonomic nervous system:	St. John's wort
	• Adrenergic	Caffeine
	• Cholinergic	
5.	Drug acting on CNS	Caffiene
6.	Antispasmodic	Lavender
7.	Anticancer	Taxusbrevifolia
8.	Antirheumatic	Nux vomica
9.	Astringent	Catechu
10.	Galactogogue	Shatavari
11.	Antiepileptic	Bacopamonnieri
12.	Antidiabetic	Gudmar
13.	Anti-inflammatory	Curcuma
14.	Analgesic	White willow bark
15.	Antioxidant	Amla
16.	Hypolipidemic	Garlic
17.	Anti-ulcer	Liquorice

TABLE 1.1 *(Continued)*

Sl. No.	Pharmacological Category	Herbs
18.	Anti-acne	Neem
19.	Oxytocic	Ergot
20.	Detoxification	Amla
21.	Thyroid	Amla
22.	Antituburcular	Chaulmoogra oil
23.	Wound healing	Curcuma

- **Merits:** If a drug is unavailable at a specific location or time, this categorization system can be used to recommend alternatives.
- **Demerits:** Drugs with distinct physiological effects are categorized into multiple groups, leading to uncertainty and disarray. Due to quinine's antimalarial properties, cinchona falls under the category of medications that affect the heart because of quinidine's antiarrhythmic properties.

1.1.3.5 CHEMICAL CLASSIFICATION

Crude drugs are categorized based on their active ingredients. Numerous components, including alkaloids, glycosides, tannins, carbohydrates, and saponins, are present in the plants. Medications with comparable chemical constituents are grouped together regardless of taxonomy or morphological characteristics. Table 1.2 displays the examples [34].

TABLE 1.2 Various Chemical Groups of Herbs

Sl. No.	Chemical Group	Examples
1.	Alkaloids	Cinchona, datura, ipecac nux vomica, vinca
2.	Carbohydrates and its derived products	Acacia, starch, isabgol, tragacanth
3.	Glycosides	Aloe, senna, ginseng, digitalis, glycyrrhiza
4.	Volatile oils	Coriander, clove, cumin, cinnamon, fennel
5.	Resin and resin combination	Tolu balsam, benzoin, balsam of Peru
6.	Lipids	Beeswax, lanolin, kokum butter
7.	Enzymes	Casein, papain, trypsin
8.	Tannins	Tea, catechu

- **Merits:** It is a widely used methodology in phytochemical research.
- **Demerits:** When specific drugs contain multiple compounds from various compound groups, ambiguities occur.

1.1.3.6 CHEMOTAXONOMICAL CLASSIFICATION

This taxonomy system is predicated on a taxon's chemical similarity or the presence of a bond between ingredients in different plants. Definite classes of plants are characterized by particular types of chemical constituents. This introduces a completely new idea in chemotaxonomy: the use of chemical facts and characteristics to comprehend the relationships, taxonomy, and evolutionary history of plants [35].

Tropane alkaloids, for instance, are typically found in Solanaceae members and function as a chemotaxonomic marker. Similarly, the categorization of crude medications can be based on other secondary plant metabolite systems. Some examples include the berberine alkaloid found in Berberis and Argemone, rutin in members of the Rutaceae family, alkaloids found in members of the Ranunculaceae family, and so forth.

It is the most recent classification scheme that provides greater flexibility for comprehending the interactions between chemical components, their biosynthesis, and potential actions [36].

1.1.3.7 SEROTAXONOMICAL CLASSIFICATION

One way to define serotaxonomy is as the study of how serology is applied or useful in resolving taxonomical issues. The study of the antigen-antibody response is known as serology. Antigens are substances that have the ability to induce the production of antibodies. The immune system's plasma cells produce highly specific protein molecules known as antibodies. Proteins serve as both common antigens in serotaxonomy and carriers of taxonomical information [37].

It conveys the similarities and differences between various taxa, and taxonomy benefits from these facts. It determines the mark of likeness among species, genera, families, and so on by contrasting the antibodies present against a particular taxon with the response to antigens from different plant taxa.

1.2 OTHER CLASSIFICATION

1.2.1 CLASSIFICATION OF HERBS

Herbal medications can be categorized according to a number of factors, including their chemical composition, medicinal effects, and traditional/ cultural applications. This is a fundamental classification:

1. **Based on Therapeutic Effects:**
   - **Adaptogens:** Help the body adapt to stress.
   - **Analgesics:** Pain-relieving herbs.
   - **Antipyretics:** Reduce fever.
   - **Diuretics:** Increase urine production.
   - **Sedatives:** Calming or sleep-inducing herbs.
2. **Based on Parts Used:**
   - **Leaves:** Examples include tea made from dried leaves.
   - **Roots:** Often used for medicinal properties.
   - **Bark:** Can have therapeutic compounds.
   - **Flowers:** Used for various remedies.
   - **Seeds:** Some herbs have medicinal seeds.
3. **Based on Chemical Constituents:**
   - **Alkaloids:** Plants with alkaline properties.
   - **Flavonoids:** Compounds with antioxidant effects.
   - **Essential Oils:** Oils with aromatic properties.
   - **Glycosides:** Compounds with sugar molecules.
4. **Cultural/Traditional Classification:**
   - **Ayurvedic Herbs:** Used in traditional Indian medicine.
   - **Traditional Chinese Medicine (TCM) Herbs:** Follows principles of TCM.
   - **Native/Indigenous Remedies:** Specific to certain regions or cultures.

5. **Based on Regulatory Perspective:**
    - **Over-the-Counter (OTC):** Available without a prescription.
    - **Prescription Herbal Medicines:** Require a prescription.

Although herbal remedies have been used historically, it is important to remember that their effectiveness and safety can vary. Before using herbal remedies, always seek medical advice, especially if you are taking other medications or already have a medical condition.

1.2.2 UNDERSTANDING THE CATEGORIES OF HERBS

Herbs are categorized in many ways:

i. As per usage;
ii. As per active constituents; and
iii. As per the period of life.

1.2.2.1 AS PER USAGE

As per usage, the herbs are defined in four parts:

1. **Medicinal Herbs:** Because of their therapeutic qualities, medicinal herbs are utilized to make medicines.
2. **Ornamental Herbs:** Because decorative herbs, such as lavender and chives, have vividly colored flowers and foliage, they are used as decorations.
3. **Culinary Herbs:** Because culinary herbs have strong flavors like mint, parsley, and basil, they are probably the most commonly used herbs in cooking.
4. **Aromatic Herbs:** The term "aromatic herbs" refers to the pleasant scent that many of these herbs possess. They are widely used in medicine as well as flavorings and fragrances. Stimulant herbs and nervine herbs are the two subcategories of aromatic herbs:

    i. Stimulant Herbs: Such as fennel, ginger, garlic, and lemongrass, generally influence the respiratory, digestive, and circulatory systems and increase energy and actions of the body or organs or their parts.

ii. **Nervine Herbs:** These are known to restore and calm the nervous system and also normally have an impact on the digestive, circulatory, and respiratory systems. They are frequently used in teas or in capsule form, such as catnip or ginger.

1.2.2.2 AS PER ACTIVE CONSTITUENTS

As per active constituents present, the herbs are divided into five major categories: essential (volatile oils), astringents (tannins), bitter (phenolic compounds, alkaloids, or saponins), mucilaginous (polysaccharides), and nutritive (foodstuffs).

1. **Essential Oils Herbs:** As implied by the name, many of these herbs have a pleasant scent. They are widely used in medicine as well as flavorings and fragrances. Stimulants and nerviness are the two subcategories of aromatic herbs.
2. **Astringent Herbs:** Tannins found in astringent herbs have the ability to cause proteins to precipitate, which contracts or tightens living tissue and aids in stopping discharges. They have an adverse effect on the circulatory, urinary, and digestive systems and are hepatotoxic in large doses. Examples of these include peppermint and red raspberry. They are also astringent, emmenagogue, hemostatic, styptic, antiseptic, and antiabortive.
3. **Bitter Herbs:** These are classified into four subcategories: diuretic herbs, laxative herbs, saponin-containing herbs, and alkaloid-containing herbs. The names of the subcategories stem from the occurrence of phenols and phenolic glycosides, alkaloids, or saponins.

    i. **Laxative Bitter Herbs:** These include licorice, aloe, barberry, cascara, licorice, senna, pumpkin, yucca, yellow dock, gentian, safflowers, and golden seal. They are also anticatarrhal, antipyretic, cholagogue, purgative, hepatonic, sialagogue, and vermifuge.

    ii. **Diuretic Herbs:** These cause the body to lose fluid over the urinary system. The water expelled aids in liver, kidney, and vascular system cleansing. When found in nature, such as in asparagus, butcher's broom, burdock, blessed thistle, chaparral, buchu, cornsilk, chickweed, dandelion, dog grass, grapevine, and parsley, they are alterative, anticatarrhal, antiseptic, antibiotic, antipyretic, blood purifier, and lithotriptic.

iii. **Saponin-Containing Herbs:** These are well known for their capacity to foam or create froth when dissolved in water. The Latin word for soap is where the term "saponin" originates. Their primary function in the digestive system is to improve the body's absorption of additional active compounds by emulsifying fat-soluble molecules.

It is possible for saponins to efficiently break down and dissolve red blood cell membranes. In nature, they have altered antispasmodic, emmenagogue, aphrodisiac, cardiac stimulant, and longer lifespan properties. For example, blue cohosh, licorice, ginseng, gotu kola, yucca, alfalfa, black cohosh, yam root, and schizandra.

4. **Mucilaginous Herbs:** The polysaccharides that mucilaginous herbs contain are responsible for their slippery, mild flavor that tastes sweet when diluted. In one way or another, plants make mucilage to hold water for later use as food. Generally used topically as knitting agents and poultices, as well as in the digestive tract, these herbs are most effective when applied topically [38]. Since very few mucilages are not broken down by the human gut, they absorb contaminants from the bowel and provide bulk to the stool. They have a soothing effect on the throat when taken as lozenges or extracts.

   They shorten the time it takes for the bowel to transit, help to regulate, and clear toxins from the intestine. They function as a detoxifier, culinary agent, demulcent, emollient, antibiotic, and antacid in nature. For example, aloe, althea, comfrey, burdock, dandelion, dulse, fenugreek, psyllium, echinacea, kelp, slippery elm, glucomannan from konjac root, Irish moss, and mullein.

5. **Nutritive Herbs:** The nutritional value that these herbs add to the diet is the source of both their name and their classification. They are real foods that have some therapeutic benefits, such as fiber, mucilage, and diuretic action. Primarily, they offer the essential nutrients—protein, carbohydrates, fats, and the vitamins and minerals required for sufficient nourishment. Rose hips, for

instance, acerola, apple, asparagus, barley grass, banana, bilberry, grapefruit, hibiscus, lemon, onion, oat straw, orange, papaya, pineapple, red clover, spirulina, wheat germ, and stevia are a few examples.

1.2.2.3 AS PER PERIOD OF LIFE

Herbs can also be categorized as annuals, biennials, or perennials based on their life cycle. Once a season, annuals bloom before dying. Biennials only bloom in their second season of life. Perennials survive the winter once they are established and bloom all year long.

The following is a list of commonly grown herbs, many of which are cultivated as annuals depending on climate and growing conditions.

Herbs that endure beyond a single growing season comprise parsley, sweet marjoram, thyme, mint, sage, and chives. Except for parsley, the majority can be initiated from seedlings.

Herbs classified as only bloom in their second year of life:

- **Anise:** Seeds of this plant show similarity with licorice in taste and smell.
- **Basil:** This is an herb belonging to the Lamiaceae family.
- **Borage:** This is an annual herb belonging to the family Boraginaceae; the whole aerial part of the plant is edible.
- **Calendula (Pot Marigold):** This is a flowering plant in the marigold family.
- **Chamomile:** This is an evergreen plant of the daisy family.
- **Chervil:** This herb is used in French cooking.
- **Cilantro/Coriander:** This is essential for Indian cuisines.
- **Dill Bouquet:** This is a culinary herb.
- **Dill Dukat:** This herb is excellent for pickles.
- **Fennel, Smoky:** It is an aromatic herb used as an expectorant as well.
- **Marjoram:** This has a camphoraceous scent.

- **Parsley:** This herb is used for adding flavor and fragrance.
- **Shiso:** This is an Asian herb with a complicated flavor profile.
- **Saffron:** This is used for flavor and fragrance.
- **Summer Savory:** This is used for seasoning grilled meat and barbecues.

Herbs that endure beyond a single growing season comprise sweet marjoram, parsley, mint, sage, thyme, and chives. Except for parsley, most can be started from young plants:

- **Alfalfa:** It is a flowering plant of the legume family.
- **Allspice:** This is a pepper spice.
- **Aloe Vera:** This is used for cosmetic and medicinal purposes.
- **Angelica**: This is an edible herbal medicine of China.
- **Agrimony:** It is a plant of the rose family.
- **Asafetida:** This is a carminative.
- **Avens:** This belongs to the rose family.
- **Bee Balm:** It is used for respiratory and digestive ailments.
- **Bay Leaves:** These leaves are used for culinary purposes.
- **Catnip:** This plant belongs to the mint family.
- **Chamomile:** This plant is used for age-defying.
- **Common Thyme:** This is used for respiratory ailments.
- **Dill:** It is used as a digestive aid.
- **Echinacea:** This plant belongs to the daisy family.
- **Fennel:** It is used for culinary purposes.
- **Lavender:** It is used for flavor and fragrance.
- **Lemon Balm:** This is used for insecticidal activity.
- **Mint:** Spearmint/peppermint/applemint/orangemint: This is used for fragrance purposes.

- **Marjoram Sweet:** This is a culinary herb.
- **Mitsuba:** It is a Japanese herb.
- **Rosemary:** It is used as a condiment and food preservative.
- **Stevia:** It is used as a substitute for sugar.
- **Salad Burnet:** This plant has a nutty flavor.
- **Sage:** This is a culinary herb.
- **Tarragon:** This herb is rich in minerals.
- **Thyme:** This is used as a condiment.
- **Watercress:** This has antioxidant potential.
- **Yarrow:** This herb is used in various treatments.

Herbs classified as biennials only bloom in their second year of life:

- **Caraway Seeds:** This is used for culinary purposes.
- **Primrose:** This plant is used for combating PCOD.
- **Bai Zhu:** This plant is used in traditional Chinese medicine.
- **Mullein:** This tea is used to cure respiratory troubles.
- **Teasel:** This is a flowering plant of the genus Dipsacus.
- **Viper's Bugloss:** This plant belongs to the Borage family and is native to Eurasia.

1.3 CONCLUSION

Herbal drugs have been used worldwide for centuries. The scientific and systematic arrangement of sources of drugs for better recognition and evaluation of herbal medicine is now available. The use of organized and unorganized drugs to achieve full therapeutic potential, along with the classification of herbal drugs based on various factors, aids in the search and management of data relevant to herbs for understanding phytochemistry and phytotherapeutics.

KEYWORDS

- **herbal drugs**
- **medicinal plants**
- **pharmacognosy**
- **plant extracts**
- **therapeutic compounds**
- **traditional medicine**

REFERENCES

1. Singh, S., & Agrawal, A. (2022). Ethnopharmacological, phytochemistry and pharmacological activities of *Psoralea corylifolia*: A review. *International Research Journal of Ayurveda & Yoga, 5*(5), 115–124.
2. Cheng, J. T., Liu, I. M., & Shen, S. C. (2022). *Plant Therapeutics*. MDPI–Multidisciplinary Digital Publishing Institute. Retrieved from: https://www.mdpi.com/books/book/6395 (accessed on 22 March 2025).
3. Sahoo, N., Manchikanti, P., & Dey, S. (2010). Herbal drugs: Standards and regulation. *Fitoterapia, 81*(6), 462–471.
4. Shah, B., & Seth, A. (2012). *Textbook of Pharmacognosy and Phytochemistry* (E-Book). Elsevier Health Sciences. Retrieved from: https://books.google.com/books?hl=en&lr=&id=obWBB_-ke38C&oi=fnd&pg=PT9&ots=ZjjJKA7fw3&sig=GS5R_Kkuste0TLgR1oymDcOZdu0 (accessed on 22 March 2025).
5. Shah, B. N. (2009). *Textbook of Pharmacognosy and Phytochemistry*. Elsevier India. Retrieved from: https://books.google.com/books?hl=en&lr=&id=UmOoJ0kQo74C&oi=fnd&pg=PA3&ots=OB-jTzJJ3b&sig=ZM1YuNSL6CjzEShWkO8lRH8Rfpc (accessed on 22 March 2025).
6. Ahad, B., Shahri, W., Rasool, H., Reshi, Z. A., Rasool, S., & Hussain, T. (2021). Medicinal plants and herbal drugs: An overview. In T. Aftab & K. R. Hakeem (Eds.), *Medicinal and Aromatic Plants* (pp. 1–40). Springer International Publishing. Retrieved from: https://link.springer.com/10.1007/978-3-030-58975-2_1 (accessed on 22 March 2025).
7. Vasil, I. K., & Thorpe, T. A. (2013). *Plant Cell and Tissue Culture*. Springer Science & Business Media. Retrieved from: https://books.google.com/books?hl=en&lr=&id=BCX-CAAAQBAJ&oi=fnd&pg=PR7&dq=Plant+cell+and+tissue+culture,+vasil&ots=YzYvnydDZu&sig=lYP05F-v_v4YtmWjbzom_gFHoL8 (accessed on 22 March 2025).
8. Thorpe, T. (2012). History of plant tissue culture. In V. M. Loyola-Vargas & N. Ochoa-Alejo (Eds.), *Plant Cell Culture Protocols* (pp. 9–27). Humana Press.

Retrieved from: http://link.springer.com/10.1007/978-1-61779-818-4_2 (accessed on 22 March 2025).

9. Caponetti, J. D., Gray, D. J., & Trigiano, R. N. (2018). History of plant tissue and cell culture. In *Plant Tissue Culture Concepts and Laboratory Exercises* (pp. 11–17). Routledge. Retrieved from: https://www.taylorfrancis.com/chapters/edit/10.1201/9780203743133-2 (accessed on 22 March 2025).
10. Samadelli, M., Zink, A. R., Roselli, G., Gabrielli, S., Tabandeh, S., & Fernicola, V. C. (2019). Development of passive controlled atmosphere display cases for the conservation of cultural assets. *Journal of Cultural Heritage, 35*, 145–153.
11. Effros, R. B. (1998). Replicative senescence in the immune system: Impact of the Hayflick limit on T-cell function in the elderly. *American Journal of Human Genetics, 62*(5), 1003–1007.
12. Rattan, S. I. S. (2016). Origins of the Hayflick system, the phenomenon, and the limit. In S. I. S. Rattan & L. Hayflick (Eds.), *Cellular Ageing and Replicative Senescence* (pp. 3–14). Springer International Publishing. Retrieved from: http://link.springer.com/10.1007/978-3-319-26239-0_1 (accessed on 22 March 2025).
13. Park, H. W. (2016). Constructing failure: Leonard Hayflick, biomedicine, and the problems with tissue culture. *Annals of Science, 73*(3), 303–327.
14. Wolman, S. R. (1986). Cytogenetic heterogeneity: Its role in tumor evolution. *Cancer Genetics and Cytogenetics, 19*(1, 2), 129–140.
15. Effros, R. B., & Walford, R. L. (1984). T cell cultures and the Hayflick limit. *Human Immunology, 9*(1), 49–65.
16. Bhojwani, S. S., & Dantu, P. K. (2013). Culture media. In S. S. Bhojwani & P. K. Dantu (Eds.), *Plant Tissue Culture: An Introductory Text* (pp. 27–37). Springer. Retrieved from: https://doi.org/10.1007/978-81-322-1026-9_3 (accessed on 22 March 2025).
17. Murashige, T. (1973). Nutrition of plant cells and organs *in vitro*. *In Vitro, 9*(2), 81–85.
18. Brito, A., Areche, C., Sepúlveda, B., Kennelly, E., & Simirgiotis, M. (2014). Anthocyanin characterization, total phenolic quantification and antioxidant features of some Chilean edible berry extracts. *Molecules, 19*(8), 10936–10955.
19. Jaiswal, P., Singh, A. V., Yadav, V. K., Kumar, A., & Kumari, N. (2022). Phytochemical studies in the field of plant tissue culture. In *Advances in Plant Tissue Culture* (pp. 395–405). Elsevier. Retrieved from: https://linkinghub.elsevier.com/retrieve/pii/B9780323907958000229 (accessed on 22 March 2025).
20. Devi, J., Kumar, R., Singh, K., Gehlot, A., Bhushan, S., & Kumar, S. (2021). *In vitro* adventitious roots: A non-disruptive technology for the production of phytoconstituents on the industrial scale. *Critical Reviews in Biotechnology, 41*(4), 564–579.
21. Khan, S., Ullah, M. W., Siddique, R., Nabi, G., Manan, S., Yousaf, M., et al. (2016). Role of recombinant DNA technology to improve life. *International Journal of Genomics.* Retrieved from: https://www.hindawi.com/journals/ijg/2016/2405954/abs/ (accessed on 22 March 2025).
22. Pappu, H. R., Niblett, C. L., & Lee, R. F. (1995). Application of recombinant DNA technology to plant protection: Molecular approaches to engineering virus resistance in crop plants. *World Journal of Microbiology and Biotechnology, 11*(4), 426–437.

23. Kneifel, W., Czech, E., & Kopp, B. (2002). Microbial contamination of medicinal plants—A review. *Planta Medica, 68*(1), 5–15.
24. Alamgir, A. N. M. (2017). Classification of drugs, nutraceuticals, functional food, and cosmeceuticals; proteins, peptides, and enzymes as drugs. In *Therapeutic Use of Medicinal Plants and their Extracts: Volume 1* (pp. 125–175). Cham: Springer International Publishing. Retrieved from: http://link.springer.com/10.1007/978-3-319-63862-1_5 (accessed on 22 March 2025).
25. Alamgir, A. N. M. (2017). Pharmacognostical botany: Classification of medicinal and aromatic plants (MAPs), bostanical taxonomy, morphology, and anatomy of drug plants. In *Therapeutic Use of Medicinal Plants and their Extracts: Volume 1* (pp. 177–293). Cham: Springer International Publishing. Retrieved from: http://link.springer.com/10.1007/978-3-319-63862-1_6 (accessed on 22 March 2025).
26. Alamgir, A. N. M. (2017). *Therapeutic Use of Medicinal Plants and their Extracts: Volume 1*. Cham: Springer International Publishing. Retrieved from: http://link.springer.com/10.1007/978-3-319-63862-1 (accessed on 22 March 2025).
27. Rajak, H. (2018). *Classification of herbs*. Retrieved from: https://hmhub.in/classification-of-herbs/ (accessed on 22 March 2025).
28. Mir, S. R. (2008). *Different Systems of Classification of Crude Drugs*. Retrieved from: http://nsdl.niscpr.res.in/bitstream/123456789/710/1/corrected%20different%20Systems%20of%20Classification%20of%20crude%20drugs.pdf.
29. Harte, V. J., O'Hanrahan, M. T., & Timoney, R. F. (1978). Microbial contamination in residues of ophthalmic preparations. *International Journal of Pharmaceutics, 1*(3), 165–171.
30. Bhosale, V. V., & Banerjee, D. (2020). Scientific validation of herbal medicine. In S. Sen & R. Chakraborty (Eds.), *Herbal Medicine in India* (pp. 573–579). Singapore: Springer Singapore. Retrieved from: http://link.springer.com/10.1007/978-981-13-7248-3_34 (accessed on 22 March 2025).
31. Mali, S., Yadav, R., Gauttam, V., & Sawale, J. (2023). An updated review on taxonomy and chemotaxonomy. *Toxicology International*, 121–129.
32. Lee, S. M., Kim, H., & Jang, Y. P. (2012). Chemometric classification of morphologically similar Umbelliferae medicinal herbs by DART-TOF-MS fingerprint. *Phytochemical Analysis, 23*(5), 508–512.
33. Dimpfel, W. (2013). Pharmacological classification of herbal extracts by means of comparison to spectral EEG signatures induced by synthetic drugs in the freely moving rat. *Journal of Ethnopharmacology, 149*(2), 583–589.
34. Ahmad, I., Aqil, F., & Owais, M. (2006). *Modern Phytomedicine: Turning Medicinal Plants into Drugs* (1st ed.). Wiley. Retrieved from: https://onlinelibrary.wiley.com/doi/book/10.1002/9783527609987 (accessed on 22 March 2025).
35. Singh, R. (2016). Chemotaxonomy: A tool for plant classification. *Journal of Medicinal Plants Studies, 4*(2), 90–93.
36. Singh, R. (2018). Chemotaxonomy of medicinal plants: Possibilities and limitations. In *Natural Products and Drug Discovery* (pp. 119–136). Elsevier. Retrieved from: https://www.sciencedirect.com/science/article/pii/B978008102081400006X (accessed on 22 March 2025).

37. Lee, Y. S. (1984). Serotaxonomy: A promising approach to systematic problems. *Korean Journal of Plant Taxonomy, 14*(1), 59–69. Retrieved from: http://www.e-kjpt.org/upload/pdf/0i800105.pdf (accessed on 22 March 2025).
38. Shaheen, S., Ramzan, S., Khan, F., & Ahmad, M. (2019). History, classification, worldwide distribution, and significance of herbal plants. In S. Shaheen, S. Ramzan, F. Khan, & M. Ahmad (Eds.), *Adulteration in Herbal Drugs: A Burning Issue* (pp. 35–49). Cham: Springer International Publishing. https://doi.org/10.1007/978-3-030-28034-5_4.

CHAPTER 2

Quality Control of Herbal Drugs

SURABHI SHAKYA,[1] PRADEEP SINGH,[2] JITENDRA KUMAR,[1] and AMIT KUMAR VERMA[1,*]

[1]*Department of Pharmacy, MJP Rohilkhand University, Bareilly, Uttar Pradesh, India*

[2]*Department of Pharmacy, College of Health Sciences, Debre Tabor University, Ethiopia*

*Corresponding author

ABSTRACT

With scientific development and advancements in modernization, people are also becoming more aware of health and associated issues. The consumption of natural products (NPs) is increasing day by day; therefore, there is a great need to divert attention toward high-quality natural medicinal products, which have enormous potential to deal with various ailments. The size of the herbal market globally is about 62 billion dollars, with the European share being the largest, contributing about 45% of the total. The increase in consumption has also raised the issue of adulteration in herbal products to meet demand. The practice of adulteration raises questions about the quality of NPs, as there is a lack of strict guidelines regarding safety parameters and the determination of quality and purity. Various pharmacopoeias and the World Health Organization (WHO) have provided evaluation parameters for NPs. The different parameters include quality evaluation through organoleptic studies, chemical and physical methods, biological methods for evaluating activity, and many more. Additionally, other parameters like quantitative microscopy are used in cases where organoleptic, physical, or chemical methods for

The Essentials of Herbal Drugs. Varsha Tiwari, Abhishek Tiwari, and Ajay Sharma (Eds.)

DOI: 10.1201/9781998511778-2

evaluation are inapplicable. Accurate identification of NPs is of paramount importance for their correct use in phytomedicines. Furthermore, various chromatography and analytical techniques, such as spectroscopy, DNA fingerprinting, or DNA profiling, serve as beneficial tools for the standardization of NPs. This book chapter provides detailed information about the methods affecting the quality of NPs and how to evaluate them for safety and efficacy.

2.1 INTRODUCTION

The world is changing day by day, and in reference to this, our lifestyle is also changing. With the change in the living scenario, our bodies also face many health issues due to various reasons. To keep the body healthy and stress-free, people are encouraging the use of herbal products. The universal trend is shifting from synthetic to herbal medicine and herbal products. Most of the phytoconstituents are extracted from plants and used in the treatment of many acute and chronic diseases, and after so much investigation, plants are still the source of many essential and new components [1].

The Indian medicinal system has been dealing with traditional medicines since ancient times. Different systems such as Ayurveda, Siddha, Unani, and so forth, have a close relationship with herbal products, as their treatment methodologies are purely based on plants and their natural products (NPs). During the last few years, efforts have been made to introduce the cultivation of medicinal plants at a commercial level by farmers [2].

Lots of health benefits are associated with NPs. Medicinal plants and their NPs are gaining popularity in the herbal market because of their tremendous properties. One of the reasons for the popularity of herbal products is that they are cost-effective and safer than synthetic products. The emergence of various health-related products like nutraceuticals, hygiene products, natural cosmetic products, and Ayurvedic medicines has increased the demand for herbal products manyfold [3]. Without a prescription, people are consuming herbal products on a large scale because they consider them safe, as they are natural in origin. The World Health Organization (WHO) also estimates that a major portion of the world population depends on natural medicinal herbs and herbal products to fulfill their health needs. Different parts of medicinal plants, like seeds, leaves, stems, roots, bark, and tubers, have different proportions of phytoconstituents in them. Medicinal plants show various pharmacological activities, such as anti-cancer, anti-inflammatory, anti-arthritis, anti-emetic, anti-viral, hepatoprotective, cardioprotective, anti-rheumatic, anti-depressant, antioxidant, anti-microbial, anti-aging, bacteriostatic, anti-HIV, anti-spasmodic, anti-anxiety, anti-fertility, anti-depressant, and many more. Medicinal herbs not only cure diseases but are also used in the management of symptoms like dryness in the mouth, which generally occurs due to the overuse of allopathic medicines, nausea, and indigestion. Persons with compromised immune systems can improve their condition by using medicinal herbs [4].

The WHO reported in a survey that generally three kinds of herbal medicines are used, that is, herbal products, processed plant material, and plant material in raw form. For primary health care and fitness, about 80% of the world population consumes traditional products and herbs. In the present condition, the assessment of the quality of drugs and the standardization of herbal products seem to be important for assessing the concentration of active ingredients [5]. The high demand for medicinal plants for various purposes is not only threatening the existence of many rare and wild species but also leading to their degradation. The trade of raw medicinal plants around the globe is skyrocketing, and the destructive, early, and over-harvesting of endemic medicinal species raises questions about their existence in the future. The collection and trade of 1500 tons of aromatic and medicinal plants have been conducted annually, and most of the trade is done illegally, as mentioned in a 2003 report. A large proportion, that is, 75%, of medicinal plants were collected from the wild in India [6].

India is the largest producer of medicinal plants after China. The herbal products and their medicinal value are known all over the world. Medicinal plants are collected not only from wild sources but also on a commercial level. The secondary metabolites present in the plants show valuable effects on the human body. Based on their chemical properties, they can be categorized into three distinct groups: that is, sulfur and nitrogen-containing compounds (such as alkaloids, non-protein amino acids, cyanogenic glucosides, alliin, thionins, etc.), terpenes (such as polyterpenes, triterpenes, diterpenes, sesquiterpenes, and monoterpenes), and phenolics (such as coumarin, lignin, flavonoids, tannins, etc.) [7]. According to the presence of the secondary metabolites, different parts of plants are used for medicinal purposes. Some examples are the seeds of *Thymus vulgaris* (Ajwain), used as an antiseptic and antispasmodic; the fruits and leaves of *Datura stramonium* (Dhatura), used to cure cardiac pains and asthma; the leaves of *Ocimum sanctum* (Tulsi), used as an antidiabetic and antiallergic; the root, flower, and bark of *Azadirachta indica* (Neem), used in the treatment of diabetes, bronchitis, arthritis, and cough; the fruits of *Phoenix dactylifera* (Khajoor), used to cure diarrhea and genitourinary ailments; and the bark, fruits, seeds, leaves, and latex of *Ficus religiosa* (Peepal), used in the treatment of various diseases such as gynecological diseases, neuralgia, skin diseases, and constipation, and so forth [8].

Many of the medicinal herbs used for trade are distributed according to their habitats. The northern fold includes the area of the Kashmir Valley and the Himalayan region, with areas in Kashmir such as Sonamarg, Lolab Valley, Gulmarg, Pahalgam, Khilanmarg, and Tilail Valley, which are known for the abundance of species like *Picrorhiza kurroa*, *Dioscorea adeltoidea*, *Saussurea* spp., *Rheum emodi*, *Hyoscyamus niger*, *Arnebia benthamii*, *Hypericum perforatum*, *Inula racemosa*, *Juniperus macropoda*, *Podophyllum hexandrum*, *Aconitum heterophyllum*, *Artemisia* spp., and so forth. The aromatic plants that grow in the high-altitude regions of Kashmir include the following species: *Foeniculum vulgare* (Fennel), *Trigonella foenum-graecum* (Hare's foot), *Crocus sativus* (Saffron), *Carum carvi* (Caraway), *Baniumpersicum* (Siyazira), and so forth [9]. The southern part of India is rich in biodiversity and provides favorable climatic conditions for the growth and development of various species. The cultivation of different species such as *Moringa oleifera* (Drumstick tree), *Ricinus communis* (Castor bean), *Gloriosa superba* (Agnishikha), *Zingiber officinale* (Ginger), *Tamarindus indica* (Tamarind), *Curcuma longa* (Turmeric), *Aloe vera* (Ghritkumari), *Sesamum indicum* (Sesame), *Azadirachta indica* (Neem), *Phyllanthus emblica* (Indian gooseberry), *Solanum americanum* (American Black Nightshade), *Eucalyptus tereticornis* (Forest red gum), and *Sesbania grandiflora* (Agati) are being practiced by farmers in the southern districts on a mass level [10].

The changes in climatic conditions also challenge the cultivation of different species. Due to several factors, climatic changes are directly or indirectly affecting aromatic and medicinal plants all over the world. Mostly, the endemic species of medicinal and aromatic plants are at high risk due to these changes. These changes can also cause great variation in the amount of phytoconstituents present in them, the timing of flowering and fruiting, and their quality. The decline of important medicinal plants is a broad area of concern, as it is reported that *Taxus wallichiana*, *Picrorhiza kurroa*, *Coscinium fenestratum*, *Saraca asoca*, and *Aconitum heterophyllum* are six species that are declining at a rapid rate. These species are currently being used in large amounts by the herbal industries because of their medicinal properties, and they are used to treat many different ailments and diseases. The extinction of these species ultimately affects the industrial sector as well as our environment because once the species disappear, it will become difficult for us to obtain them back. These are only a few examples, but there are several species that are becoming vulnerable either due to over-exploitation or climatic conditions [11].

In India, the environmental information system (ENVIS) Centre in Floral Diversity, sponsored by the Botanical Survey of India (BSI), Calcutta, recently estimated that there are 26 medicinal plant species that are now extinct, 124 are critically endangered, 71 are at intermediate risk, 41 are possibly unknown or extinct, 108 are vulnerable, and 248 are rare medicinal plant species. The lack of adequate supply due to high demand has created a crisis that fuels the potential for product adulteration in the absence of effective regulation, quality control, or standardization of herbal products [12].

2.2 ADULTERATION OF HERBAL SPECIES

In herbal raw material trade, adulteration is the most common malpractice, which is done either intentionally or unintentionally. Adulteration is described as the process of mixing the original and genuine drug with some inferior variety that has low activity or no activity at all. The adulterant used in the process can be either a part of the same plant or a different plant; many morphologically similar substances are involved, and in the case of volatile substances, the adulterants are the exhausted ones. Adulterants are basically the inferior, defective, useless, spurious, and spoiled parts of the same or different plants. Faith in herbal drugs is declining due to the process of adulteration [13].

Different conditions involved in adulteration are [14]:

1. **Deterioration:** Means impairment in the drug's quality.
2. **Sophistication:** An act done deliberately or intentionally.

3. **Inferiority:** Addition of a substituted drug in the original sample.
4. **Spoilage:** Drug product attacked by microorganisms.
5. **Substitution:** In place of the original drug, totally different substances are added.
6. **Admixture:** Due to carelessness and ignorance, any unwanted substance is added to the main sample.

When adulterated and poor-quality drugs are supplied in the market, they cause harmful effects on our health, resulting in adverse effects or drug resistance. In developing countries where the regulatory systems are inappropriate and weak, adulteration and substitution are major issues. The proportion of sales of counterfeit drugs is 10% in developing countries, and in online purchases, the proportion is greater than 50%. Sometimes, the adulteration of herbal products becomes life-threatening for the consumer. Many examples are present in the surrounding area, as adulteration is not an issue of a particular country or area; almost every part of the world experiences these types of processes. In Southeast Asia, 50% of Artesunate tablets were reported to be of poor quality. Artesunate, a phytoconstituent extracted from the plant *Artemisia annua* L., is used to treat malaria [15].

2.2.1 REASONS FOR ADULTERATION

Availability of poor-quality products is decreasing consumer faith in herbal products. Adverse events have occurred due to the consumption of unintended herbs present in genuine products. Traders and producers have adulterated the main herbal products for many reasons; some actions are done knowingly, while others happen due to mistakes.

1. **Unintentional Adulteration:** Sometimes the quality of the original product is compromised due to carelessness during the collection or processing of the product. Some of the reasons are listed in sub list:

   i. **Careless Behavior of Individuals During Collection:** During the harvesting, processing, and collection of medicinal plants or their parts, adulteration can occur. *Parmelia perlata* (common name: Stone flower), which belongs to the family

Parmeliaceae, is used in Siddha, Unani, and Ayurvedic medicines. This species is often adulterated with other species like *Parmelia cirrhata* and *Parmelia perforata*.

ii. **Morphological Similarity:** Similar-looking medicinal plants often get mixed during collection. *Mucuna pruriens* (commonly known as Velvet bean), which belongs to the family Fabaceae, is adulterated with other similar-looking Papilionaceae seeds such as *Mucuna deeringiana* and *Mucuna utilis*. *M. deeringiana* has larger seeds, while *M. utilis* has white seeds.

iii. **Unavailability of Authentic Plants:** *Hypericum perforatum* generally grows in European countries and is sold in their markets. However, the availability of this plant is very limited in India; therefore, another species named *Hypericum patulum* is often sold in place of *H. perforatum*. Both species show major differences in their anatomical features, such as *H. perforatum* having no calcium oxalate crystals, while calcium oxalate crystals are present in *H. patulum*.

iv. **Insufficient Knowledge About Authentic Sources:** *Mesua ferrea*, which belongs to the family Calophyllaceae, is popularly known as Cobra saffron or Nagkesar. Nagkesar is used in the treatment of colds and coughs and is also used for asthma. It is an important species in Ayurvedic medicine. The flowers of *Calophyllum inophyllum* are used as an adulterant and are mixed with market samples of Nagkesar. Although *Mesua ferrea* is available in large quantities in different parts of the Himalayas and the Western Ghats, collectors are often unaware of the original species.

2. **Intentional Adulteration:** It is done deliberately with the aim of enhancing profit or increasing supply. This practice is common in the case of costly products whose demand is high in the market but whose supply is low. Some of the reasons for intentional adulteration are:

i. **Genuine Drugs Adulterated with Inferior Quality Material:** Drugs are mixed with inferior quality materials. Sometimes the inferior quality material either belongs to the same species with low-quality phytoconstituents or to another species. For example, senna is adulterated with dog senna.

ii. **Adulteration with Fictitious Material:** Sometimes the main drug is adulterated with harmful and totally worthless materials that are not plant parts and do not belong to the category of herbal products. Examples include lead shot mixed with opium, asafetida containing pieces of limestone as an adulterant, and synthetic products such as benzyl benzoate mixed with Balsam of Peru.

iii. **Adulteration with Exhausted Products:** This type of adulteration mainly occurs in the case of herbal products that contain volatile oils. Suppliers often extract the main volatile oil from the herbal species using different techniques and mix the exhausted product either with products that are rich in volatile oils or supply only the exhausted one, using the entire oil for other purposes. Some products that are rich in volatile oil include clove, jalap, and umbelliferous fruits.

iv. **Adulteration with Artificially Manufactured Material:** Materials are manufactured with the following points in mind: the material should closely resemble the main product in color, shape, and size. This is done so that the artificial material has a close resemblance to the genuine product. For example, beeswax can be replaced by colored paraffin wax, and basswood of the same shape and size can be used as an adulterant for nutmeg [16]. Herbal products that have medicinal importance are often adulterated with synthetic or prescription drugs such as dexamethasone, diazepam, hydrocortisone, prednisolone, diclofenac, glibenclamide, and many others [17].

An example of some commonly used adulterants that are used to replace or substitute the original drugs is mentioned in Table 2.1.

Some of the herbal medicines sold under the name of dietary supplements contain herbal ingredients identified by the US FDA, and it was found that they contain synthetic drugs. A notice was displayed against them on a public website [21], as mentioned in Table 2.2.

TABLE 2.1 Adulterants or Substitutes for Original Drugs

Sl. No.	Original Drugs	Substitute or Adulterant	References
1.	*Pterocarpus santalinus* Linn. (Rakta Chandana)	*Capsicum annuum* Linn. (Red Capsicum)	[18]
2.	*Carum carvi* Linn. (Kala Jeera)	*Centratherum anthelminticum* Kuntze (Kali Jeeri)	[19]
3.	*Saraca asoca* (Ashoka)	*Polyalthia longifolia*	[20]
4.	*Aconitum heterophyllum* (Ativisha)	*Cyperus rotundus* (Mustaka)	[18]
5.	*Gloriosa superba* (Langali)	*Costus speciosus*	[20]
6.	*Rauwolfia serpentina* (Sarpagandha)	*Rauwolfia densiflora*	[20]
7.	*Saussurea lappa* C.B. Clarke (Kustha)	*Valeriana wallichii* DC (Tagar)	[19]
8.	*Glycyrrhiza glabra* Linn. (Madhuyasthi root)	*Abrus precatorius* Linn. (Gunja Root)	[19]

TABLE 2.2 List of Products Adulterated with Synthetic Drugs

Sl. No.	Product	Synthetic Drug	Purpose
1.	Tiger King	Sildenafil	For sexual stimulation
2.	Vimax (100% natural product)	Tadalafil	Dietary supplement
3.	SexRx	Sildenafil and Tadalafil	Dietary supplement for both males and females for enhancement of sexual performance
4.	Bali Mojo	Tadalafil	Dietary supplement
5.	TINQIANGBUDOR Red Dragon	Sildenafil	Dietary supplement
6.	Weekend Warrior	Thiosildenafil	Dietary supplement
7.	Alpha Male (100% natural)	Five chemicals identified (all having similar action, found to be lethal)	Dietary supplement

2.3 STANDARDIZATION AND EVALUATION OF HERBAL PRODUCTS

Due to the increased cases of adulteration and poor-quality control parameters, there is a great need for the standardization and evaluation of herbal products. People have been consuming herbal products since ancient times.

The market for herbal products has surpassed the demand for conventional drugs. People are using herbal remedies for common problems such as digestive upset, colds, fevers, pain, cuts, and allergies, and so forth. The side effects of conventional drugs have also increased the value of herbal formulations. While it is not true that herbal medicines do not show any side effects, if used in the right amounts, they do not exhibit any unwanted symptoms. Approximately 80% of the population worldwide uses herbs, and in developing countries, this figure is about 95%. Every country has its own share in the global market, and the overall global market for herbal products is over US$ 60 billion, with the value increasing day by day [22].

Despite having such a large market for herbals in India, there is a lack of strong and rigid quality control parameters for herbals. One of the Indian governing bodies, that is, the Department of AYUSH, Government of India, deals with the pharmacopoeial standards for the manufacturing and processing of herbal products [23]. It addresses the matter of standardization and evaluation of herbal products. Standardization describes all aspects related to the life cycle of plants, from their birth to their clinical application, including the quality of herbs associated with their physical, chemical, organoleptic, and microscopic properties. It also deals with the reproducible quality of the product and the defined content of the phytoconstituents present in the products during processing. Evaluation of a drug describes the identity of the genuine drug, its purity and quality, and the nature of any adulterants present in the drug [24].

The huge demand for herbal products among the people creates the problem of a lack of quality control parameters. Herbal products are complex in nature because of the presence of a large number of phytoconstituents, and in the case of polyherbal formulations, the detection of marker compounds becomes difficult with the currently existing methods. Many of the recent advanced analytical techniques focus on the identification and tracking of marker compounds. Regulatory bodies take appropriate measures to ensure the efficacy, purity, and safety of medicinal products [25].

Some of the studies revealed the importance of standardization and the need for appropriate measures:

1. Boston University School of Medicine conducted research on Ayurvedic herbal products available online and found in their study that one-fifth of the Ayurvedic products contain high amounts of arsenic, mercury, and lead. There are many websites

featuring online Ayurvedic products; they randomly selected 163 products from different manufacturers. They found that 20.7% of the products contain detectable amounts of lead, arsenic, and mercury.

2. The UK market banned many Ayurvedic products from consumption because of the presence of heavy metals. Some of the products include Maha Sudarshan Churna powder manufactured by Zandu Pharmaceuticals, Dabur, and Chhatrisha from India, Karela capsules supplied by Himalayan Drug Co., and Sudharshan and Guggal tablets from Zandu Pharmaceuticals [26].
3. Firozian et al. [27] conducted a study to detect the existence of harmful adulterants in herbal weight loss formulations (a total of 63 formulations were used in the study). All the formulations were procured from different apothecaries in Hamadan, Iran. For the primary screening, thin-layer chromatography was employed, and the positive samples were further evaluated using high-performance liquid chromatography (HPLC). The results showed that about 26.98% of the total formulations contain sibutramine (an appetite suppressant). Sibutramine's daily dose intake is about in the range of 5–15 mg daily, while the dose in the formulation was found to be 17.76 ± 6.02 mg/cap [27].

2.4 EVALUATION PARAMETERS FOR HERBAL DRUGS

First of all, the authentication is done for each and every step, area of collection, and parts of the plant collected for study purposes and its regional situation. The WHO published quality control measures for determining the quality of herbal products by utilizing different methods. They publish a series of guidelines for assessing the quality of herbal products. The evaluation parameters for herbal formulations include organoleptic evaluation, microscopical evaluation, physical evaluation, and biological evaluation methods.

1. **Organoleptic Evaluation:** It includes the analysis of raw drugs by their shape, size, odor, taste, and color.
2. **Microscopical Character:** These characters include cell wall characteristic features, starch grains, cell contents, hairs, fibers,

vessels, and the presence or absence of calcium oxalate crystals, as well as histological parameters such as vein islet number, vein termination, stomatal number, stomatal index, palisade ratio, and so on.

3. **Physical Evaluation:** It includes swelling index, foaming index, extractive values, determination of foreign matter, total ash, acid-insoluble ash, successive extractive values, pH, viscosity, moisture content, hardness, alcohol content, flocculation rate, sedimentation rate, and so forth.
4. **Chemical Evaluation:** It includes phytochemical screening, chemical tests, and limit tests.

Other methods for the evaluation of herbal drugs are:

1. **Microbiological Assay:** It includes methods for determining microbiological loads, pesticide residue, and heavy metal determination.
2. **Chromatographic and Spectroscopic Analysis:** Many chromatographic methods are used for the separation and detection of active compounds, such as thin-layer chromatography (TLC), HPLC, gas chromatography (GC), column chromatography (CC), and analytical methods that include volumetric analysis, gravimetric determination, infrared spectroscopy (IR), nuclear magnetic resonance (NMR), UV-Vis spectroscopy, Fourier transform infrared spectroscopy (FTIR), and so forth [28].

Some of the recent advanced techniques used in standardization include supercritical fluid chromatography, which is an advanced technique that combines liquid and GC and is used in the separation of compounds that cannot be separated by either technique alone. Another technique is DNA fingerprinting, which is used for the identification of substances that differ from genuine drugs, as every organism has its unique DNA, which is the fundamental unit of every living cell. Genetic markers are also used for standardization purposes. They are small sequences of genes located on particular genes or traits. Some examples of genetic markers are variable number tandem repeat (VNTR), random amplification of polymorphic DNA (RAPD), Restriction Fragment Length Polymorphism (RFLP), and microsatellite polymorphism, and so forth [29].

2.4.1 ORGANOLEPTIC EVALUATION

When the herbal drugs evaluated by the sensory organs like eyes, nose, tongue, skin, or ear come under organoleptic evaluation. Macroscopical examination of the herbal drugs, such as their color, shape, size, texture, odor, and touch, provides insight into the sensory profile and morphological data of herbal drugs [30]. All pharmacopoeial monographs include the description of morphological parameters of herbal drugs under various headings. For example, in the United States Pharmacopeia (USP), the heading is "Botanic Characteristics;" the European Pharmacopoeia includes the heading "Identification;" and the Pharmacopoeia of the People's Republic of China and the Ayurvedic Pharmacopoeia of India include the heading "Description." The details included in these headings provide information about the size, form, shape, and physical appearance of crude drugs. The plant identity is revealed by the presence of significant characteristics associated with the main plant. These characteristics include aroma, flavor, color, and intensity. They give an idea about the quality of the herbal drugs. The presence of visually detectable adulterants or any other foreign matter can easily be recognized through visual inspection [31].

Some of the important characteristics of herbal species:

- Cinchona, Cascara, and Quillia bark have a fractured surface.
- An aromatic odor is present in umbelliferous fruits.
- Nux vomica, having a disc shape, shows its characteristic feature [29].
- The brown color of cinnamon bark [32].
- The sweet flavor of liquorice [29].
- Different drugs have their characteristic shapes: sarsaparilla (cylindrical), podophyllum (subcylindrical), aconite (conical), jalap (fusiform) [29].

2.4.2 MICROSCOPICAL EVALUATION

The detailed study of the crude drug can be done by microscopical examination. The study of thin sections of specific drugs includes histological studies in which different characteristics are examined. The identifying features of leaves and bark are specific, and their identification can provide insight into the specific plant species. For leaf powder microscopy, the following identification parameters are included: stone cells, fibers, calcium oxalate crystals, medullary rays, epidermis, starch grains, xylem vessels, sclereids, trichomes, lactiferous canals, and stomata [33]. In the case of powdered bark microscopy, the identifying features are medullary rays, starch grains, tubular lactiferous canals, cork, secretory canals, stone cells, and many others [33]. The starch is present in powdered clove fruits but not in the whole fruit part. The powdered clove stalks contain calcium oxalate crystals or sclereids. The powdered forms of rhubarb and ginger showed the presence of non-lignified vessels. The histological or microscopical characters are the same for crude drugs with slight differences; this difference forms the basis for the identification of a particular drug. The presence of any other objectionable structure indicates adulteration in the authentic drug. For roots, bark, stems, and leaves, transverse sections are used for preparation, and for roots and stems, longitudinal sections can also be prepared. Longitudinal sections are also prepared for bark. The quantitative microscopy of herbs includes various histological characters for study and leaf constants such as stomatal index, stomatal number, vein termination number, vein-islet number, palisade ratio, and the Lycopodium spore method, especially for the detection of adulteration in powdered drugs.

Qualitative characters include the types of microscopical structures, such as the different types of stomata present in herbs, which indicate the diagnostic factors. The types of stomata (Table 2.3) are parallel-celled or rubiaceous or paracytic stomata, cross-celled or caryophyllaceous or diacytic stomata, unequal-celled or cruciferous or anisocytic stomata, and irregular-celled or ranunculaceous stomata or anomocytic stomata [34].

TABLE 2.3 Examples for Types of Stomata Present in Herbal Drugs [34]

SL. No.	Types of Stomata	Examples
1.	Stomata with parallel-celled	Coca and Senna
2.	Stomata with cross-celled	Peppermint and Vasaka
3.	Stomata having unequal-celled	Belladona and Datura
4.	Stomata with irregular shape	Lobelia and Digitalis

Another histological feature of herbal drugs is that trichomes are outgrowths from the epidermal cells in tubular form, providing protection to the herbs and secreting essential oil. Different types and their subtypes of trichomes are mentioned in Table 2.4 [34].

TABLE 2.4 Different Types of Trichomes

Sl. No.	Types of Trichomes	Examples
1.	Non-glandular or covering trichomes: • Sharp pointed, curved, lignified • Strongly shrunken, conical, large • Lignified trichomes • Warty, conical, large	*Cannabis*, *Strophanthus*, *Lobelia*, *Nux-vomica*, *Senna*
2.	Covering trichomes (multicellular)	*Pyrethrum*, *Artemisia*
3.	Glandular trichomes: • Unicellular • Multicellular	*Vasaka*, *Cannabis*
4.	Covering unbranched trichomes: • Conical bi-cellular • Three celled long • Four to five celled long	*Belladonna*, *Datura*, *Stramonium*

Calcium oxalate crystals form due to the accumulation of calcium and other environmental factors in various plant species. The size and crystal habit of the crystals differ in crude drugs. Different types of crystals include sphaerocrystals (*Tribulus terrestris*), prismatic crystals (*Aegle marmelos*), acicular crystals (*Boerhavia diffusa*), rosette crystals (*Carissa spinarum*), and microcrystals (*Datura innoxia*) [35].

Diagnostic characters of leaves, also referred to as leaf constants, are studied for the determination of herbal drugs.

1. **Palisade Ratio:** The term palisade ratio was introduced by Wallis and Dewar in 1933. The palisade ratio is defined as the number of palisade cells (average palisade cells) present beneath each epidermal cell [36]. To determine the palisade ratio, a light microscope is used to study the leaf area treated with chloral hydrate. A camera lucida is utilized for the study of epidermal cells and is hence marked. The traced epidermal cells are focused on for the intersection of palisade cells, and the average number is calculated (Table 2.5). The palisade cells covering half of the area are included, and the rest are excluded from the study [37].

TABLE 2.5 List of Some Drugs with the Range of Their Palisade Ratio

SL. No.	Plant Name	Range	References
1.	*Digitalis purpurea*	3.7–4.2	–
2.	*Malva parviflora* L.	1–2	[37]
3.	*Adhatoda vasica* Nees	2.25–3.25	[36]
4.	*Andrographis elongata* T. Anders.	3.75–4.75	[36]
5.	*Cassia angustifolia*	4–7.4 (lower)	–
		5.5–10 (upper)	
6.	*Elytraria acaulis* (L.f) Lindau	7.75–12.5	[36]
7.	*Ocimum sanctum*	2–3.5	–

2. **Stomatal Number:** Stomata are referred to as the minute openings present in the aerial part of the epidermis. Stomatal number is defined as the average number of stomata present per square mm of the epidermis of a leaf.

3. **Stomatal Index:** Stomatal index is defined as the percentage of the total number of stomata (each stoma referred to as a single cell) present to the total number of epidermal cells in a per unit area. The formula used for the calculation:

$$\text{Stomatal Index} = S/S + E \times 100$$

where; S is the stomata per unit area; and E is the epidermal cells in same per unit area.

Clean and washed pieces of leaf are taken for calculating the stomatal index. Using forceps, peel off the lower and upper epidermis of the leaf for a clear visual appearance of the stomata present per unit area. Observe the number of stomata present under the microscope and calculate the stomatal index [37].

4. **Vein Islet Number:** The total number of conducting strands present per square mm of the leaf surface, midway between the margin and the midrib. The vein islet number is a characteristic feature for the identification of leaf drugs, and it is constant for particular species of plants [38].

5. **Vein Termination Number:** The free termination of veinlets is referred to as vein termination. The average number of vein terminations present per square mm of the leaf surface, midway

between the margin and the midrib, is referred to as the vein termination number [38].

The leaf under study is boiled in chloral hydrate solution for clarification. The camera lucida is adjusted, and a 1 mm line is drawn on the board with the help of a stage micrometer to form a square. Similarly, four squares of the same size are drawn adjacently. The leaf under observation is set on the stage, and the vein terminations or islets in the square are traced to detect the vein islet or vein termination number [39].

2.4.3 PHYSICAL METHOD OF EVALUATION

The quality of the herbal drugs is determined by physiochemical analysis, evaluating the herbal drugs through different parameters such as optical rotation, swelling index, foaming index, melting point, viscosity, specific gravity, moisture content, ash value, extractive values, solubility, volatile oil content, and foreign matter detection. The WHO specified the procedures for the physical evaluation of herbal drugs to assess quality and detect adulteration in herbal drugs [38].

1. **Viscosity:** At a given temperature, the viscosity of a liquid is constant, making it an important parameter for the standardization of liquid drugs. For example, liquid paraffin has a kinematic viscosity of not less than 64 centistokes [40].
2. **Moisture Content:** Moisture in crude drugs can lead to microbial contamination and sometimes chemical modification of active constituents, so moisture content is detected to prevent the drug from degradation. Accurately weigh the herbal sample and heat it in hot air at a temperature of 105°C until a constant weight is attained. Weigh the sample again, and the difference in weight indicates the moisture present in the sample. Three methods are commonly used for the determination of moisture content:

    i. **Volumetric Method:** Azeotropic distillation.

    ii. **Gravimetric Method:** Loss on drying.

    iii. **Instrumental Method:** NMR, GC [41].

3. **Optical Rotation:** The ability of the sample (either in solution form or in pure state) to rotate the plane polarized light from its original path is referred to as the property of optical rotation, and the compounds known to be optically active. The rotation of plane polarized light is either towards the left, known as laevo rotatory, or towards the right, known as dextro rotatory. Sodium light is used as a light source in the study for the determination of optical rotation at a temperature of 25°C. Alfikri et al. [42] measured the optical rotation of clove oil using a polarimeter and found it to be 1?63 ± 1?10 in the budding stage.

4. **Melting Point:** The melting point of a particular substance gives an idea about the purity of that substance. The apparatus used in melting point determination provides readings in a particular range, but in the case of a pure compound, the range is very narrow, that is about 1°C for pure drugs [43]. The temperature at which the solid substance melts and changes into liquid form is referred to as its melting point. For example, agar melts at 85°C, and wool fat melts in a range of about 34–44°C [38].

5. **Ash Value:** On ignition of an herbal drug, the remaining material after incineration is referred to as ash. The ash generally contains inorganic salts like calcium, magnesium, carbonates, silicates, phosphates, sodium, and so forth. The presence of inorganic salts in the ash gives an idea about adulteration in herbal drugs [44]. Different types of ash values are:

    i. **Total Ash:** When the sample is treated at very high temperatures (500–600°C), the residues remaining after incineration are called ash. At high temperatures, all the organic matter present in the sample degrades into ions and is released in the form of gas. The minerals remain in the residue in the form of ash.

    ii. **Water-Soluble Ash:** The herbal drugs are subjected to extraction by various solvents. The residues remaining after the extraction are incinerated to determine the ash value of the exhausted drug. The ash is boiled in water and further filtered using ashless filter paper. Water-soluble ash is calculated by the difference between the total ash and the residue left after washing.

iii. **Acid-Insoluble Ash:** The portion of ash insoluble in dilute hydrochloric acid is referred to as acid-insoluble ash. Sand-like particles and silica are not soluble in acid [37, 45].

iv. **Sulfated Ash:** Sulfated ash is determined by treating the sample with sulfuric acid before incineration. This process ensures that all organic matter is fully oxidized, and it converts metals to their sulfate forms. The residue, after incineration in the presence of sulfuric acid, represents the sulfated ash. This method is particularly useful for determining the total amount of inorganic substances present in the form of stable sulfates and helps detect impurities such as heavy metals or extraneous matter.

6. **Extractive Values:** When the herbal drug is kept in contact with the solvent for a definite time interval, the phytoconstituents present in it are extracted into that solvent, resulting in the extractive value [46]. Different solvents are used for the extraction of herbal drugs, and based on this extractive value, they are classified as alcohol soluble extractive values, water soluble extractive values, ether soluble extractive values, and so forth.

   i. **Alcohol Soluble Extractive Value:** Alcohol, being polar in nature, is a suitable solvent for the extraction of a number of phytoconstituents like resins, tannins, and so forth. A 90–95% alcohol solution is used for the extraction of herbal drugs. Dilute alcohol is also used if the solubility of the crude drug is higher in alcohol. A coarsely powdered sample (air dried) is weighed accurately and macerated with 100 ml of alcohol (90–95%) for a specific time interval with occasional shaking. After 24 hours, filter the solution with no loss of solvent, concentrate the filtrate, and dry it at 105°C. Then weigh the dried extract obtained to determine the percentage of extractive value in reference to the air-dried sample taken for extraction [46].

   ii. **Water Soluble Extractive Value:** This method is used when the drug contains active constituents that are readily soluble in water, such as mucilage, glycosides, and so forth. For example, the water-soluble extractive value of glycyrrhiza is not less than 20 [38].

7. **Foreign Organic Matter:** Foreign organic matter refers to any unwanted material present in the authentic sample. It is referred to as foreign matter if the substance falls into the following categories:

   i. Any contamination including insects, molds, and other animal waste products.

   ii. Any material not related to the original source.

   iii. Any part or organ not mentioned in the description of the original drug.

   iv. Any organ that is not related to the description of the authentic drug.

   Weigh the specific amount of sample (as specified in the monograph), spread the sample on a white-colored tile, and observe it with the naked eye or with the help of a magnifying lens. Identify and separate the foreign organic matter, if present in the sample, and weigh it. Then calculate the % w/w of foreign organic matter present in the sample [47].

8. **Volatile Oil Content:** Volatile oils are present in aromatic plants; they are referred to as volatile because, upon increasing the temperature, these oils evaporate easily. They are also known as essential oils due to the presence of fragrance. The volatile oil content is determined by the extraction of oil from the sample through the apparatus known as "Clevenger." The sample in the round-bottom flask is boiled at a specific temperature with either water or a solvent like hexane or any other. The oil, due to its volatile nature, evaporates with the water and gets collected in the side arm at the upper portion. The collected oil is later separated from the water. The percentage yield can be calculated [48]. For example, clove contains not less than 10% w/w of volatile.

9. **Foaming Index:** Herbal drugs contain a number of phytoconstituents, but the presence of saponins has the ability to produce foam when shaken with an aqueous solution. Saponins form persistent foam while shaking due to their detergent-like properties. According to the WHO [46], foaming ability is defined as the ability of a plant extract or its aqueous decoction to form foam, and it is measured in terms of the foaming index [47].

Coarsely powdered herbal sample (1 g in weight) is taken in a conical flask (500 ml). Pour boiling water into it (100 ml) and boil the mixture for about 30 minutes. After that, filter it and transfer the extract into a volumetric flask (100 ml), adjusting the volume if needed. Now pour the sample into tubes covered with stoppers in the proportions of 1 ml, 2 ml, 3 ml, 4 ml, 5 ml, 6 ml, 7 ml, 8 ml, and so on. Adjust the volume up to 10 ml in all the tubes. Shake the tubes in such a manner that there are two shakes in one second. Observe the foam produced in different test tubes and record the results as follows:

i. If in each tube the height of the foam after shaking is found to be below 1 cm, then the foaming index is indicated as less than 100.

ii. If any of the tubes has a foam height above 1 cm, then prepare a serial dilution to obtain more accurate results.

iii. If all the tubes show a foam height greater than 1 cm, then the foaming index is greater than 1000. Prepare the dilution and repeat the experiment.

$$\text{Foaming Index} = 1000/a$$

where; a is when the height of foam produced observed above 1 cm, then the decoction volume used for dilution is denoted as "a" [48].

10. **Swelling Index:** Under specified conditions, 1 g of the sample absorbs the volume of solution (any swelling agent) or water, and the resulting swelling is referred to as the swelling index. The determination of the swelling index is important for herbal drugs that contain mucilage, as it provides an idea about the mucilage content.

A sample of about 1 g is taken in a measuring cylinder (25 mL), and then water or any other solution is added according to the requirement. Shake the measuring cylinder occasionally for about 24 hours. Keep it aside for an hour, then measure the volume occupied by the swollen sample. Example: *Isabgol* seeds – swelling factor not less than 10 [47].

2.4.4 CHEMICAL METHOD OF EVALUATION

Chemical evaluation methods involve the phytochemical screening of herbal drugs to detect the presence of phytoconstituents in herbal extracts. The phytochemical screening is carried out for alkaloids, flavonoids, proteins, saponins, tannins, steroids, carbohydrates, and glycosides as per standard methods.

1. **Test for Alkaloids:**
   - **Dragendorff's Reagent:** 2–3 mL of extract was taken, and a few drops of Dragendorff's reagent were added; the formation of an orange-brown precipitate indicates the presence of alkaloids.
   - **Mayer's Reagent (Potassium Mercuric Iodide Reagent):** A few drops of Mayer's reagent were added to the plant extract; the formation of a yellow-colored precipitate indicates the presence of alkaloids.
2. **Test for Saponins:**
   - **Froth Formation Test:** 2–3 mL of extract was taken in a test tube along with water; after shaking, stable foam formation indicates the presence of saponins.
3. **Test for Tannins:**
   - **Ferric Chloride Test:** To 2–3 mL of extract, 3–4 drops of ferric chloride solution were added. The formation of a bluish-black color indicates the presence of phenolic compounds [45].
4. **Test for Flavonoids:**
   - **Shinoda Test:** A few magnesium turnings were added to the test solution, and concentrated hydrochloric acid was added dropwise; the formation of an orange, pink, red, or purple color indicates the presence of flavonoids.
   - **Sulfuric Acid Test:** To saffron extract, sulfuric acid was added. The formation of a deep yellow solution indicates the presence of flavones and flavonoids.
5. **Test for Proteins:**
   - **Millon's Test (Mercuric Nitrate Solution):** To 3 mL of plant extract, a few drops of Millon's reagent were added; the

formation of a white precipitate that slowly changes to pink upon warming indicates the presence of proteins [45].

6. **Test for Carbohydrates:**
   - **Molisch Test:** 2–3 mL of extract was taken, and a few drops of alpha-naphthol solution in alcohol were added. Then concentrated sulfuric acid was added from the side of the test tube. The formation of a violet ring at the junction of the two liquids indicates the presence of sugars.
7. **Test for Steroids:**
   - **Salkowski Test:** To 2–3 mL of extract, 2 mL of chloroform and 2 mL of concentrated sulfuric acid were added from the side of the test tube. The chloroform layer appears red, and the acid layer shows greenish-yellow fluorescence, indicating the presence of steroids.
8. **Test for Glycosides:**
   - **Keller-Kiliani Test (Test for Deoxy Sugars):** 2–3 mL of chloroform extract was taken, and 1 drop of glacial acetic acid was added, followed by the addition of trace amounts of ferric chloride. Then, 2–3 drops of concentrated sulfuric acid were added. A blue-green color indicates the presence of glycosides.

2.4.5 BIOLOGICAL METHOD OF EVALUATION

Different evaluation parameters, such as organoleptic, physical, microscopical, macroscopical, or chemical, are important for the standardization of herbal drugs. However, the biological or pharmacological evaluation of crude drugs is necessary when the above parameters are not sufficient for complete standardization and determination of the therapeutic activity of herbal drugs. Pharmacological screening of drugs or preclinical studies follows the CPCSEA guidelines. From the selection of animals, their handling, choice of model, experimentation, and evaluation of biological activity through various screening models (Table 2.6), all are important parameters for the pharmacological study of drugs. Rodents, non-rodents, and miscellaneous are the three categories of animals used in experiments.

Rodents include guinea pigs, rats, mice, hamsters, and so forth.; non-rodents include dogs, monkeys, cats, rabbits, and so forth; and pigeons, chickens, and frogs fall into the miscellaneous category [49].

TABLE 2.6 Different Models for the Pharmacological Screening of Herbal Drugs

Sl. No.	Pharmacological Screening Model	*In Vivo* Model	*In Vitro* Model	References
1.	For anti-diabetic drugs	• Streptozotocin-induced diabetic model • Alloxan-induced diabetic model • Goldthioglucose obese diabetic model • Dithizone-induced diabetic model	• α-Glucosidase inhibition assay • α-Amylase inhibition assay • Glucose uptake assay by adipocyte cell line	[50]
2.	For anti-inflammatory drugs	• Carrageenan-induced paw edema • Serotonin-induced paw edema in rats • Croton oil-induced ear edema in rats • Granuloma model induced by cotton • Pleurisy in rat model • Air pouch technique	• Phospholipase A_2 enzyme assay • Prostaglandin synthase assay • Electrophoretic mobility shift assay	[51]
3.	Memory and learning	• Morris water maze test • Radial arm test • Elevated plus maze model • Step-through and step-down passive avoidance test • Chemically-induced amnesia • Shock-induced amnesia	–	[52]
4.	For anti-parkinsonian drugs	• Tremorine and oxotremorine antagonism • Catalepsy induced by haloperidol • MPTP model in monkeys • Chemically-induced models such as lipopolysaccharide, methamphetamine	• Cell transplantation	[53]

TABLE 2.6 *(Continued)*

Sl. No.	Pharmacological Screening Model	*In Vivo* Model	*In Vitro* Model	References
5.	For analgesic drugs	• Hot plate test • Tail flick test • Tail pressure test • Formalin test • Writhing test induced by acetic acid	–	[54]
6.	For antioxidant drugs	–	• DPPH assay • Nitric oxide radical scavenging assay • Hydrogen peroxide radical scavenging assay • Lipid peroxidation assay • Aspartate aminotransferase assay • Superoxide dismutase assay • Trolox equivalent antioxidant capacity assay	[55]
7.	For anti-cancer drugs	• Ehrlich ascites carcinoma induction	• Trypan blue dye exclusion assay • Sulforhodamine B assay • Lactic dehydrogenase assay	[56]

2.5 QUANTITATIVE MICROSCOPY OF CRUDE DRUGS

2.5.1 *LYCOPODIUM SPORE METHOD*

Wallis introduced this method to detect the adulteration in powdered drugs and it was later officially accepted in the Indian Pharmacopoeia (1996).

Lycopodium clavatum Linn., also known as club moss, belongs to the family Lycopodiaceae and contains yellow-colored lycopodium spores. The spores have a reticulate surface and are tetrahedral and somewhat spheroidal in shape. The average diameter of Lycopodium spores is 25 microns. A total of 94,000 spores is equal to 1 milligram in weight. The spores show resistance to pressure and have a similar weight due to the presence of uniform moisture content.

The evaluation of powdered drugs by this technique is possible if it contains: (i) objects having uniform thickness so that the actual area or length can be measured through suitable magnification; (ii) tissues having a single layer or cells that can be evaluated so that the actual area can be calculated under magnification; and (iii) countable particles like pollen grains or starch grains. The authentic ginger powder was evaluated for its percent purity for the detection of adulterants in powdered form by using the formula:

$$(N \times W \times 94{,}000 \times 100)/(S \times M \times P) = \%\text{ purity of drug}$$

where; N is the characteristics structure in 25 or 26 fields; W is the lycopodium weight (mg); S is the lycopodium spores present in 25 or 26 fields which was taken for study of characteristic structure; M is the sample weight (mg); and P is 2,86,000 (for ginger starch grains powder) [37].

2.6 DNA FINGERPRINTING TECHNIQUES FOR IDENTIFICATION OF NATURAL DRUGS

The genetic identity of the herbal species, cultivars, or the genetic makeup of the herbal drug can be determined by the DNA fingerprinting technique. The Ayurvedic formulation *Rasayana Churna* contains three main ingredients: *Tinospora cordifolia* (stem), *Emblica officinalis* (dried fruit), and *Tribulus terrestris* (dried fruit) in powder form. RAPD DNA analysis was performed to establish the presence of these herbs [57]. DNA fingerprinting is an advanced technique for the standardization of herbal drugs. The identification of samples is done at the molecular level, that is, by identifying the genetic characteristics. DNA is the basic component of all cells, whether they belong to plants or animals. DNA comprises nucleotide base pairs (guanine, cytosine, thymine, adenine) and sugar linked by phosphate bonds. Each plant species has its specific DNA sequence pattern or gene located on the chromosome, referred to as DNA markers. They may be short in length [58].

2.6.1 MAJOR STAGES OF DNA FINGERPRINTING

DNA fingerprinting involves three important steps:

1. **Isolation of DNA from Plant Parts:** In the procedure of DNA fingerprinting, the DNA is isolated from the plant cells by digesting the cell wall with a suitable enzyme and then removing the nuclear membrane present around the DNA. Other cellular components, such as RNA, proteins, lipids, and other cell debris, are also separated from each other. A fresh part of the plant is generally preferred for the isolation of DNA.

2. **Quantification of Isolated DNA and Its Quality Assessment:** The quantification of isolated DNA is performed using analytical instruments like a UV-Visible spectrophotometer.

3. **Polymerase Chain Reaction:** Isolated DNA is further amplified through polymerase chain reaction (PCR) from a specific single or duplex amount of DNA template into millions of copies [59].

2.6.2 GENETIC MARKERS USED IN DNA FINGERPRINTING TECHNIQUES

The genetic markers used in DNA fingerprinting techniques are:

1. **Random Amplification of Polymeric DNA (RAPD):** The RAPD technique is based on the PCR technique. The short fragments of isolated DNA (up to 10 bases long) are amplified by the PCR under low annealing temperatures. The amplified fragments are further separated on agarose gel after staining with ethidium bromide. A huge number of genetic markers are obtained by the RAPD technique, which requires a small amount of DNA with no additional requirements for sequencing, cloning, or any other molecular characterization [60].

2. **Restriction Fragment Length Polymorphism (RFLP):** By cutting sequences of Variable Number of Tandem Repeats of up to 30 sequences with restriction enzymes, unequal lengths of DNA fragments are obtained, which are known as RFLP. The cutting of DNA at specific sites is performed by the restriction enzymes. The amplification of DNA by PCR is not necessary for this method [61].

3. **Variable Number Tandem Repeat (VNTR):** These are the repeated sequences of DNA present in an individual. The RFLP technique analyzes the variable number of tandem repeats and further amplifies them by PCR. This genotypic tool provides data in a simple and repetitive format [62].
4. **Short Tandem Repeats (STR):** These are also known as Short Sequence Repeats or Microsatellites. DNA lengths of up to 1–6 base pairs are present repetitively and can form up to 100 nucleotide-long series. Microsatellites make up about 3% of the total genome, with about 8% present in coding regions and the remaining in non-coding regions. Dinucleotide repeats are a common example of short tandem repeats [63].
5. **Amplified Fragment Length Polymorphism (AFLP):** It is the modified form of RFLP, which relies on the PCR methodology. Restriction enzymes cut the DNA at specific sites, then adaptors ligate to the fragment's sticky ends. The selected sequence is amplified and then separated by electrophoresis.
6. **Single Nucleotide Polymorphism (SNP):** Nucleotides like adenine, cytosine, guanine, and thymine are present in the genomic DNA. Plant species differ in the single nucleotide sequence in their genomic DNA, which is used to analyze by this technique [58].

KEYWORDS

- **adulteration**
- **amplified fragment length polymorphism**
- **DNA fingerprinting**
- **herbal drugs**
- **quantitative microscopy**
- **short tandem repeats**
- **single nucleotide polymorphism**
- **Wallis method**

REFERENCES

1. Gunjan, M., Naing, T. W., Saini, R. S., Ahmad, A. B., Naidu, J. R., & Kumar, I. (2015). Marketing trends and future prospects of herbal medicine in the treatment of various diseases. *World Journal of Pharmaceutical Research, 4*(9), 132–155.
2. Arya, R., Singh, D. C., Tiwari, R. C., & Tripathi, B. M. (2016). An overview of ethnomedicine and future aspect of ethnomedicinal plants. *International Journal of Ayurveda and Pharmaceutical Research, 4*(5), 29–33.
3. Nirmal, S. A., Pal, S. C., Otimenyin, S. O., Aye, T., Elachouri, M., Kundu, S. K., Thandavarayan, R. A., & Mandal, S. C. (2013). Contribution of herbal products in the global market. *The Pharmaceutical Review*, 95–104.
4. Sonaye, H. V., Pund, L. G., Chilate, V., & Doifode, C. A. (2017). Opportunities and challenges in recent trends in herbal medicines. *World Journal of Pharmaceutical and Medical Research, 3*(6), 138–143.
5. Srivastava, A. K. (2018). Chapter 1–Significance of medicinal plants in human life. In *Synthesis of Medicinal Agents from Plants* (pp. 1–24). Elsevier. https://doi.org/10.1016/B978-0-08-102071-5.00001-5.
6. Raghu, A. V., & Amruth, M. (2018). Cultivation of medicinal plants: Challenges and prospects. In *Prospects in Conservation of Medicinal Plants* (Chapter 8, pp. 85–94). KSCSTE-KFRI.
7. Pagare, S., Bhatia, M., Tripathi, N., Pagare, S., & Bansal, Y. K. (2015). Secondary metabolites of plants and their role: Overview. *Current Trends in Biotechnology and Pharmacy, 9*(3), 293–304.
8. Gangola, S., Khati, P., Bhatt, P., Parul, & Sharma, A. (2017). India as the heritage of medicinal plants and their use. *Current Trends in Biomedical Engineering & Biosciences, 4*(4), 0050–0051.
9. Ahmad, D. R., Shahnawaz, M., & Qazi, P. H. (2017). General overview of medicinal plants: A review. *Journal of Phytopharmacology, 6*(6), 349–351.
10. Rajendran, K., Balaji, P., & Basu, M. J. (2008). Medicinal plants and their utilization by villagers in southern districts of Tamil Nadu. *Indian Journal of Traditional Knowledge, 7*(3), 417–420.
11. Das, M., Jain, V., & Malhotra, S. K. (2016). Impact of climate change on medicinal and aromatic plants: Review. *Indian Journal of Agricultural Sciences, 86*(11), 1375–1382.
12. Shanmughanandhan, D., Ragupathy, S., Newmaster, S. G., Mohana, S. S., & Sathish, R. (2016). Estimating herbal product authentication and adulteration in India using a vouchered, DNA-based biological reference material library. *Drug Safety, 39*(2), 1211–1227. https://doi.org/10.1007/s40264-016-0459-0.
13. Prakash, O., Jyoti, Kumar, A., Kumar, A., & Manna, N. K. (2013). Adulteration and substitution in Indian medicinal plants: An overview. *Journal of Medicinal Plants Studies, 1*(4), 127–132.
14. Kumar, N. N., & Ruba, K. (2018). Identification of adulterants by pharmacognostical evaluation in selected medicinal plants. *World Journal of Pharmaceutical and Medical Research, 4*(2), 67–70.

15. Han, J., Pang, X., Liao, B., Yao, H., Song, J., & Chen, S. (2016). An authenticity survey of herbal medicines from markets in China using DNA barcoding. *Scientific Reports, 6*, 18723. https://doi.org/10.1038/srep18723.
16. Agarwal, P., & Goyal, A. (2021). A comprehensive review on adulteration and substitution of crude drugs. *Asian Journal of Pharmaceutical and Clinical Research, 14*(4), 33–38.
17. Posadzki, P., Watson, L., & Ernst, E. (2013). Contamination and adulteration of herbal medicinal products (HMPs): An overview of systematic reviews. *European Journal of Clinical Pharmacology, 69*, 295–307. https://doi.org/10.1007/s00228-012-1353-z.
18. Raviraja, S. G., & Harsha, R. (2021). Adulteration in medicinal plants and herbal drugs. *International Journal of Agricultural Sciences, 12*(1), 12–17.
19. Rathore, B. S., Kotecha, M., Chaudhary, K., & Manjula. (2022). Adulteration and substitution in Indian medicinal plants: A review article. *International Research Journal of Ayurveda & Yoga, 5*(5), 72–78.
20. Sreelekshmi, M., Vimala, K. S., Paul, R. P., Chandran, N., Shine, P. A., & Salam, N. A. (2017). Drug adulteration: A threat to efficacy of Ayurveda medicine. *Journal of Medicinal Plants Studies, 5*(4), 1–6.
21. Sarker, M. R. (2014). Adulteration of herbal medicines and dietary supplements with undeclared synthetic drugs: Dangerous for human health. *International Journal of Pharmacy and Pharmaceutical Sciences, 6*(4), 1–2.
22. Khan, S. A., & Ahmad, I. (2019). Herbal medicine: Current trends and future prospects. In *New Look to Phytomedicine* (pp. 3–13). https://doi.org/10.1016/B978-0-12-814619-4.00001-X.
23. Patel, C. J., Tyagi, S., Patel, K. J., Patel, T., Patel, H. K., & Patel, P. H. (2014). Standardization of herbal medicine: A concise review. *Indian Journal of Pharmaceutical and Biological Research, 2*(1), 97–101.
24. Yadav, P., Mahour, K., & Kumar, A. (2011). Standardization and evaluation of herbal drug formulations. *Journal of Advanced Laboratory Research in Biology, 2*(4), 161–166.
25. Kunle, F. O., Egharevba, O. H., & Ahmadu, O. P. (2012). Standardization of herbal medicines: A review. *International Journal of Biodiversity and Conservation, 4*(3), 101–112.
26. Aneesh, T. P., Hisham, M., Sonal, S. M., Manjushree, M., & Deepa, T. V. (2009). International market scenario of traditional Indian herbal drugs: India declining. *International Journal of Green Pharmacy, 3*(3), 184–190.
27. Firozian, F., Nili-Ahmadabadi, A., Moradkhani, S., Moulaei, M., Fasihi, Z., & Ahmadimoghaddam, D. (2021). Adulteration of the herbal weight loss products by the illegal addition of synthetic antiobesity medications: A pilot study. *Journal of Obesity, 2021*, 1–3. https://doi.org/10.1155/2021/9968730.
28. Rasheed, A., Reddy, S. B., & Roja, C. (2012). A review on standardization of herbal formulation. *International Journal of Phytotherapy Research, 2*(2), 74–88.
29. Bijauliya, R. K., Sashi, A., Chanchal, D. K., & Kumar, M. (2017). A comprehensive review on standardization of herbal drugs. *International Journal of Pharmaceutical Sciences and Research, 8*(9), 3663–3677.
30. Kamboj, A. (2012). Analytical evaluation of herbal drugs. In *Drug Discovery Research in Pharmacognosy* (pp. 23–60).

31. Upton, R., David, B., Gafner, S., & Glas, S. (2020). Botanical ingredient identification and quality assessment: Strengths and limitations of analytical techniques. *Phytochemistry Reviews, 19*, 1157–1177. https://doi.org/10.1007/s11101-019-09625-z.
32. Patil, S. G., Wagh, A. S., Pawar, R. C., & Ambore, S. M. (2013). Standard tools for evaluation of herbal drugs: An overview. *Pharma Innovation, 2*(9), 60–65.
33. Aeri, V. (2020). *Powdered Crude Drugs: Microscopy for Leaves and Bark. Microscopic Identifying Features for Bark and Leaves* (pp. 21–30).
34. Alamgir, A. N. M. (2021). Microscopy in pharmacognosy. In *Therapeutic Use of Medicinal Plants and Their Extracts* (Vol. 73). Springer, Cham. https://doi.org/10.1007/978-3-319-63862-1_11.
35. Krishnan, V., Munuswamy, E., Nandhagopal, K., & Amerjothy, S. (2018). Micromorphology of calcium oxalate crystals in selected medicinal plants. *World Journal of Pharmaceutical Research, 7*(11), 751–758.
36. Simon, T. K. (2018). Systematic significance of palisade ratio in pharmacognostic applications. *Journal of Pharmaceutical and Biological Sciences, 13*(2), 1–8.
37. Akbar, S., Hanif, U., Ali, J., & Ishtiaq, S. (2014). Pharmacognostic studies of stem, roots and leaves of *Malva parviflora* L. *Asian Pacific Journal of Tropical Biomedicine, 4*(5), 410–415.
38. Shah, B., & Seth, A. K. (2010). *Textbook of Pharmacognosy & Phytochemistry* (1st ed.). Elsevier.
39. Kumar, D., Kumar, K., Kumar, S., Kumar, T., Kumar, A., & Prakash, O. (2012). Pharmacognostic evaluation of leaf and root bark of *Holoptelea integrifolia* Roxb. *Asian Pacific Journal of Tropical Biomedicine, 2*(3), 169–175.
40. Prakash, K. D., Shivaji, G. S., Rohidas, K. P., Patel, V., & Bhalke, R. (2017). Current quality control methods for standardization of herbal drugs. *International Journal of Pharmaceutical and Drug Analysis, 5*(3), 82–95.
41. Pradhan, N., Gavali, J., & Waghmare, N. (2015). World Health Organization (WHO) guidelines for standardization of herbal drugs. *International Ayurvedic Medical Journal, 3*(8), 2238–2243.
42. Alfikri, F. N., Pujiarti, R., Wibisono, M. G., & Hardiyanto, E. B. (2020). Yield, quality, and antioxidant activity of clove (*Syzygium aromaticum* L.) bud oil at different phenological stages in young and mature trees. *Scientifica, 2020*(4), 1–8.
43. Young, J. C. O. C. (2013). True melting point determination. *Chemical Educator, 18*, 203–208.
44. Mukherjee, P. K. (2019). Qualitative analysis for evaluation of herbal drugs. In P. K. Mukherjee (Ed.), *Quality Control and Evaluation of Herbal Drugs* (pp. 79–149). Elsevier. https://doi.org/10.1016/b978-0-12-813374-3.00004-1.
45. Khandelwal, K. R. (2010). *Practical Pharmacognosy* (20th ed.). Nirali Prakashan.
46. Ahmed, S., & Hasan, M. M. (2015). Standardization of crude drugs: A precise review. *World Journal of Pharmaceutical Research, 4*(10), 155–174.
47. Hait, M. (2021). Physicochemical analysis of herbal drugs. In *Recent Advances in Pharmaceutical Sciences* (Vol. 3, pp. 29–53). AkiNik Publications.
48. World Health Organization. (1998). *Quality Control Methods for Medicinal Plant Materials*. Geneva, Switzerland: World Health Organization.

49. Uthirapathy, S., Ahamad, J., Albert, J., & Dubey, G. P. (2020). Pharmacological evaluation of herbal medicine. In *Bioactive Phytochemicals: Drug Discovery to Product Development* (Chapter 6, pp. 100–120). Bentham Science.
50. Vijayaraj, R., Kumaran, N. S., & Swarnakala. (2019). *In vivo* and *in vitro* models for biological screening of anti-diabetic drugs. *International Journal of Pharmaceutical and Biological Sciences, 9*(2), 294–298.
51. Eze, F. I., Philip, F. U., Peter, I., Bonaventure, C. O., & Patience, O. O. (2019). *In vitro* and *in vivo* models for anti-inflammation: An evaluative review. *INNOSC Theranostics and Pharmacological Sciences, 2*(2), 3–15.
52. Narwal, S., Saini, D. R., Kumari, K., Narwal, S., Singh, G., Negi, R. S., & Sarin, R. V. (2012). Behavior and pharmacological animal models for the evaluation of learning and memory condition. *Indo Global Journal of Pharmaceutical Sciences, 2*(2), 121–129.
53. Kanase, V. G., Pandagale, P. M., & Dani, S. M. (2022). Screening models of anti-parkinsonian agents. *International Journal of Pharmaceutical Sciences & Research, 13*(6), 2230–2241. https://doi.org/10.13040/IJPSR.0975-8232.13(6).2230-41.
54. Deshmukh, A. S., Morankar, P. G., & Kumbhare, M. R. (2014). Review on analgesic activity and determination methods. *PhTechMed, 3*(1), 425–428.
55. Sharma, A., Bhardwaj, S., Mann, A. S., & Jain, K. M. D. (2007). Screening methods of antioxidant activity: An overview. *Pharmacognosy Reviews*, 1 (2), 1–7.
56. Chanda, S., & Nagani, K. (2013). *In vitro* and *in vivo* methods for anticancer activity evaluation and some Indian medicinal plants possessing anticancer properties: An overview. *Journal of Pharmacognosy and Phytochemistry, 2*(2), 140–152.
57. Joshi, D. D. (2012). Herbal drugs and DNA fingerprints. In *Herbal Drugs and Fingerprints* (pp. 231–245). Springer India. https://doi.org/10.1007/978-81-322-0804-4_13.
58. Minoch, S. (2017). Short review on DNA-fingerprinting and standardization of herbal drugs. *International Journal of Medical and Biomedical Studies, 1*(2), 1–9.
59. Gharde, P. R., Chothe, D. S., & Shekokar, S. (2019). Herbal drug standardization and application of DNA fingerprinting: A review. *European Journal of Pharmaceutical and Medical Research, 6*(1), 202–208.
60. Bardakci, F. (2001). Random amplified polymorphic DNA (RAPD) markers. *Turkish Journal of Biology, 25*, 185–196.
61. Singla, K., Rani, Y., Panchal, K., Singh, R. K., & Chouksey, V. (2017). DNA fingerprinting. *European Journal of Pharmaceutical and Medical Research, 4*(8), 244–246.
62. Mansoor, S. K., Hussein, E. F., & Ibraheem, A. K. (2021). Use of variable number tandem repeats (VNTR) in DNA fingerprinting and its application in biological sciences. *Eurasia Journal of Biosciences, 14*, 2835–2839.
63. Fan, H., & Chu, J. Y. (2007). A brief review of short tandem repeat mutation. *Genomics, Proteomics & Bioinformatics, 5*(1), 7–14.

CHAPTER 3

Cultivation, Collection, and Processing of Drugs of Natural Origin: The Quality Perceptions

SANYAM SHARMA,[1] SUBH NAMAN,[1,2] VARINDER SINGH,[1] MANSOUR GHORBANPOUR,[3] JITENDER MADAN,[4] M. S. ASHAWAT,[5] and ASHISH BALDI[1,*]

[1]*Pharma Innovation Lab, Department of Pharmaceutical Sciences and Technology, Maharaja Ranjit Singh Punjab Technical University, Bathinda, Punjab, India*

[2]*Faculty of Pharmaceutical Sciences, ICFAI University, Himachal Pradesh, India*

[3]*Department of Medicinal Plants, Faculty of Agriculture and Natural Resources, Arak University, Iran*

[4]*Department of Pharmaceutics, National Institute of Pharmaceutical Education and Research, Hyderabad, Telangana, India*

[5]*Laureate Institute of Pharmacy, Kathog, Kangra, Himachal Pradesh, India*

*Corresponding author

ABSTRACT

Medicinal plants contain various secondary metabolites or bioactive components responsible for their therapeutic properties. It is crucial to employ straightforward methods that preserve the therapeutic qualities of natural products (NPs) during the cultivation, harvesting, and storage

The Essentials of Herbal Drugs. Varsha Tiwari, Abhishek Tiwari, and Ajay Sharma (Eds.)

DOI: 10.1201/9781998511778-3

of medicinal herbal plants. The pharmacological attributes of medicinal plants largely depend on the presence of diverse bioactive phytochemicals, including volatile oils, alkaloids, glycosides, tannins, and resins. Modern agricultural techniques like hybridization, polyploidy, and mutation may enhance the production of these secondary metabolites. Various environmental factors such as sunlight, temperature, rainfall, and soil composition significantly impact the development and growth of medicinal plants, as well as the concentration of bioactive components. Geographical location and seasonal variations can also influence the quality of aromatic and medicinal plants by altering the levels of these bioactive constituents. The present chapter will focus on quality risk management during the cultivation and collection of medicinal plants. Critical materials encompass any agricultural materials that affect the quality of raw medicinal plants, including soil, water, seeds, site, and fertilizers. Similarly, the processes involved in agricultural practices such as soil preparation, sowing, manure addition, irrigation, protection from weeds and pests, harvesting, and storage is critical for maintaining quality. Understanding the interplay between natural conditions, agricultural techniques, and environmental factors is essential to ensure the production of high-quality medicinal plants. Implementing effective quality risk management practices throughout the cultivation and collection process, as detailed here, will provide deep insights for adopting optimum cultivation practices and environments for farm-level production of herbal drugs.

3.1 INTRODUCTION

In the realm of medicinal plants and their therapeutic properties, these botanical wonders have served as remedies for diverse ailments for centuries. Various cultures worldwide have acknowledged and harnessed the therapeutic potential inherent in medicinal plants. In contemporary times, there is a renewed interest in medicinal plants as organic alternatives to synthetic drugs, driven by their perceived efficacy and minimal side effects. Medicinal plants, alternatively known as medicinal herbs or herbal medicines, encompass plants or plant parts (leaves, stems, flowers, roots, etc.) valued for their therapeutic properties. These plants harbor a myriad of chemical compounds, including alkaloids, flavonoids, terpenoids, and phenolic compounds, which contribute to their medicinal prowess.

Essential to traditional medicine systems such as Ayurveda, Traditional Chinese Medicine (TCM), and indigenous healing practices, the significance of medicinal plants lies in their potential to deliver a broad spectrum of therapeutic benefits. They have historically been instrumental in treating various ailments, spanning infections, digestive disorders, respiratory conditions, skin afflictions, and even chronic diseases like diabetes and cardiovascular disorders. Furthermore, medicinal plants can manifest antioxidant, anti-inflammatory, antimicrobial, and anticancer properties.

India stands as a prominent producer of raw materials in South Asia. Export data from 1992 to 1995 reveals that the country exported approximately 32,600 tons of crude drugs valued at US$ 46 million. The commercial significance of these plant-derived medicines is evident in their annual value, reaching around US$ 14 billion in the USA and US$ 40 billion worldwide. Notably, Americans expended an estimated US$ 21.2 billion on services offered by alternative medicine practitioners [1]. Estimating the number of plant species utilized for medicinal purposes poses a challenge, with the WHO's late 1970s enumeration listing 21,000 medicinal species. However, in China alone, 4941 out of 26,092 native species are employed as drugs in TCM, constituting a remarkable 18.9% [2]. Extrapolating this proportion to other renowned medicinal floras and applying it to the global total of 422,000 flowering plant species, it is reasonable to estimate that the number of plant species [3] used for medicinal purposes exceeds 50,000.

3.1.1 THERAPEUTIC PROPERTIES OF MEDICINAL PLANTS

Traditional medicine represents the accumulated healing knowledge derived from generations of practicing physicians within an indigenous system of healthcare [4]. While conventional preparations incorporate medicinal and aromatic plants, minerals, and other organic substances, herbal drugs specifically refer to traditional medicines predominantly utilizing medicinal plant preparations for therapeutic purposes. Traditional medicine encompasses the collective knowledge, skills, and practices rooted in the theories, beliefs, and experiences indigenous to diverse cultures. It is applied for maintaining health, as well as in the prevention, diagnosis, improvement, or treatment of both physical and mental illnesses, regardless of their universal applicability [5]. As per a 1983 estimation by the World Health Organization (WHO), a significant portion of the population in developing countries relies on traditional and herbal medicines as their primary means of healthcare.

The majority of people globally rely on traditional medicine, which mostly uses herbal remedies. Herbal medicine is not only in high demand, but it is also growing. Ayurvedic medicine sales in India are expected to rise at a 20% annual pace, while during the past 10 years, the number of medicinal plants in many countries has increased tenfold [6]. The increasing demand for traditional medicine can be attributed to several causes, such as the growing global population and the limited availability of Western (allopathic) treatment in developing countries. Complementary and alternative medicine is the term for non-traditional medical practices that are widely used in industrialized nations in conjunction with traditional medicine for conditions including cancer therapy. This trend may be influenced by worsening physical symptoms, undesirable side effects of prescription drugs, and diminishing hope. Examples abound of patients with chronic diseases like cancer and HIV exploring various forms of alternative medicine [7]. In southeastern Rajasthan, India, 400 medicinal plants from 97 families are presently employed in ethnomedicine, with claims from folklore about natural drugs undergoing verification through modern scientific methods. The WHO advocates increased efforts in this direction [8, 9]. Table 3.1 comprises the data of some popular medicinal and aromatic plants used in India.

3.2 BIOACTIVE PHYTOCHEMICALS IN MEDICINAL PLANTS

In the enduring saga of the alliance between humanity and medicinal plants, a rich tapestry unfolds, woven with written records and monumental evidence. The annals of our ancestral history bear witness to the integral role played by medicinal plants in addressing diverse disorders, with knowledge passed down through the corridors of civilizations. Human exploration and migration further unveiled new botanical allies with therapeutic properties [39, 40]. Turning attention to secondary metabolites in medicinal herbal plants and their ecological significance, these bioactive compounds are hailed as "chemical goldmines." They serve as reservoirs of valuable substances indispensable for the production of cosmetics, dyes, insecticides, medicines, and perfumes [41]. Emerging as by-products or

TABLE 3.1 Popular Medicinal and Aromatic Herbal Plants in India

Sl. No.	Name of Plant	Part of Plant Used	Active Constituent	Annual Trade (Metric Tons) [10]	Uses	References
1.	Ajwain (*Hyoscyamus niger*)	Seed	Thymol, γ-terpinene, *p*-cymene	>10,000	Asthma, loose motion	[11]
2.	Amla (*Embelica officinalis*)	Fruit	Emblicanin A and B, phyllembein, quercetin, ascorbic acid	>10,000	Liver tonic, immunity booster	[12]
3.	Ashwagandha (*Withania somnifera*)	Root	Withanolides	2000–5000	Joint pain, skin diseases	[13, 14]
4.	Bach (*Acorus calamus*)	Rhizomes	Asarone	500–1000	Carminative, bronchitis, remittent fever	[15, 16]
5.	Brahmi (*Bacopa monnieri*)	Plant	Bacosides, bacopasides	500–1000	Nerve tonic, memory enhancer	[17, 18]
6.	Catechu (*Acacia catechu*)	Heartwood	Catechin, catechuin	200–500	Leprosy, sore mouth, chest pain, bronchial asthma	[19, 20]
7.	Ghritkumari (*Aloe vera*)	Leaves	Emodin	>10,000	Anthelmintic, blood purifier	[21–23]
8.	Giloe (*Tinospora cordifolia*)	Root, stem, leaf, fruit	Alkaloids, glycosides, steroids, phenolics, aliphatic compounds	2000–5000	Leprosy, jaundice	[24, 25]
9.	Haldi (*Curcuma longa*)	Rhizomes	Curcumin	1000–2000	Anti-inflammatory	[26, 27]
10.	Kalmegh (*Andrographis paniculata*)	Plant	Andrographolide	2000–5000	Psoriasis, malaria	[28]
11.	Kesar (*Crocus sativus*)	Dried stigma and top of style	Crocin, carotene, crocetin	>1000	Nerve sedative, stimulant	[29]
12.	Mentha (*Mentha* species)	Oil	Flavonoids	>10,000	Irritable bowel syndrome	[30]

TABLE 3.1 *(Continued)*

Sl. No.	Name of Plant	Part of Plant Used	Active Constituent	Annual Trade (Metric Tons) [10]	Uses	References
13.	Mulethi (*Glycyrrhiza glabra*)	Underground stem	Saponin glycoside, glycyrrhizin	2000–5000	Heartburn, bloating	[31, 32]
14.	Nagarmotha (*Cyperus scariosus*)	Rhizomes	Polyphenol, flavonol, glycoside	200–500	Heart diseases	[33]
15.	Neem (*Azadirachta indica*)	Whole plant	Nimbidin, nimbin, azadirone	>1000	Antileprotic, piles, urinary infection	[34, 35]
16.	Safed Musali (*Chlorophytum borivilianum*)	Rhizome root	Saponins, alkaloids, flavonoids, phenolic acids	>1000	Main ingredient of *Chyawanprash*	[36]
17.	Shatavari (*Asparagus racemosus*)	Root	Asparagines, diosgenin	2000–5000	Antioxidant, anti-inflammatory, immunity booster	[37]
18.	Tulsi (*Ocimum sanctum*)	Leaves, seed	Eugenol	2000–5000	Immunity booster	[38]

intermediates in the biosynthetic pathways of primary metabolites, the fundamental structures of major secondary metabolite classes—alkaloids, phenylpropanoids, and terpenoids, and so forth—are crafted through carbon and nitrogen biosynthesis. Other secondary metabolites, such as cyanogenic glycosides, polyketides, quinones, alkylamides, and glucosinolates, derive from fatty acid and sulfur metabolism, and so forth [42]. The vast repertoire of plant bioactive secondary metabolites, exceeding 200,000, far surpasses the limited count of primary metabolites, capped at 10,000. While primary and secondary metabolites share a common biosynthetic pathway, secondary metabolites primarily absorb and store surplus carbon and nitrogen produced during primary metabolism. In times of need, these stored reservoirs, in the form of secondary metabolites, undergo disintegration and are reintegrated into primary metabolism. This intricate interplay establishes an effective balance between primary and secondary metabolism [41]. Categorically, based on biosynthetic pathways, three primary types of secondary metabolites prevail: terpenes, phenolic compounds, and nitrogen-containing compounds [43].

3.3 MODERN AGRICULTURAL TECHNIQUES FOR ENHANCING METABOLITES IN MEDICINAL PLANTS

Global surge in the popularity of herbal medicines underscores the need for prioritizing safety considerations. This heightened usage has brought to light various safety concerns, many of which are attributed to the suboptimal quality of raw materials [44]. Different types of herbal medicines present distinct challenges in terms of quality. The quality issues are categorized into two main groups: external and internal.

External challenges include adulteration, misidentification, and contamination (from microorganisms, pesticide residues, and hazardous metals). Conversely, internal challenges have to do with the intricacy and variation of the components found in herbal remedies. External quality issues in medicinal plant agriculture pose significant risks to patient health, primarily stemming from contamination, adulteration, and misidentification. Contaminants, such as toxic heavy metals, pesticides, microbes, and mycotoxins, are prevalent concerns, particularly in Asian countries [45]. Heavy metals are found in Chinese patent medicines and Indian Ayurvedic medicines. Pesticide residues, including organochlorines and modern compounds like pyrethroids, contribute to contamination, affecting both domestic and imported herbal materials. Microbial contamination, involving pathogenic organisms and mycotoxins, is widespread, especially in tropical regions with conducive climates [46]. Addressing these external issues requires stringent adherence to quality standards, including the establishment of regulatory frameworks and the implementation of Good Agricultural and Collection Practices (GACP) globally [47].

On the other hand, enhancing secondary metabolite production is crucial for obtaining plants rich in desirable active compounds. To achieve this, various agronomic techniques are employed, including genetic improvement through crosses and hybridization [48]. Hybrid cultivars offer advantages such as increased yield and seed protection. Additionally, mutation induction, a promising breeding approach using chemicals or radiation, contributes to the development of superior genotypes. However, its limited application is attributed to the lack of efficient screening methods. Induced polyploidy, involving autoploidy and alloploidy, provides another avenue for genetic enhancement. Autoploidy involves increasing the chromosome number within a species, while alloploidy results from hybridization between two species. Figure 3.1 represents how hybridization, polyploidy, and mutation work in plants.

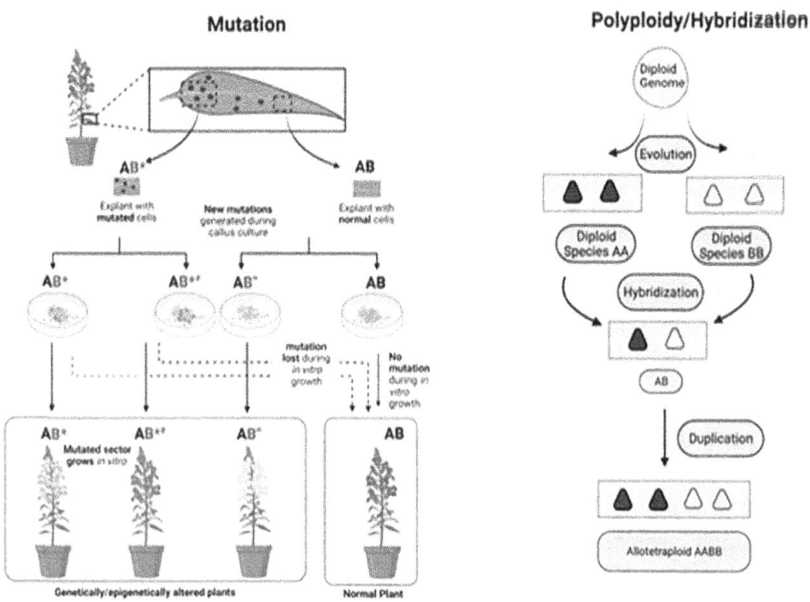

FIGURE 3.1 Diagrammatic representation of mutation and polyploidy/hybridization in plants.

This method is particularly valuable for plants with limited genetic variability. Overall, integrating these techniques into cultivation practices ensures the production of standardized, high-quality raw material for medicinal use, contributing to the conservation of valuable germplasm. Despite the limited focus on agronomic studies, advancements in breeding methods underscore the potential for sustainable and improved medicinal plant cultivation [49]. Table 3.2 summarizes the experimental manipulations and their outcomes on various medicinal plants, providing valuable insights into the potential enhancement of bioactive compounds through different techniques.

TABLE 3.2 Applications of Polyploidy, Mutation, and Hybridization on Medicinal and Aromatic Plants

Sl. No.	Name of Medicinal Plant	Phenotype	Outcomes	References
		Polyploidy		
1.	*Artemisia annua*	Delayed growth	Increase in artemisinin (a sesquiterpene) by 38% and decrease in essential oils (monoterpenes) by 32%.	[50]
2.	*Carum carvi*	Delayed flowering	Increase of 35.6% in the concentration of essential oil.	[51]
3.	*Cichorium intybus*	Loss of explant	Leaves exhibit a remarkable rise of 185% in total phenolic compounds and a substantial surge of 96.5% in chlorogenic acid content.	[52]
4.	*Catharanthus roseus*	Greater quantity of branches and foliage	Increase in vindoline by 130.9%, catharanthine by 188.6%, and vinblastine by 122.6%.	[53]
5.	*Dioscorea zingiberensis*	Loss of explant by oxidation	Increase of diosgenin up to 80%.	[54]
6.	*Glycyrrhiza glabra*	Delayed growth	Glycyrrhizic acid content increased up to 12%.	[55]
7.	*Hyoscyamus niger*	Enlarged leaves, flowers, pollen, seeds, and epidermal cells; reduced chloroplast counts; heightened stomatal guard cell numbers	Tropane alkaloid concentration improved by 22.5%.	[56]

TABLE 3.2 *(Continued)*

Sl. No.	Name of Medicinal Plant	Phenotype	Outcomes	References
8.	*Papaver somniferum*	Delayed growth	Increased morphine content by 25% to 50%.	[57]
9.	*Panax ginseng*	Increased biomass with thicker, less branched roots	22% increase in ginsenosides.	[58]
10.	*Stevia rebaudiana*	Loss of explant	Stevioside content increased by up to 66%.	[59]
		Mutation		
SL. No.	**Name of Medicinal Plant**	**Mutagen Used**	**Outcomes**	**References**
11.	*Catharanthus roseus*	Chemical mutagen	Salt-tolerant with bare inflorescence and heightened flower abundance.	[60]
12.	*Curcuma longa*	Gamma rays	Curcumin levels in rhizomes and crop yields increased up to 4.2%.	[61]
13.	*Cymbopogon citratus*	UV and gamma rays	Increased oil cell production alters essential oil quality, percentage, and physical attributes.	[62]
14.	*Chamomilla recutita*	Gamma rays	Plant height, flower quantity, and oil yield increased.	[63]
15.	*Mentha piperita*	Gamma rays	More abundant oil components: menthol and menthone.	[64]
16.	*Papaver somniferum*	Gamma rays	Increased seed yield and elevated morphine levels.	[65, 66]
17.	*Plantago ovata*	Ionizing radiation	Seed yield increased.	[67]
18.	*Trigonella foenum-graecum*	Gamma rays	Increased yield and higher diosgenin content.	[68]
		Hybridization		
SL. No.	**Name of Medicinal Plant**	**Method and Gene**	**Outcomes**	**References**
19.	*Curcuma longa*	PCR, sequencing; 5S gene spacer	Genetic markers served as a quality control measure for different species.	[69]
20.	*Datura metel*	PCR, sequencing; microarray; 5S gene spacer	Quality control and safety monitoring.	[70]
21.	*Digitalis obscura*	Random amplified polymorphic DNA	Used to check genetic diversity within populations.	[71]

TABLE 3.2 *(Continued)*

Sl. No.	Name of Medicinal Plant	Phenotype	Outcomes	References
22.	*Hyoscyamus niger*	PCR, sequencing; microarray; 5S gene spacer	Quality control and safety monitoring.	[70]
23.	*Rheum officinale*	PCR, sequencing; trnL-trnF	Used to check adulteration.	[72]
24.	*Rheum reticulatum*	PCR, sequencing; trnL-trnF	Used to check adulteration.	[72]
25.	*Rheum wittrockii*	PCR, sequencing; trnL-trnF	Used to check adulteration.	[72]
26.	*Swertia angustifolia*	PCR, sequencing; allele-specific diagnostic PCR; rpl16; ITS	Used to check molecular authentication.	[73]
27.	*Swertia macrosperma*	PCR, sequencing; allele-specific diagnostic PCR; rpl16; ITS	Used to check molecular authentication.	[73]
28.	*Swertia punicea*	PCR, sequencing; allele-specific diagnostic PCR; rpl16; ITS	Used to check molecular authentication.	[73]
29.	*Typhonium divaricatum*	PCR, sequencing; microarray; 5S gene spacer	Quality control and safety monitoring.	[70]
30.	*Trifolium pratense*	PCR, sequencing; ITS	Used to identify both primary and contaminating plant material.	[74]

3.4 OTHER METHODS FOR ENHANCING SECONDARY METABOLITE PRODUCTION

The techniques used for enhancing secondary metabolite production are crucial for various industries, including pharmaceuticals, nutraceuticals, and cosmetics. In this context, *in vitro* strategies, tissue culture, hydroponics, plant-microbe interactions, and bioreactors play pivotal roles. This comprehensive approach involves manipulating plant metabolism, optimizing growth conditions, and exploring the synergistic effects of plant-microbe interactions.

In vitro metabolic engineering stands out as a promising biological tool for the continuous production of commercially important secondary metabolites. By manipulating the metabolic profile of plants through undifferentiated organogenic and callus culture, *in vitro* strategies can yield enormous amounts of target chemicals. Stress induction and elicitor application further enhance metabolite production, making these strategies valuable for industries relying on natural molecules for pharmacological or dietary purposes [75].

Tissue culture methods have transformed the synthesis of plant secondary metabolites by providing tailored nutrient formulations, genetic and epigenetic modifications, stress stimulation, and sustainable cultivation setups. Rigorous oversight of growth parameters, stress application, and the implementation of cell suspension or organ cultures in bioreactors guarantee a consistent and expandable output of secondary metabolites. Various *in vitro* culture strategies, including callus, hairy roots, shoot, and suspension cultures, offer diverse avenues to enhance the yield of valuable plant compounds [75–77].

Meeting the consumer demand for fresh, crisp, and uniform medicinal and aromatic plant products presents a challenge to producers. Hydroponics emerges as a viable solution, offering a cultivation system characterized by controlled nutrient availability and environmental conditions. This method minimizes pest and pathogen incidence, enhances nutritional content, and ultimately leads to higher yields compared to traditional cultivation techniques. Moreover, hydroponics enables off-season crop production, thereby contributing to the generation of high-quality bioactive compounds [78, 79].

Plant secondary metabolites play diverse roles in environmental stress response, defense against pathogens, and interactions with other organisms. Plant microbiomes influence secondary metabolite metabolism, impacting plant phenotype and stress tolerance. The interplay between plants and microbes involves complex molecular mechanisms, and understanding these interactions can lead to enhanced metabolite synthesis. Microbial influences on plant metabolomes and transcriptomes can result in the accumulation of specific plant secondary metabolites [80, 81].

Bioreactors are now recognized as valuable instruments for cultivating secondary metabolites in plants. These systems offer a regulated environment conducive to the growth of plant tissues submerged in liquid nutrient media. Different modes of bioreactor operation, such as batch, fed-batch, chemostat, or continuous perfusion, offer flexibility in optimizing growth conditions and enhancing metabolite production. Bioreactors have been used to increase the secondary metabolite yield, contributing to the sustainable and controlled production of valuable compounds [82, 83].

Understanding the molecular basis of plant metabolite synthesis involves unraveling complex responses to abiotic and biotic stressors. Transcription factors play a crucial role in regulating gene expression in response to stress. Plant stress response mechanisms include signal perception, intracellular signal transduction, activation of phytohormones, and the coordination of various pathways leading to the activation or repression of stress-responsive genes. In conclusion, the integration of these techniques provides a holistic approach to enhancing secondary metabolite production in plants [84, 85]. The collaboration of *in vitro* strategies, tissue culture, hydroponics, plant-microbe interactions, and bioreactors open up avenues for sustainable and scalable production of valuable compounds with applications across diverse industries. Ongoing exploration in this domain has the capacity to drive additional progress in the production of plant metabolites and the creation of innovative applications for these valuable compounds.

3.5 PHYTO HORMONES AND THEIR APPLICATIONS

Plant hormones act as chemical messengers, originating in one tissue followed by influencing cellular processes by binding to specific proteins which serve as receptors linked to cellular transduction pathways. Hormones are synthesized in one tissue but exert their effects on specific target sites in distant tissues at minimal concentrations. Endocrine hormones travel to sites far from their origin, while paracrine hormones affect nearby cells. Six major hormone groups like auxins, cytokinins, gibberellins, abscisic acid, ethylene, and brassinosteroids which modulate plant growth and development [86]. Additionally, signaling compounds like jasmonic acid, salicylic acid, small polypeptides, and strigolactone play roles in pathogen resistance and herbivore protection [86, 87]. Flavonoids, among other compounds, act as regulators of signal transduction pathways, highlighting the expanding list of factors influencing plant growth and development [88, 89].

Plant hormones play a crucial role in optimizing the production of bioactive compounds with therapeutic properties in medicinal and aromatic plants. Auxins, for instance, find application in the cultivation of medicinal herbs by promoting cell enlargement and stem growth, enhancing overall biomass and the concentration of active compounds [87, 90]. Additionally, the use of auxins facilitates root initiation in cuttings, aiding the propagation of specific plant varieties with desirable medicinal properties [91]. Gibberellins contribute to the cultivation of medicinal plants by promoting stem growth, thus influencing the overall yield of plant material. Moreover, they play a role in breaking seed dormancy, a factor significant in the cultivation of medicinal plants from seeds [92]. Cytokinins, known for their role in cell division, are employed in tissue culture to induce cell proliferation, a technique valuable in the mass production of plant clones for consistent medicinal compound content [93]. Brassinosteroids, with their impact on cell division and elongation, influence the overall growth of medicinal plants, ensuring optimal development of plant tissues rich in bioactive compounds [94]. Ethylene, though primarily associated with responses such as fruit abscission, also contributes to the overall development of plants, influencing the synthesis of secondary metabolites. Abscisic acid, by regulating stomatal closure, assists in water management and affects the quality and quantity of medicinal compounds synthesized [95, 96].

Jasmonates and salicylic acid, integral to plant defense mechanisms, are used for enhancing the medicinal value of plants by inducing the production of secondary metabolites with protective and therapeutic properties [97]. Signal peptides, which regulate various aspects of plant growth and development, can be harnessed to modulate the biosynthesis of medicinal compounds in specific plant tissues. Polyamines, useful for growth and development, contribute to the overall health of medicinal plants, impacting the synthesis of bioactive compounds [98]. In conclusion, the strategic application of plant hormones in medicinal plant cultivation offers a means to optimize the production of valuable compounds, ensuring the efficacy of medicinal herbs and plants in traditional and modern medicine. Figure 3.2 depicts various plant hormones that are essential for plant growth and other functions within the plants.

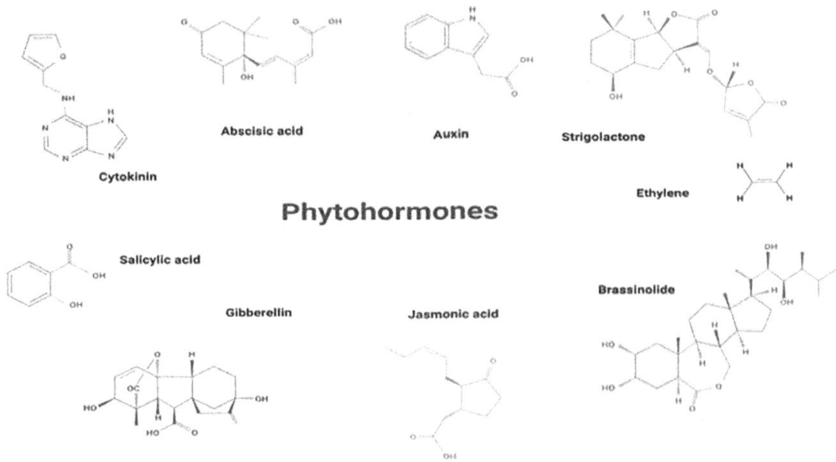

FIGURE 3.2 Various plant hormones.

3.6 FACTORS AFFECTING CULTIVATION OF MEDICINAL PLANTS

The cultivation of medicinal and aromatic plants is intricately linked to the understanding of plant habits and the favorable climatic conditions necessary for their growth. Various factors influencing plant cultivation include soil quality, altitude, temperature, humidity, precipitation or irrigation patterns, fertilizers, and nutrients, as well as considerations for pests and their control. Each of these elements is important in the successful farming of these plants, requiring careful attention and management to optimize their growth and maximize medicinal and aromatic qualities [43].

1. **Soil:** It is defined as the Earth's surface layer resulting from the erosion of rocks, is shaped through the collaborative actions of weathering agents, including plants and microorganisms. Soil must contain adequate nutrients, organic matter, and other crucial components. Optimal soil characteristics, such as texture, drainage, water retention, fertility, and pH, are determined based on the specific requirements of the chosen medicinal plant. The application of compost is often indispensable for achieving high yields. The type of soil significantly influences various aspects of plants, including seed germination, plant posture, vigor, stem hardness, root depth, and flower abundance. There are different soil types such as clay, loamy, silt loam, sandy loam, sandy soil,

and chalky soil. Clay soil, with its tiny particles, tends to become quickly waterlogged, affecting plant water absorption. Sandy soil, characterized by larger particles, drains water rapidly, leading to deep root growth but lower nutrient content. Loam soil, a balanced mixture of clay and silt, is highly fertile, providing essential nutrients for robust plant growth. Silt loam, rich in organic substances, is considered the most fertile soil. Sandy loam is a blend of silt and clay, combining the beneficial properties of both soil types. Understanding and managing these soil conditions are crucial for cultivating medicinal plants and ensuring their optimal growth [99–101].

2. **Altitude, Temperature, and Humidity:** Environmental factors, such as day length, precipitation, and temperature, significantly impact the physical, chemical, and biological characteristics of medicinal plants. Parameters like daylight duration, average rainfall, minimal temperature, and diurnal temperature fluctuations also play a crucial role in influencing the biochemical processes within the plant. These climatic conditions are essential considerations for understanding and optimizing the quality and composition of medicinal plants [102, 103].

3. **Rainfall and Irrigation:** Medicinal plants typically necessitate well-managed irrigation systems or adequate rainfall to support optimal growth and development. The regulation of irrigation and drainage is crucial, tailored to the specific requirements of each medicinal plant species at different stages of its growth. The water employed for irrigation must adhere to local, regional, and/or national quality standards [104]. Diligent supervision is essential to ensure that medicinal plants under cultivation receive the necessary and appropriate watering. Examples of xerophytic plants, such as Aloe and Acacia, highlight species that thrive without relying on irrigation or rainfall, presenting an added advantage in their cultivation [105].

4. **Fertilizer and Nutrients:** Fertilizers play a vital role in enhancing soil fertility for the cultivation of medicinal plants, comprising a mix of organic and inorganic materials. Various types of fertilizers cater to different needs. Biotic origin fertilizers, derived from biological sources, are utilized to

supplement elements like nitrogen in nutrient-poor soils. Green leaf manures, a blend of fertile material and clay, provide essential nutrients, contributing to increased medicinal plant productivity [106–108]. Farmyard manure combines livestock muck, plant remnants, and husk, enriching the soil. Composite manure comprises decomposed flora and fauna components. Green manure involves plowing non-woody plants into the soil, offering an organic and nitrogen-rich blend that prevents erosion and enhances curative plant mass by 30–50%. Bio-fertilizers, derived from microorganisms like bacteria, algae, and fungi, aid nutrient delivery to the soil, with examples including nitrogen-fixing bacteria and cyanobacteria [109]. Chemical fertilizers supply macronutrients to support plant growth, that is, nitrogen, phosphorus, potassium, calcium, magnesium, sulfur, and micronutrients such as iron, manganese, zinc, boron, copper, molybdenum, carbon, and oxygen [107, 108]. Low macronutrient levels lead to the accumulation of esters in roots [110]. Phenolic compounds in sesquioxide's inhibit phosphate adsorption, enhancing inorganic phosphorus availability. Nitrogen deficiency alters secondary metabolism, increasing total phenolic content in plants [111].

5. **Pest and Pest Management:** A pest refers to an unwanted species, be it animal or plant, and pesticides are substances derived synthetically from chemical or natural sources that are effective in small concentrations against these pests [112]. Various insects can transmit serious diseases like malaria and typhus, while others can cause significant damage to valuable medicinal plants such as *Zea mays*, *Gossypium*, *Triticum aestivum*, and *Oryza sativa.* Additionally, common pests encompass bacteria, fungi, *Rattus rattus*, and weeds like *Ambrosia artemisiiflora* and *Toxicodendron radicans*. Understanding the origin of pest-related issues is crucial in devising and implementing effective pest control strategies that incorporate substances of natural origin [113]. Globally, the traditional pesticide industry constitutes a significant business, with the majority of synthetic pesticides being utilized for agricultural and other purposes [114].

3.7 ABIOTIC AND BIOTIC STRESS

Plants, including medicinal ones, face various challenges from abiotic and biotic stressors, impacting their growth, productivity, and overall health. Abiotic stresses like drought, salt, cold, heat, and toxins significantly affect medicinal plant yield. Drought, driven by unpredictable rainfall patterns and exacerbated by climate change, restricts water availability, leading to stunted growth and reduced metabolic activity. Salt stress arises from the accumulation of salts in the soil, causing osmotic stress and ion toxicity, consequently hindering crop growth and yield [115]. Cold stress poses a threat, especially during reproductive growth, affecting crop quality and post-harvest life. Similarly, rising global temperatures contribute to heat stress, diminishing seed germination, photosynthetic efficiency, and overall yield. Toxins, often introduced into agricultural soils through chemical fertilizers and industrialization, further challenge medicinal plants. Toxic metals gradually infiltrate plants, impacting their metabolic processes and compromising the quality of medicinal compounds [116]. On the biotic front, medicinal plants contend with various living organisms, including fungi, viruses, bacteria, nematodes, and insects. These biotic stressors induce diseases, infections, and physical damage, leading to a decline in agricultural yields. Genetic modification has emerged as a strategic approach to developing resistant crop varieties, offering a promising solution against biotic stressors [117].

In response to abiotic stresses, medicinal plants deploy botanical defenses such as the cuticle, composed of hydrophobic waxes, acting as a protective barrier against environmental challenges [118]. Unsaturated fatty acids in membranes play a crucial role in maintaining fluidity, adapting to temperature fluctuations. Reactive species scavengers, including reactive oxygen species (ROS) and reactive carbonyl species (RCS), form part of a sophisticated defense system against abiotic stress-induced bursts. Molecular chaperones, such as heat shock proteins, aid in protein folding and prevent cellular damage under stressful conditions. Additionally, medicinal plants accumulate compatible solutes, acting as osmoprotectants and stabilizers against dehydration and oxidative stress [119]. Understanding and harnessing these defense mechanisms is crucial for ensuring the resilience and productivity of medicinal plants under diverse environmental conditions, ultimately influencing the quality of medicinal compounds derived from these plants.

3.8 GEOGRAPHICAL AND SEASONAL INFLUENCES

Geographical and seasonal influences play a vital role in shaping the impact on aromatic and medicinal plants, leading to alterations in the levels of bioactive components. The quest for evidence-based traditional plants as a promising and alternative source for safe and effective drug development is gaining traction globally [40]. This pursuit is particularly crucial in both developed and developing countries, aiming to address acute and chronic diseases. The limitations and diverse side effects associated with mainstream allopathic medicines underscore the need for alternative remedies. To achieve the goal of harnessing the therapeutic potential of traditional plants, it becomes imperative to cultivate a diverse array of these plants under uniform environmental conditions. This involves selecting favorable geographical and climatic settings to optimize plant metabolite yield and enhance production rates. A conducive climate, high-quality soil, and advantageous geographical conditions contribute to the cultivation of medicinal plants with optimal growth. Adhering to such cultivation protocols empowers farmers and cultivators to provide standardized phytoconstituents in crude extracts for herbal drug discovery [120]. Furthermore, the global shift in climate patterns is modifying weather conditions within the same geographical regions, significantly impacting the production rates and composition of secondary metabolites in organized medicinal plant extracts. Variables such as rainfall and humidity exhibit variability in different geographical locations, leading to differences in phytometabolite composition and yield when cultivating the same species of medicinal plants in diverse areas. These variations are exacerbated by disparities in soil quality, collection times, and processing methods employed for extracting secondary metabolites from cultivated medicinal plants. As a result, these changes contribute to substantial discrepancies in the reproducibility of bioactive phytometabolite extraction yield and composition from identical species of medicinal plants. This inconsistency poses a challenge, as patients may not experience consistent and optimized bioactivity from identical herbal formulations produced in different batches. To address these challenges, there is an urgent need for the implementation of various standardization techniques and characterization methods, including optimized fingerprinting technology based on marker compounds. These measures are essential to ensure the reliability and consistency of bioactive phytometabolite extracts from traditional plants, promoting uniform efficacy in herbal formulations across different batches. Table 3.3 presents information on various medicinal plants, their important compounds, optimal harvest seasons, and key findings from various prior studies.

TABLE 3.3 Seasonal Impact of Some Medicinal and Aromatic Herbal Plants

Sl. No.	Medicinal Plants	Important Compounds	Inference	References
1.	*Achillea filipendulina*	Volatile oil	Early summer harvest boosts yield.	[121]
2.	*Clinopodium pulegium*	Essential oil	Optimal development stage enhances oil content; summer is preferable.	[122]
3.	*Sclerocarya birrea*	Volatile oil	Cold season (August) enhances oil yield.	[123]
4.	*Origanum cyrenaicum*	Monoterpenes, hydrocarbon, oxygenated sesquiterpene hydrocarbon	Spring season is suitable for oil collection.	[124]
5.	*Eucalyptus citriodora*	Citronellal, citronellol, citronellyl acetate	Harvest in high-temperature months (autumn, winter, spring).	[125]
6.	*Santolina chamaecyparissus*	Limonene, pinene, caryophyllene oxide	Summer enhances *Santolina* oil.	[126]
7.	*Laurus nobilis*	% yield of extract	Summer or vegetative period enhances oil yield.	[127]
8.	*Plectranthus amboinicus*	Volatile oil	Spring yields highest oil content.	[128]
9.	*Mentha longifolia*	Volatile oil	Summer yields highest oil content.	[129]
10.	*Artemisia annua*	% yield of volatile oil	Summer boosts *Artemisia annua* yield.	[130]
11.	*Micromeria fruticosa*	Limonene, menthone, menthol	Summer and spring yield richer oil composition.	[131]
12.	*Cistus monspeliensis*	Essential oil	Oil content is richer in autumn and winter.	[132]
13.	*Ocimum gratissimum*	Volatile oil	Spring yields optimal eugenol potency.	[133]
14.	*Pistacia atlantica*	Volatile oil	Spring (September) is favorable for higher yield.	[134]
15.	*Pelargonium graveolens*	Volatile oil (geranium)	Optimal harvest in cool seasons, i.e., summer and winter.	[135]

TABLE 3.3 *(Continued)*

Sl. No.	Medicinal Plants	Important Compounds	Inference	References
16.	*Thymbra spicata*	Volatile oil	Harvest in summer yields best quantity of volatile oil.	[136]
17.	*Melittis melissophyllum*	Flavonoid	Harvest in spring enriches medicinal value.	[137]
18.	*Adhatoda vasica*	Vasicine, deoxyvasicine	Vasicine peaks in August.	[138]
19.	*Catharanthus roseus*	Flavonoids	Best harvest in winter, summer, and rainy seasons.	[139]
20.	*Ipomoea pes-caprae*	Total phenolic content of flavonoids	Summer, spring, and winter are best for harvesting.	[140]
21.	*Apis mellifera*	Phenolic	Optimal harvest in dry season, preferably in winter.	[141]
22.	*Parkia biglobosa*	Flavonoids	Spring season is best for good yield.	[142]
23.	*Phyllanthus amarus*	Total alkaloids and flavonoids	Summer season favors highest metabolite production.	[143]
24.	*Prunus amygdalus*	Phenolic content (stems and leaves)	Summer and spring are favorable seasons.	[144]

3.9 QUALITY RISK MANAGEMENT-BASED RISK ASSESSMENT FOR QUALITY PRODUCTION OF MEDICINAL AND AROMATIC PLANTS

Quality risk management plays a crucial role in the production of medicinal plants, ensuring the safety, efficacy, and overall quality of the final products. The assessment encompasses a thorough evaluation of potential risks associated with various stages of production, spanning cultivation, harvesting, processing, and storage of medicinal plants. Factors such as environmental conditions, cultivation practices, pest and disease control, and post-harvest handling are scrutinized to identify potential risks that could compromise the desired quality attributes of the medicinal plants [145]. Moreover, the assessment takes into account potential contamination by pesticides, heavy metals, microorganisms, or other impurities that might negatively impact the medicinal properties of the plants [146]. Conducting a comprehensive quality risk assessment enables producers to implement suitable control measures. This involves adopting GACP and establishing robust quality assurance systems. These measures are essential for ensuring the production of high-quality medicinal plants that not only meet regulatory requirements but also align with consumer expectations [47]. Figure 3.3 illustrates the various factors that influence the quality of medicinal plants and related phytochemicals.

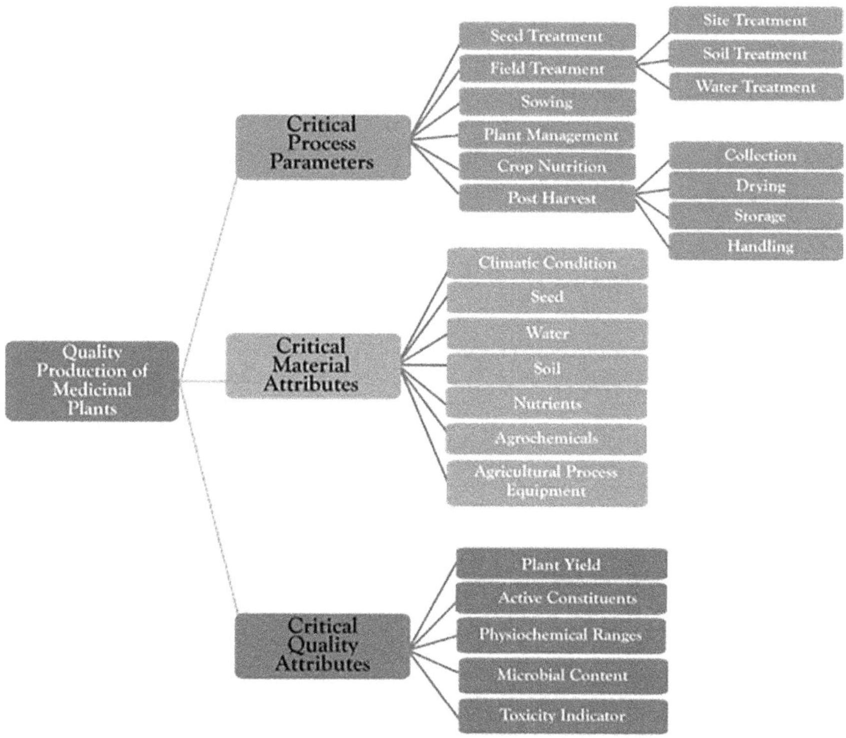

FIGURE 3.3 Critical attributes during large-scale production of medicinal plants.

3.9.1 IDENTIFICATION OF THE RISK FACTORS

Recognizing and managing risk factors is a pivotal aspect of comprehending and addressing potential challenges in the cultivation of medicinal plants. This process involves a systematic approach to identify and categorize elements that may adversely affect the cultivation process or desired outcomes. In the realm of medicinal plant cultivation, these risk factors extend across various domains, encompassing environmental conditions, pest and disease threats, market fluctuations, operational hurdles, and socio-economic considerations [147, 148].

Farmers, agricultural experts, and pertinent stakeholders play a crucial role in discerning these risk factors, drawing on their knowledge, experience, and observations [149]. Additionally, a comprehensive literature review, engaging in discussions and consultations, and analyzing historical data contribute valuable insights for identifying potential risks specific to the cultivation of medicinal plants [150]. This meticulous identification of risk factors lays a robust foundation for subsequent risk assessment and the development of mitigation strategies. Such strategies enable proactive measures to be implemented, addressing and minimizing potential risks and enhancing the likelihood of successful cultivation of medicinal plants.

3.9.2 DEVELOPING A QUALITY RISK MANAGEMENT STRATEGY BASED ON CRITICAL VARIABLES FOR MEDICINAL PLANTS

The implementation of quality risk management is essential to mitigate the potential risks associated with obtaining substandard medicinal plant produce. This involves a systematic evaluation of quality risks, utilizing both scientific knowledge and inputs from farmers to identify critical material attributes (CMA) and critical process parameters (CPP). The establishment of a critical quality risk scale for agricultural materials or processes affecting the quality of medicinal plants is crucial [151]. This risk scale is developed by assessing the consequences of agricultural materials or processes on the quality attributes of medicinal plants, relying on thorough literature exploration. The critical quality risk scale categorizes materials or processes based on the degree of risk they pose to the quality of medicinal plants, with classifications: "high," "moderate," and "low." The selection of Critical Quality Attributes is guided by empirical data, considering their industrial significance and supported by comprehensive literature research. Within this scientific design, three sets of variables are outlined:

1. **Critical Material Attributes (CMA):** These factors include fundamental physical, biological, or chemical properties associated with input materials like water, soil, seeds, fertilizers, pesticides, and biological elements. These variables directly influence the quality of medicinal products.
2. **Critical Process Parameters (CPP):** Ensuring the quality of medicinal plants requires the oversight and regulation of essential processes. In herb production, vital process parameters encompass

key stages such as plant identity verification, soil and water treatment methods, site selection, sowing, harvesting, fertilizer application, harvest collection, drying, and storage. The variations in these processes significantly impact the quality of medicinal plants. To reduce risks in subsequent stages of plant production and uphold predetermined quality standards, thorough monitoring and control of these critical variables are essential [152, 153].

3. **Critical Quality Attributes (CQA):** These refer to physical, biological, or chemical attributes that must fall within a specific range or limit to ensure the quality of the raw material. Quality parameters are crucial for various aspects of the raw material, including active chemical constituents, toxicity indicators (such as limits for heavy metals and pesticides), microbial load (including aflatoxin levels and microbial contamination associated with diseases), physicochemical ranges (such as ash values and extractives), and overall medicinal plant productivity. These attributes hold significant importance for the herbal and related industries, as well as during trade, as they determine the overall quality and safety of the raw materials. Table 3.4 depicts the CPP, CMA, and CQA for the cultivation of medicinal plants.

TABLE 3.4 Process Parameters, Material Attributes, and Quality Attributes for the Cultivation of Medicinal Plants

Process Parameters	Material Attributes	Quality Attributes
• Seed treatment	• Climatic condition	• Plant yield
• Site treatment	• Seed	• Active constituents
• Soil treatment	• Water	• Physicochemical ranges
• Water treatment	• Soil	• Microbial content
• Sowing	• Nutrients	• Toxicity indicator
• Plant management	• Agrochemicals	
• Crop nutrition	• Agricultural process equipment	
• Harvest		
• Collection		
• Drying		
• Storage		
• Handling		

3.9.3 DEFINING THE RELATIONSHIP BETWEEN THE CPP-CQA AND CMA-CQA FOR RISK ANALYSIS FOR MEDICINAL AND AROMATIC PLANTS

In risk analysis for medicinal plant cultivation, a comprehensive understanding of the interplay between CPP, CQA, and CMA is imperative for effective risk management. These three components are intricately linked and exert mutual influence throughout the cultivation process [154]. CPPs serve as pivotal variables or parameters directly impacting the growth, development, and yield of medicinal plants. The dynamic relationship among CPP, CQA, and CMA unfolds as follows: CPPs wield a direct influence on the cultivation process, subsequently affecting the CQAs of the medicinal plants. The quality attributes, or CQAs, play a vital role in gauging the overall quality and efficacy of the cultivated medicinal plants. Furthermore, CMAs, encompassing the manufacturing processes, are shaped by the combined influence of both CPPs and CQAs. Through the optimization of CPPs and the assurance of desired CQAs, cultivators can proficiently manage CMAs, consistently producing high-quality medicinal plant products. In the risk analysis framework, a nuanced understanding of the interrelationship between CPP, CQA, and CMA empowers cultivators and stakeholders to pinpoint potential risks at each stage. An evaluation of the impact of risk factors on CPPs, CQAs, and CMAs facilitates the development and implementation of tailored risk mitigation strategies. This approach ensures a controlled cultivation process, attainment of desired quality attributes, and optimization of manufacturing processes, ultimately reducing potential risks, and elevating the success of medicinal plant cultivation.

Developing a risk analysis structure for the cultivation and processing of medicinal and aromatic plants necessitates a thorough and methodical approach to guarantee the excellence and security of the end products. This comprehensive framework includes CPP, CMA, and CQA at different phases of the growing and processing process. The process of cultivating medicinal plants starts with seed treatment, in which the quality of seeds assumes crucial significance. Factors to be taken into account include the origin and genetic integrity of the seeds, techniques used for disinfection and priming, and suitable storage conditions, including meticulous control of temperature and humidity. At this early stage, they are designated as CPPs. Simultaneously, CMAs such as seed viability and germination rate play a crucial role in guaranteeing effective culture [102, 155].

Regarding site treatment, behaviors including soil preparation and site cleanliness are designated as CPPs. The soil composition and pH levels are essential factors in determining the general health and fertility of the soil, making them critical manufacturing attributes. The presence of pollutants in the soil is recognized as a CQA. Soil treatment includes the use of fertilizers and soil additives. Soil treatment refers to the specific processes of fertilization and nutrient application, while CMAs comprise the amounts of nutrients and the structure of the soil [156]. Water treatment is an essential phase in the agricultural process. The characteristics of water, such as its level of purity and origin, as well as the techniques used for irrigation, are recognized as CPPs. Water purity and mineral content are identified as crucial manufacturing attributes, guaranteeing the absence of pollutants carried by water in industrial facilities [102, 157]. The process of sowing, which involves planting seeds, has its own distinct set of crucial factors. Planting depth and spacing are considered to be crucial control points, whereas seed placement and planting density are regarded as critical manufacturing attributes. The resultant CQAs pertain to the consistency in plant development and the lack of diseases.

Plant management is a phase focused on supervising the vitality and welfare of the developing plants. Pest and disease management strategies, together with pruning procedures, are designated as CPPs. The plant's general health and its ability to fight pests are considered critical manufacturing attributes [116]. Medicinal crop nutrition includes the planning of fertilization programs and the implementation of nutrient application strategies [158]. Once the plants have fully grown, the harvest stage brings out a distinct set of crucial factors.

Harvesting techniques and timing are designated as critical control points, while the calibration of harvesting equipment is recognized as a CQA [159]. Collection entails the accurate identification and use of appropriate means to gather the harvested plants. These processes are recognized as important critical points, whereas the cleanliness of collecting equipment is classified as CQAs. At this step, it is crucial to ensure that the genetic makeup is genuine and that there is no presence of alien substances [114]. Drying, an essential stage in the cultivation of plants, involves the management of drying techniques and temperature regulation. Controlling moisture content is a crucial aspect of manufacturing. CQAs include the maintenance of bioactive components and the lack of fungal growth or decomposition [160]. Storage is an essential phase in preserving the quality of harvested and dried plants. The important factors are determined to be the storage conditions, which include factors such as temperature and humidity. Temperature and humidity regulation are identified as crucial factors in manufacturing, whereas maintaining quality over time and preventing contamination are considered essential quality factors [160].

Handling refers to the implementation of appropriate packing and transportation methods. The packaging's integrity is classified as a critical quality attribute, while the overall integrity of the product and its protection from harm during handling are considered important factors. During all phases of cultivation, the climatic conditions have a significant impact on several components of the process. Effective regulation and surveillance of climatic circumstances, encompassing temperature, humidity, and other ecological elements, are crucial for guaranteeing the achievement of every phase [161]. The interconnection between these CPP, CMA, and CQAs creates a strong risk analysis framework. This framework is specifically developed to detect, manage, and oversee possible hazards during the production and processing of medicinal and aromatic plants. Through comprehending and overseeing these connections, growers and producers may minimize hazards, comply with quality requirements, and generate superior, secure items for customers.

3.10 INTERPLAY OF NATURAL CONDITIONS, AGRICULTURAL TECHNIQUES, AND ENVIRONMENTAL FACTORS: ESSENTIAL UNDERSTANDING FOR HIGH-QUALITY MEDICINAL PLANT PRODUCTION

The complex interaction of natural circumstances, agricultural techniques, and environmental variables is fundamental to the development of high-quality medicinal plants. This requires comprehensive knowledge that encompasses many aspects of plant biology, cultivation methods, and ecological dynamics. Within the domain of natural circumstances, the genetic variability of medicinal plants has great significance, impacting not only their inherent ability to withstand challenges but also the makeup of bioactive substances that are crucial for therapeutic effectiveness. The selection of plant types and the implementation of cultivation techniques are guided by adaptability to certain ecological niches and a deep understanding of the life cycle and growth habits of these plants. Within the realm of agricultural practices, the careful curation and processing of seeds signify the beginning of a process that encompasses the choice of location and the preparation of the soil. At this juncture, the arrangement of soil particles, acidity levels, and nutrient composition are adjusted to provide an ideal setting for plants to thrive. Water and nutrient management procedures maintain the long-term health of the plants, while integrated pest and disease control measures protect against possible risks. The quality of the final product is heavily influenced by the harvesting processes that are synchronized with the growth phases of the plants. Plant growth is significantly influenced by environmental variables, which include climatic conditions, seasonal fluctuations, and microclimates. Comprehending and adjusting to these elements is crucial for enhancing development and increasing the production of secondary metabolites. As these components come together, a holistic approach to crop planning develops, including information from other fields of study. Continuous surveillance and adjustment, driven by scientific investigation and advancement, optimize agricultural techniques in alignment with the dynamic interaction of natural, agricultural, and environmental factors. This comprehensive understanding guarantees not only the amount but, more importantly, the excellence and strength of bioactive substances, establishing the basis for the creation of secure, efficient, and top-notch medicinal plants that align with both traditional knowledge and modern scientific standards.

3.11 IMPLEMENTING EFFECTIVE QUALITY RISK MANAGEMENT

It is crucial to implement efficient quality risk management in the cultivation of medicinal plants to guarantee the manufacture of superior herbal medications. The procedure entails a comprehensive strategy that combines knowledge of the best growing techniques with the establishment of an ideal farming environment. Effective risk management in terms of quality requires a thorough understanding of the whole cultivation process, including seed selection, harvesting, and processing [162]. Thorough risk assessments determine crucial control points, possible dangers, and the likelihood and severity of risks linked to each step. Having this information allows for the creation and execution of plans to reduce risks, guaranteeing that the farming methods are in line with quality standards and regulatory demands. Understanding the most effective methods for cultivating crops involves considering several elements such as the quality of seeds, preparing the soil, managing water resources, and controlling pests. The process includes choosing appropriate cultivars, using sustainable farming methods, and regulating nutrient levels to maximize the yield of bioactive chemicals. Establishing an ideal setting for agricultural output at the farm level goes beyond cultivation techniques and takes into account elements such as weather conditions, soil quality, and ecological viability. Adopting organic farming techniques, minimizing the use of chemicals, and integrating environmentally friendly activities all contribute to a more sustainable ecosystem and improve the quality of medicinal plants. Consistent observation and adjustment, guided by new knowledge and technological progress, enhance the precision of farming methods. The incorporation of contemporary technology, such as precision farming and data analytics, facilitates the immediate surveillance of environmental factors, crop condition, and any hazards. By using data, this method enables proactive decision-making and prompt execution of remedial actions. The collaboration among farmers, agronomists, and researchers enables the sharing of information, promoting a culture of ongoing improvement in agricultural techniques. Furthermore, farmer education and training programs have a crucial function in spreading knowledge and optimal methods. Effective quality risk management in medicinal plant production is a dynamic and collaborative process that includes risk assessment, mitigation measures, and ongoing enhancement of cultivation procedures [155]. Through the strategic alignment of cultivation techniques with favorable environmental circumstances and the use of risk management insights, farmers may successfully grow medicinal plants that adhere to rigorous quality requirements for the manufacturing of herbal drugs. This comprehensive method guarantees both the long-term viability and financial success of cultivating medicinal plants. Additionally, it aids in the creation of herbal medications that possess exceptional therapeutic effectiveness and safety, therefore satisfying the increasing need for natural and traditional therapies in healthcare [163].

3.12 CONCLUSION

The global demand for high-quality medicinal plants underscores their increasing importance in natural and traditional healthcare.

The therapeutic potential of these plants relies on a myriad of bioactive phytochemicals, including volatile oils, alkaloids, glycosides, tannins, and resins. Preserving the therapeutic qualities of natural products (NPs) throughout the cultivation, harvesting, and storage processes is essential to harness their pharmacological attributes effectively. Modern agricultural techniques, such as hybridization, polyploidy, and mutation, contribute significantly to enhancing the production of secondary metabolites in medicinal plants. Additionally, *in vitro* strategies, tissue culture, and plant-microbe interactions play pivotal roles in optimizing growth conditions and increasing the yield of bioactive compounds. These approaches are crucial for meeting the rising global demand for high-quality herbal medicines. Environmental factors, geographical location, and seasonal variations have a substantial impact on the growth, development, and quality of aromatic and medicinal plants. Soil quality, altitude, temperature, humidity, precipitation, fertilizers, and pest management are critical considerations that require careful attention to optimize plant growth and maximize medicinal qualities. Abiotic and biotic stresses pose challenges to medicinal plant cultivation, and understanding plant defense mechanisms is essential for ensuring resilience and productivity under diverse environmental conditions. Geographical and seasonal influences contribute to variations in bioactive components and yield, emphasizing the need for standardization techniques to ensure consistent and reliable bioactive phytometabolite extracts. Quality risk management is paramount in the cultivation and collection of medicinal plants. Thorough risk assessments, based on factors such as environmental conditions, cultivation practices, and potential contamination, lead to the implementation of suitable control measures. The interplay of natural conditions, agricultural techniques, and environmental factors is fundamental to high-quality medicinal plant production.

Effective quality risk management involves the identification of risk factors, the development of risk mitigation strategies, and a nuanced understanding of the interrelationship between CMA, CPP, and CQA. Implementing efficient quality risk management guarantees the manufacture of superior herbal medications that meet both traditional knowledge and modern scientific standards. Continuous surveillance, adjustment, and collaboration among stakeholders contribute to ongoing improvement in agricultural techniques, ensuring the long-term viability and financial success of cultivating medicinal plants. The comprehensive approach outlined in this chapter provides deep insights into adopting optimum cultivation practices and creating an optimal environment for farm-level production of herbal drugs, ultimately contributing to the delivery of high-quality medicinal plants to meet the evolving needs of global healthcare.

ACKNOWLEDGMENT

The project is funded by the Indian Council of Social Science Research under the Research Program scheme (Project Grant No. G-39/21/ICSSR/RP) to Prof. Ashish Baldi as Project Director.

KEYWORDS

- **agricultural techniques**
- **bioactive compounds**
- **cultivation practices**
- **herbal medications**
- **medicinal plants**
- **plant growth hormones**
- **quality risk management**

REFERENCES

1. Eisenberg, D. M., Davis, R. B., Ettner, S. L., Appel, S., Wilkey, S., Van Rompay, M., et al. (1998). Trends in alternative medicine use in the United States, 1990–1997: Results of a follow-up national survey. *JAMA, 280*(18), 1569–1575.
2. Liu, Y., Dao, Z., Yang, C., Liu, Y., & Long, C. (2009). Medicinal plants used by Tibetans in Shangri-La, Yunnan, China. *Journal of Ethnobiology and Ethnomedicine, 5*(1), 1–10.
3. Govaerts, R. (2001). How many species of seed plants are there? *Taxon, 50*(4), 1085–1090.
4. Sharma, S., Sharma, R., Goyal, K., & Jindal, S. (2021). Potential of herbal treatment of psoriasis: A laconic review. *Asian Journal of Research in Pharmaceutical Sciences, 11*(1), 51–57.

5. Ved, D. K., & Goraya, G. S. (2007). Demand and supply of medicinal plants in India. *National Medicinal Plants Board, New Delhi & FRLHT, Bangalore, India, 18*(85), 210–252.
6. Maikhuri, R. K., Phondani, P. C., Rawat, L. S., Jha, N. K., Maletha, A., Bahuguna, Y. M., et al. (2017). Conservation and management strategies of medicinal plant resources through action research approaches in Indian Himalaya. *Iranian Journal of Science and Technology, Transactions A: Science, 41*, 771–777.
7. Crone, C. C., & Wise, T. N. (1998). Use of herbal medicines among consultation-liaison populations: A review of current information regarding risks, interactions, and efficacy. *Psychosomatics, 39*(1), 3–13.
8. World Health Organization. (1978). *The Promotion and Development of Traditional Medicine: Report of a WHO Meeting (Geneva, 28 Nov–Dec 1977)*. World Health Organization.
9. Bodeker, G., & Willcox, M. (2000). The first international meeting of the Research Initiative on Traditional Antimalarial Methods (RITAM). *Journal of Alternative and Complementary Medicine, 6*(2), 195–207.
10. Ved, D. K., Begum, S. N., & Kumar, K. R. (2017). Trade in Indian medicinal plants. *Ethnobotany of India, Vol 5: Indo-Gangetic Region & Central India, 321*.
11. Al-Snafi, A. E. (2018). Therapeutic importance of *Hyoscyamus* species grown in Iraq (*Hyoscyamus albus, Hyoscyamus niger*, and *Hyoscyamus reticulatus*): A review. *IOSR Journal of Pharmacy, 8*(6), 18–32.
12. Dasaroju, S., & Gottumukkala, K. M. (2014). Current trends in the research of *Emblica officinalis* (Amla): A pharmacological perspective. *International Journal of Pharmaceutical Sciences Review and Research, 24*(2), 150–159.
13. Meher, S. K., Das, B., Panda, P., Bhuyan, G. C., & Rao, M. M. (2016). Uses of *Withania somnifera (Linn) Dunal* (Ashwagandha) in Ayurveda and its pharmacological evidence. *Research Journal of Pharmacology and Pharmacodynamics, 8*(1), 23–29.
14. Umadevi, M., Rajeswari, R., Rahale, C. S., Selvavenkadesh, S., Pushpa, R., Kumar, K. P. S., et al. (2012). Traditional and medicinal uses of *Withania somnifera*. *Pharma Innovation, 1*(9, Part A), 102.
15. Singh, R., Sharma, P. K., & Malviya, R. (2011). Pharmacological properties and Ayurvedic value of Indian buch plant (*Acorus calamus*): A short review. *Advances in Biological Research, 5*(3), 145–154.
16. Rajput, S. B., Tonge, M. B., & Karuppayil, S. M. (2014). An overview on traditional uses and pharmacological profile of *Acorus calamus Linn.* (Sweet flag) and other *Acorus* species. *Phytomedicine, 21*(3), 268–276.
17. Ghibhela, B., Mishra, A., & Sharma, D. (2022). Brahmi: A memory booster medicinal herb. In *Medicinal Plants and Their Benefits* (Chapter 3, pp. 43–48).
18. G. K. S., & Bharath, M. M. S. (2011). Exploring the role of "Brahmi" (*Bacopa monnieri* and *Centella asiatica*) in brain function and therapy. *Recent Patents on Endocrine, Metabolic & Immune Drug Discovery, 5*(1), 33–49.
19. Alambayan, J., Vats, M., Sardana, S., & Sehrawat, R. (2015). Evaluation of antiulcer activity of roots of *Acacia catechu* Willd. (Mimosoideae). *Journal of Pharmacognosy and Phytochemistry, 3*(5), 79–84.

20. Kumari, M., Radha, Kumar, M., Zhang, B., Amarowicz, R., Puri, S., et al. (2022). *Acacia catechu (Lf) Willd.*: A review on bioactive compounds and their health-promoting functionalities. *Plants, 11*(22), 3091.
21. Rajeswari, R., Umadevi, M., Rahale, C. S., Pushpa, R., Selvavenkadesh, S., Kumar, K. P. S., et al. (2012). *Aloe vera*: The miracle plant, its medicinal and traditional uses in India. *Journal of Pharmacognosy and Phytochemistry, 1*(4), 118–124.
22. Sánchez, M., González-Burgos, E., Iglesias, I., & Gómez-Serranillos, M. P. (2020). Pharmacological update properties of *Aloe vera* and its major active constituents. *Molecules, 25*(6), 1324.
23. Gupta, A., & Rawat, S. (2017). Clinical importance of *Aloe vera*. *Research Journal of Topical and Cosmetic Sciences, 8*(1), 30.
24. Sharma, P., Dwivedee, B. P., Bisht, D., Dash, A. K., & Kumar, D. (2019). The chemical constituents and diverse pharmacological importance of *Tinospora cordifolia*. *Heliyon, 5*(9), e02437.
25. Modi, B., Kumari Shah, K., Shrestha, J., Shrestha, P., Basnet, A., Tiwari, I., et al. (2020). Morphology, biological activity, chemical composition, and medicinal value of *Tinospora cordifolia* (Willd.) Miers. *Advances in Journal of Chemistry B, 2020*, 36–54.
26. Razavi, B. M., Ghasemzadeh Rahbardar, M., & Hosseinzadeh, H. (2021). A review of therapeutic potentials of turmeric (*Curcuma longa*) and its active constituent, curcumin, on inflammatory disorders, pain, and their related patents. *Phytotherapy Research, 35*(12), 6489–6513.
27. Niranjan, A., & Prakash, D. (2008). Chemical constituents and biological activities of turmeric (*Curcuma longa* L.)—A review. *Journal of Food Science and Technology, 45*(2), 109.
28. Gupta, C., Prakash, D., Bakar, M. F. A., & Kitdamrongtham, W. (2022). Phytopharmaceuticals from *Andrographis paniculata*: An ambrosia for immortality. *Indian Journal of Agricultural Biochemistry, 35*(1), 1–14.
29. Rios, J. L., Recio, M. C., Giner, R. M., & Manez, S. (1996). An update review of saffron and its active constituents. *Phytotherapy Research, 10*(3), 189–193.
30. Haber, S. L., & El-Ibiary, S. Y. (2016). Peppermint oil for treatment of irritable bowel syndrome. *American Journal of Health-System Pharmacy, 73*(2), 22–31.
31. Bandi, V. J. R., Sanampudi, N., Velamuri, S. K. R., & Maddi, R. (2022). A detailed review of herbal formulations marketed and available in India for the treatment and management of gastric acidity. *International Journal of Pharmacognosy and Chemistry, 2022*, 34–52.
32. Verma, S., Arya, S., & Aman, R. (2022). A review on medicinal plants in the north region of India: Traditional use in Vedic culture and their pharmacological properties. *TMR Integrative Medicine, 6*, e22026.
33. Srivastava, R. K., Singh, A., Srivastava, G. P., Lehri, A., Niranjan, A., Tewari, S. K., et al. (2014). Chemical constituents and biological activities of promising aromatic plant Nagarmotha (*Cyperus scariosus* R. Br.): A review. *Proceedings of the Indian National Science Academy, 80*(3), 525–536.
34. Joseph, B., & Raj, S. J. (2011). A comparative study on various properties of five medicinally important plants. *International Journal of Pharmacology, 7*(2), 206–211.

35. Reddy, I. V., & Neelima, P. (2022). Neem (*Azadirachta indica*): A review on medicinal *Kalpavriksha*. *International Journal of Economic Plants, 9*(1), 59–63.
36. Vijaya, K., & Chavan, P. (2009). *Chlorophytum borivilianum* (Safed musli): A review. *Pharmacognosy Reviews, 3*(5), 154.
37. Singh, A. K., Srivastava, A., Kumar, V., & Singh, K. (2018). Phytochemicals, medicinal and food applications of *Shatavari* (*Asparagus racemosus*): An updated review. *Natural Products Journal, 8*(1), 32–44.
38. Kumar, R., Saha, P., Lokare, P., Datta, K., Selvakumar, P., & Chourasia, A. (2022). A systematic review of *Ocimum sanctum* (Tulsi): Morphological characteristics, phytoconstituents and therapeutic applications. *International Journal of Research in Applied Sciences and Biotechnology, 9*(2), 221–226.
39. Petrovska, B. B. (2012). Historical review of medicinal plants' usage. *Pharmacognosy Reviews, 6*(11), 1.
40. Inoue, M., & Craker, L. E. (2014). Medicinal and aromatic plants—Uses and functions. In *Horticultural Plants, People, and Places, Vol. 2: Environmental Horticulture* (pp. 645–669).
41. Nair, G., Raja, S. S. S., & Vijayakumar, R. (2022). Introductory chapter: Secondary metabolites—An overview. In *Secondary Metabolites: Sources and Applications*.
42. Böttger, A., Vothknecht, U., Bolle, C., Wolf, A., Böttger, A., Vothknecht, U., et al. (2018). Plant secondary metabolites and their general function in plants. In *Lessons from Caffeine, Cannabis, and Co: Plant-Derived Drugs and Their Interactions with Human Receptors* (pp. 3–17).
43. Verma, N., & Shukla, S. (2015). Impact of various factors responsible for fluctuation in plant secondary metabolites. *Journal of Applied Research on Medicinal and Aromatic Plants, 2*(4), 105–113.
44. Qadir, S. U., & Raja, V. (2021). Herbal medicine: Old practice and modern perspectives. In *Phytomedicine* (pp. 149–180). Elsevier.
45. Jeet, K., & Baldi, A. (2021). Trending microbiologicals and their role to enhance growth and essential oil content of dill (*Anethum graveolens*). *System, 2*, 3.
46. Jeet, K., & Baldi, A. (2021). Potential of microbes-containing formulations to alter growth and phytochemicals of medicinal aromatic plant—*Foeniculum vulgare*. *International Journal of Life Science and Pharma Research, 11*(1), P34–P51.
47. Zhang, J., Wider, B., Shang, H., Li, X., & Ernst, E. (2012). Quality of herbal medicines: Challenges and solutions. *Complementary Therapies in Medicine, 20*(1–2), 100–106.
48. Bashir, T., Chandra Mishra, R., Hasan, M. M., Mohanta, T. K., & Bae, H. (2018). Effect of hybridization on somatic mutations and genomic rearrangements in plants. *International Journal of Molecular Sciences, 19*(12), 3758.
49. Palevitch, D. (1991). Agronomy applied to medicinal plant conservation. *Conservation of Medicinal Plants*, 167–178.
50. Wallaart, T. E., Pras, N., Beekman, A. C., & Quax, W. J. (1999). Seasonal variation of artemisinin and precursors in *Artemisia annua*. *Planta Medica, 57*, 57–62.
51. Dijkstra, H., & Speckmann, G. J. (1980). Autotetraploidy in caraway (*Carum carvi* L.) for the increase of the essential oil content of the seed. *Euphytica, 29*(1), 89–96.
52. Ghotbi Ravandi, E., Rezanejad, F., Zolala, J., & Dehghan, E. (2013). The effects of chromosome doubling on selected morphological and phytochemical characteristics

of *Cichorium intybus* L. *Journal of Horticultural Science and Biotechnology, 88*(6), 701–709.

53. Xing, S. H., Guo, X. B., Wang, Q., Pan, Q. F., Tian, Y. S., Liu, P., et al. (2011). Induction and flow cytometry identification of tetraploids from seed-derived explants through colchicine treatments in *Catharanthus roseus* (L.) G. Don. *Biomedical Research International, 2011*, 1–7.
54. Heping, H., Shanlin, G., Lanlan, C., & Xiaoke, J. (2008). *In vitro* induction and identification of autotetraploids of *Dioscorea zingiberensis*. *In Vitro Cellular & Developmental Biology–Plant, 44*, 448–455.
55. Bernard, F., Moghbel, N., & Hassannejad, S. (2012). Treatment of licorice seeds with colchicine: Changes in seedling DNA levels and anthocyanin and glycyrrhizic acid contents of derived callus cultures. *Natural Product Communications, 7*(11), 1–4.
56. Lavania, U. C., & Srivastava, S. (1991). Enhanced productivity of tropane alkaloids and fertility in artificial autotetraploids of *Hyoscyamus niger* L. *Euphytica, 52*, 73–77.
57. Mishra, B. K., Pathak, S., Sharma, A., Trivedi, P. K., & Shukla, S. (2010). Modulated gene expression in newly synthesized auto-tetraploid of *Papaver somniferum* L. *South African Journal of Botany, 76*(3), 447–452.
58. Kim, Y. S., Hahn, E. J., Murthy, H. N., & Paek, K. Y. (2004). Effect of polyploidy induction on biomass and ginsenoside accumulation in adventitious roots of ginseng. *Journal of Plant Biology, 47*, 356–360.
59. Yadav, A. K., Singh, S., Yadav, S. C., Dhyani, D., Bhardwaj, G., Sharma, A., et al. (2013). Induction and morpho-chemical characterization of *Stevia rebaudiana* colchiploids. *Indian Journal of Agricultural Sciences, 83*(2), 159–165.
60. Kumar, S., Rai, S. P., Kumar, S. R., Singh, D., Srivastava, S., & Mishra, R. K. (2007). Plant variety of *Catharanthus roseus* named "Ili." *Google Patents*.
61. Kolakar, S. S., Nadukeri, S., Jakkeral, S. A., Lakshmana, D., Hanumanthappa, M., & Gangaprasad, S. (2018). Role of mutation breeding in improvement of medicinal and aromatic crops. *Journal of Pharmacognosy and Phytochemistry, 7*(3S), 425–429.
62. Kumari, R., Agrawal, S. B., & Sarkar, A. (2009). Evaluation of changes in oil cells and composition of essential oil in lemongrass (*Cymbopogon citratus* (DC) Stapf.) due to supplemental ultraviolet-B irradiation. *Current Science, 97*(8), 1137–1142.
63. Lal, R. K., Chanotiya, C. S., Singh, V. R., Dhawan, S. S., Gupta, P., Shukla, S., et al. (2019). Induced polygenic variations through γ-rays irradiation and selection of novel genotype in chamomile (*Chamomilla recutita* [L.] Rauschert). *International Journal of Radiation Biology, 95*(9), 1242–1250.
64. Mohamed, W. M., & El-Shimi, I. (2014). The effect of gamma rays on the pharmaceutical products of essential oils for peppermint (*Mentha piperita* L.). *International Journal of Farming and Allied Sciences, 3*(8), 884–894.
65. Floria, F., & Ichim, M. C. (2006). High yielding opium poppy (*Papaver somniferum* L.) mutant lines. *Plant Mutation Reports, 4*, 28–29.
66. Sharma, J. R., Lal, R. K., Gupta, A. P., Misra, H. O., Pant, V., Singh, N. K., et al. (1999). Development of non-narcotic (opiumless and alkaloid-free) opium poppy, *Papaver somniferum*. *Plant Breeding, 118*(5), 449–452.

67. Jain, D. K., & Nagar, R. K. (2018). Induced variability by gamma irradiation in Isabgol (*Plantago ovata* Forsk). *International Journal of Agricultural Sciences Research, 8*, 73–78.
68. Floria, F., & Ichim, M. C. (2006). Valuable fenugreek (*Trigonella foenum-graecum* L.) mutants induced by gamma rays and alkylating agents. *Plant Mutation Reports, 4*, 30.
69. Xia, Q., Zhao, K. J., Huang, Z. G., Zhang, P., Dong, T. T. X., Li, S. P., et al. (2005). Molecular genetics and chemical assessment of *Rhizoma Curcumae* in China. *Journal of Agricultural and Food Chemistry, 53*(15), 6019–6026.
70. Carles, M., Cheung, M. K. L., Moganti, S., Dong, T. T. X., Tsim, K. W., Ip, N. Y., et al. (2005). A DNA microarray for the authentication of toxic traditional Chinese medicinal plants. *Planta Medica, 71*(6), 580–584.
71. Nebauer, S. G., del Castillo-Agudo, L., & Segura, J. (1999). RAPD variation within and among natural populations of outcrossing willow-leaved foxglove (*Digitalis obscura* L.). *Theoretical and Applied Genetics, 98*, 985–994.
72. Yang, M., Zhang, D., Liu, J., & Zheng, J. (2001). A molecular marker that is specific to medicinal rhubarb based on chloroplast *trnL/trnF* sequences. *Planta Medica, 67*(8), 784–786.
73. Xue, C. Y., Li, D. Z., Lu, J. M., Yang, J. B., & Liu, J. Q. (2006). Molecular authentication of the traditional Tibetan medicinal plant *Swertia mussotii*. *Planta Medica, 72*(13), 1223–1226.
74. Lum, M. R., Potter, E., Dang, T., Heber, D., Hardy, M., & Hirsch, A. M. (2005). Identification of botanicals and potential contaminants through RFLP and sequencing. *Planta Medica, 71*(9), 841–846.
75. Niazian, M., & Sabbatini, P. (2021). Traditional *in vitro* strategies for sustainable production of bioactive compounds and manipulation of metabolomic profile in medicinal, aromatic and ornamental plants. *Planta, 254*, 1–22.
76. Marchev, A. S., Yordanova, Z. P., & Georgiev, M. I. (2020). Green (cell) factories for advanced production of plant secondary metabolites. *Critical Reviews in Biotechnology, 40*(4), 443–458.
77. Fazili, M. A., Bashir, I., Ahmad, M., Yaqoob, U., & Geelani, S. N. (2022). *In vitro* strategies for the enhancement of secondary metabolite production in plants: A review. *Bulletin of the National Research Centre, 46*(1), 1–12.
78. Walters, K. J., & Currey, C. J. (2015). Hydroponic greenhouse basil production: Comparing systems and cultivars. *HortTechnology, 25*(5), 645–650.
79. Senizza, B., Zhang, L., Miras-Moreno, B., Righetti, L., Zengin, G., Ak, G., et al. (2020). The strength of the nutrient solution modulates the functional profile of hydroponically grown lettuce in a genotype-dependent manner. *Foods, 9*(9), 1156.
80. Finkel, O. M., Salas-González, I., Castrillo, G., Spaepen, S., Law, T. F., Teixeira, P. J. P. L., et al. (2019). The effects of soil phosphorus content on plant microbiota are driven by the plant phosphate starvation response. *PLoS Biology, 17*(11), e3000534.
81. Dastogeer, K. M. G., Tumpa, F. H., Sultana, A., Akter, M. A., & Chakraborty, A. (2020). Plant microbiome – an account of the factors that shape community composition and diversity. *Current Plant Biology, 23*, 100161.

82. Sharma, S., & Shahzad, A. (2013). Bioreactors: A rapid approach for secondary metabolite production. In *Recent Trends in Biotechnology and Therapeutic Applications of Medicinal Plants* (pp. 25–49). Springer.
83. Khan, S. A., Siddiqui, M. H., & Osama, K. (2018). Bioreactors for hairy roots culture: A review. *Current Biotechnology, 7*(6), 417–427.
84. Tolosa, L. N., & Zhang, Z. (2020). The role of major transcription factors in Solanaceous food crops under different stress conditions: Current and future perspectives. *Plants, 9*(1), 56.
85. Baillo, E. H., Kimotho, R. N., Zhang, Z., & Xu, P. (2019). Transcription factors associated with abiotic and biotic stress tolerance and their potential for crops improvement. *Genes (Basel), 10*(10), 771.
86. Davies, P. J. (2012). *Plant Hormones and Their Role in Plant Growth and Development.* Springer Science & Business Media.
87. Brewer, P. B., Dun, E. A., Ferguson, B. J., Rameau, C., & Beveridge, C. A. (2009). Strigolactone acts downstream of auxin to regulate bud outgrowth in pea and Arabidopsis. *Plant Physiology, 150*(1), 482–493.
88. Davies, P. J. (2010). The plant hormones: Their nature, occurrence, and functions. In *Plant Hormones: Biosynthesis, Signal Transduction, Action* (Vol. 1, pp. 1–15). Springer.
89. Turnbull, C. G. (1999). *Plant Hormones: Chemical Signalling in Plant Development.*
90. Naz, R., Anis, M., & Aref, I. M. (2015). Management of cytokinin–auxin interactions for *in vitro* shoot proliferation of *Althaea officinalis* L.: A valuable medicinal plant. *Rendiconti Lincei, 26*, 323–334.
91. Shekhawat, M. S., & Manokari, M. (2016). Impact of auxins on vegetative propagation through stem cuttings of *Couroupita guianensis* Aubl.: A conservation approach. *Scientifica (Cairo), 2016*(1), 1–8.
92. Sciuchetti, L. A. (1961). Influence of gibberellic acid on medicinal plants. *Journal of Pharmaceutical Sciences, 50*(12), 981–998.
93. Grzegorczyk-Karolak, I., Hnatuszko-Konka, K., Krzemińska, M., Olszewska, M. A., & Owczarek, A. (2021). Cytokinin-based tissue cultures for stable medicinal plant production: Regeneration and phytochemical profiling of *Salvia bulleyana* shoots. *Biomolecules, 11*(10), 1513.
94. Clouse, S. D., & Sasse, J. M. (1998). Brassinosteroids: Essential regulators of plant growth and development. *Annual Review of Plant Biology, 49*(1), 427–451.
95. Nazari, M., Ghasemi-Soloklui, A. A., Kordrostami, M., & Latef, A. A. H. A. (2023). Deciphering the response of medicinal plants to abiotic stressors: A focus on drought and salinity. *Plant Stress, 10*, 1–10.
96. Fonseca, J. M., Rushing, J. W., Rajapakse, N. C., Thomas, R. L., & Riley, M. B. (2006). Potential implications of medicinal plant production in controlled environments: The case of feverfew (*Tanacetum parthenium*). *HortScience, 41*(3), 531–535.
97. Bennett, R. N., & Wallsgrove, R. M. (1994). Secondary metabolites in plant defence mechanisms. *New Phytologist, 127*(4), 617–633.
98. Mustafavi, S. H., Naghdi Badi, H., Sękara, A., Mehrafarin, A., Janda, T., Ghorbanpour, M., et al. (2018). Polyamines and their possible mechanisms involved in plant physiological processes and elicitation of secondary metabolites. *Acta Physiologiae Plantarum, 40*, 1–19.

99. Darini, M. T. (2017). Studies of chemical sandy soil and physiological properties of *Aloe vera* L. plant on nutrient stress condition. *International Journal of Current Agricultural Science, 7*, 208–212.
100. Bünemann, E. K., Bongiorno, G., Bai, Z., Creamer, R. E., De Deyn, G., De Goede, R., et al. (2018). Soil quality – A critical review. *Soil Biology and Biochemistry, 120*, 105–125.
101. Meuser, H. (2010). *Contaminated Urban Soils* (Vol. *18*). Springer Science & Business Media.
102. Ashraf, M., & Foolad, M. R. (2005). Pre-sowing seed treatment—A shotgun approach to improve germination, plant growth, and crop yield under saline and non-saline conditions. In *Advances in Agronomy* (Vol. 1, pp. 223–271). Academic Press.
103. Kumar, A., Abrol, E., Koul, S., & Vyas, D. (2012). Seasonal low temperature plays an important role in increasing metabolic content of secondary metabolites in *Withania somnifera* (L.) Dunal and affects the time of harvesting. *Acta Physiologiae Plantarum, 34*, 2027–2031.
104. Rawlins, S. L., & Raats, P. A. C. (1975). Prospects for high-frequency irrigation: Uniform, frequent irrigation optimizes the root environment while drastically reducing water use. *Science, 188*(4188), 604–610.
105. Krishnamurthy, R., Chandorkar, M. S., Kalzunkar, B. G., Palsuledesai, M. R., Pathak, J. M., & Rajendra, G. (2004). Agronomic manipulations for improving the productivity of *Shatavari* (*Asparagus racemosus*) under irrigated and rainfed conditions. *Journal of Medicinal and Aromatic Plant Sciences, 26*, 740–745.
106. Smitha, G. R., Basak, B. B., Thondaiman, V., & Saha, A. (2019). Nutrient management through organics, bio-fertilizers and crop residues improves growth, yield, and quality of sacred basil (*Ocimum sanctum* Linn). *Industrial Crops and Products, 128*, 599–606.
107. Rahman, K. M., Khan, M. R. I., Haque, M. A. H., & Karim, M. R. (2015). Effect of fertilizer and manures on growth and yield of *Tulsi* (*Ocimum sanctum*). *2015*(1), 1–4.
108. Badalingappanavar, R., Hanumanthappa, M., Veeranna, H. K., Kolakar, S., & Khidrapure, G. (2018). Organic fertilizer management in cultivation of medicinal and aromatic crops: A review. *Journal of Pharmacognosy and Phytochemistry, 7*(3S), 126–129.
109. Jeet, K., & Baldi, A. (2022). Changes in growth parameters and essential oil composition of *Ajwain* (*Trachyspermum ammi*) fruits in response to various biofertilizers. *International Journal of Life Science and Pharma Research, 12*(2).
110. Gobbo-Neto, L., & Lopes, N. P. (2007). Plantas medicinais: fatores de influência no conteúdo de metabólitos secundários. *Química Nova, 30*, 374–381.
111. Hättenschwiler, S., & Vitousek, P. M. (2000). The role of polyphenols in terrestrial ecosystem nutrient cycling. *Trends in Ecology & Evolution, 15*(6), 238–243.
112. Gahukar, R. T. (2018). Management of pests and diseases of important tropical/subtropical medicinal and aromatic plants: A review. *Journal of Applied Research on Medicinal and Aromatic Plants, 9*, 1–18.
113. Kumar, J., Kashyap, N. P., & Sharma, S. D. (2001). Pests of maize and their management in Himachal Pradesh – A review. *Agricultural Reviews, 22*(1), 47–51.

114. Porwal, O., Singh, S. K., Patel, D. K., Gupta, S., Tripathi, R., & Katekhaye, S. (2020). Cultivation, collection, and processing of medicinal plants. *Bioactive Phytochemicals: Drug Discovery to Product Development* (pp. 14–30).
115. Rahman, S., Iqbal, M., & Husen, A. (2023). Medicinal plants and abiotic stress: An overview. In *Medicinal Plants: Their Response to Abiotic Stress* (pp. 1–34).
116. Shinwari, Z. K., Tanveer, F., & Iqrar, I. (2019). Role of microbes in plant health, disease management, and abiotic stress management. In *Microbiome in Plant Health and Disease: Challenges and Opportunities* (pp. 231–250).
117. Moënne-Loccoz, Y., Mavingui, P., Combes, C., Normand, P., & Steinberg, C. (2015). Microorganisms and biotic interactions. In *Environmental Microbiology: Fundamentals and Applications–Microbial Ecology* (pp. 395–444).
118. Shirokova, A. V., Dmitriev, L. B., Belopukhov, S. L., Dmitrieva, V. L., Danilova, I. L., Kharchenko, V. A., et al. (2023). The accumulation of volatile compounds and the change in the morphology of the leaf wax cover accompanied the "anti-aging" effect in *Anethum graveolens* L. plants sprayed with 6-benzylaminopurine. *International Journal of Molecular Sciences, 24*(20), 15137.
119. Zhou, X., Joshi, S., Patil, S., Khare, T., & Kumar, V. (2021). Reactive oxygen, nitrogen, carbonyl, and sulfur species and their roles in plant abiotic stress responses and tolerance. *Journal of Plant Growth Regulation, 2021*, 1–24.
120. Jeet, K., & Baldi, A. (2019). A comprehensive review on *Pistacia integerrima. Current Traditional Medicine, 5*(2), 98–113.
121. Zeinali, E., & Rahimmalek, M. (2013). Effect of seasonal variation on essential oil yield, and morpho-physiological properties of *Achillea filipendulina* Lam. *Journal of Medicinal Herbs, 3*(4), 199–208.
122. Slavkovska, V., Zlatković, B., Bräuchler, C., Stojanović, D., Tzakou, O., & Couladis, M. (2013). Variations of essential oil characteristics of *Clinopodium pulegium* (Lamiaceae) depending on phenological stage. *Botanica Serbica, 37*(2), 97–104.
123. Kpoviessi, D. S. S., Gbaguidi, F. A., Kossouoh, C., Agbani, P., Yayi-Ladekan, E., Sinsin, B., et al. (2011). Chemical composition and seasonal variation of essential oil of *Sclerocarya birrea* (A. Rich.) Hochst subsp *birrea* leaves from Benin. *Journal of Medicinal Plants Research, 5*(18), 4640–4646.
124. Elabbar, F. A., EL-Barasi, Y. M., & ALawamy, M. W. M. (2014). Seasonal variation study of the volatile oils of *Origanum cyrenaicum* in Libya. *Pelagia Research Library: Advances in Applied Science Research, 5*(1), 39–42.
125. Manika, N., Mishra, P., Kumar, N., Chanotiya, C. S., & Bagchi, G. D. (2012). Effect of season on yield and composition of the essential oil of *Eucalyptus citriodora* Hook. leaf grown in sub-tropical conditions of North India. *Journal of Medicinal Plants Research, 6*(14), 2875–2879.
126. Elsharkawy, E. R. (2014). Anticancer effect and seasonal variation in oil constituents of *Santolina chamaecyparissus. Chemistry and Materials Research, 6*(3), 85–91.
127. Marzouki, H., Elaissi, A., Khaldi, A., Bouzid, S., Falconieri, D., Marongiu, B., et al. (2009). Seasonal and geographical variation of *Laurus nobilis* L. essential oil from Tunisia. *The Open Natural Products Journal, 2*(1), 86–91.
128. El-Hawary, S. S., El-Sofany, R. H., Abdel-Monem, A. R., Ashour, R. S., & Sleem, A. A. (2013). Seasonal variation in the composition of *Plectranthus amboinicus* (Lour.)

Spreng essential oil and its biological activities. *American Journal of Essential Oils and Natural Products, 1*(2), 11–18.

129. Hussain, A. I., Anwar, F., Nigam, P. S., Ashraf, M., & Gilani, A. H. (2010). Seasonal variation in content, chemical composition, and antimicrobial and cytotoxic activities of essential oils from four *Mentha* species. *Journal of the Science of Food and Agriculture, 90*(11), 1827–1836.
130. Omer, E. A., Abou Hussein, E. A., Hendawy, S. F., Ezz, E., Azza, A., & El Gendy, A. G. (2013). Effect of soil type and seasonal variation on growth, yield, essential oil, and artemisinin content of *Artemisia annua* L. *International Research Journal of Horticulture, 1*(1), 15–27.
131. Al-Hamwi, M., Bakkour, Y., Abou-Ela, M., El-Lakany, A., Tabcheh, M., & El-Omar, F. (2011). Chemical composition and seasonal variation of the essential oil of *Micromeria fruticosa*. *Journal of Natural Products, 4*(2011), 147–149.
132. Angelopoulou, D., Demetzos, C., & Perdetzoglou, D. (2002). Diurnal and seasonal variation of the essential oil labdanes and clerodanes from *Cistus monspeliensis* L. leaves. *Biochemical Systematics and Ecology, 30*(3), 189–203.
133. Freire, C. M. M., Marques, M. O. M., & Costa, M. (2006). Effects of seasonal variation on the central nervous system activity of *Ocimum gratissimum* L. essential oil. *Journal of Ethnopharmacology, 105*(1, 2), 161–166.
134. Gourine, N., Yousfi, M., Bombarda, I., Nadjemi, B., & Gaydou, E. (2010). Seasonal variation of chemical composition and antioxidant activity of essential oil from *Pistacia atlantica* Desf. leaves. *Journal of the American Oil Chemists' Society, 87*(2), 157–166.
135. Rajeswara Rao, B. R., Kaul, P. N., Mallavarapu, G. R., & Ramesh, S. (1996). Effect of seasonal climatic changes on biomass yield and terpenoid composition of rose-scented geranium (*Pelargonium* species). *Biochemical Systematics and Ecology, 24*(7), 627–635.
136. Inan, M., Kirpik, M., Kaya, D. A., & Kirici, S. (2011). Effect of harvest time on essential oil composition of *Thymbra spicata* L. growing in flora of Adıyaman. *Advances in Environmental Biology, 5*(2), 356–358.
137. Skrzypczak-Pietraszek, E., & Pietraszek, J. (2014). Seasonal changes of flavonoid content in *Melittis melissophyllum* L. (Lamiaceae). *Chemistry & Biodiversity, 11*(4), 562–570.
138. Patil, S., Ojha, R., Kaur, G., Nepali, K., Aggarwal, S., & Lal Dhar, K. (2013). Estimation of seasonal variation of two major pyrrolo [2,1-b] quinazoline alkaloids of *Adhatoda vasica* by HPLC. *The Natural Products Journal, 3*(1), 30–34.
139. Mira, Q., Yazdani, T., Ahmad, S., & Yunus, M. (2009). Total flavonoids and phenolics in *Catharanthus roseus* L. and *Ocimum sanctum* L. as biomarkers of urban auto pollution. *Caspian Journal of Environmental Science, 7*(1), 9–16.
140. Banerjee, D., Hazra, A. K., Chakraborti, S., Ray, J., Mukherjee, A., & Mukherjee, B. (2013). Variation of total phenolic content, flavonoid, and radical scavenging activity of *Ipomoea pes-caprae* with respect to harvesting time and location. *Indian Journal of Natural Products and Resources, 42*(1), 106–109.
141. Moniruzzaman, M., Sulaiman, S. A., Azlan, S. A. M., & Gan, S. H. (2013). Two-year variations of phenolics, flavonoids, and antioxidant contents in acacia honey. *Molecules, 18*(12), 14694–14710.

142. Millogo-Kone, H., Lompo, M., Kini, F., Asimi, S., Guissou, I. P., & Nacoulma, O. (2009). Evaluation of flavonoids and total phenolic contents of stem bark and leaves of *Parkia biglobosa* (Jacq.) Benth. (Mimosaceae)—Free radical scavenging and antimicrobial activities. *Research Journal of Medical Sciences, 3*(2), 70–74.
143. Gehlot, M., & Kasera, P. K. (2013). Variability in primary and secondary metabolites during different seasons in *Phyllanthus amarus*. *Indian Journal of Plant Physiology, 18*, 169–171.
144. Sivaci, A., & Duman, S. (2014). Evaluation of seasonal antioxidant activity and total phenolic compounds in stems and leaves of some almond (*Prunus amygdalus* L.) varieties. *Biological Research, 47*(1), 1–5.
145. Deshpande, R. S., Neelakanta, N. T., & Hegde, N. (2006). Cultivation of medicinal crops and aromatic crops as a means of diversification in agriculture. *Agricultural Development and Rural Transformation Unit, Institute for Social.*
146. Vakhariya, R. R., Talokar, S. S., Dhole, A. R., & Magdum, C. S. (2015). Herbomineral formulations – A review. *International Journal of Scientific Research in Science and Technology, 3*, 161–169.
147. Dkhar, M., & Tiwari, B. K. (2020). Traditional ecological knowledge of tribal communities of North East India. *Biodiversitas Journal of Biological Diversity, 21*(7).
148. Keer, N. R., Chadha, N. K., Saini, V. P., Ojha, M. L., & Sawant, P. B. (2020). Dietary shatavari, *Asparagus racemosus* root extract promotes growth, feed conversion, and nutrient utilization in *Labeo rajasthanicus*. *Journal of Environmental Biology, 41*, 1464–1469.
149. Wood, B. A., Blair, H. T., Gray, D. I., Kemp, P. D., Kenyon, P. R., Morris, S. T., et al. (2014). Agricultural science in the wild: A social network analysis of farmer knowledge exchange. *PLoS ONE, 9*(8), e105203.
150. Tyagi, D. K. (2005). *Pharma Forestry: A Field Guide to Medicinal Plants*. Atlantic Publishers & Distributors.
151. Kunle, O. F., Egharevba, H. O., & Ahmadu, P. O. (2012). Standardization of herbal medicines—A review. *International Journal of Biodiversity and Conservation, 4*(3), 101–112.
152. Namdeo, A. G. (2018). Cultivation of medicinal and aromatic plants. In *Natural Products and Drug Discovery* (pp. 525–553). Elsevier.
153. Szakiel, A., Pączkowski, C., & Henry, M. (2011). Influence of environmental abiotic factors on the content of saponins in plants. *Phytochemistry Reviews, 10*, 471–491.
154. Kovács, B., Kovács-Deák, B., Székely-Szentmiklósi, I., Fülöp, I., Bába, L. I., Boda, F., et al. (2021). Quality-by-design in pharmaceutical development: From current perspectives to practical applications. *Acta Pharmaceutica, 71*(4), 497–526.
155. Singh, P. A., & Baldi, A. (2023). Quality risk assessment on traditional immunity booster plants cultivators in Punjab, India. *Indian Journal of Traditional Knowledge, 22*(2), 273–282.
156. Hailu, B., & Mehari, H. (2021). Impacts of soil salinity/sodicity on soil-water relations and plant growth in dry land areas: A review. *Journal of Natural Sciences Research, 12*, 1–10.
157. Hamdy, A., Abdel-Dayem, S., & Abu-Zeid, M. (1993). Saline water management for optimum crop production. *Agricultural Water Management, 24*(3), 189–203.

158. McPherson, F. (2015). Herbal therapy and nutritional. *Pharmacotherapy Advances in Practice and Nurse Prescribing, 129*.
159. Mathew, G., Joy, P. P., Skaria, B. P., & Mathew, S. (2005). Cultivation prospects of tuberous medicinal plants. In *National Seminar on Achievements and Opportunities in Postharvest Management and Value Addition in Root and Tuber Crops (NSRTC 2), Centre for Tuber Crops Research Institute (CTCRI), Thiruvananthapuram, India* (pp. 81–82).
160. Pandey, A. K., & Savita, R. (2017). Harvesting and post-harvest processing of medicinal plants: Problems and prospects. *Pharma Innovation Journal, 6*(12), 229–235.
161. Kumar, S., Yadav, M., Yadav, A., & Yadav, J. P. (2017). Impact of spatial and climatic conditions on phytochemical diversity and *in vitro* antioxidant activity of Indian *Aloe vera* (L.) Burm. f. *South African Journal of Botany, 111*, 50–59.
162. Singh, P. A., Bajwa, N., Sharma, L., & Baldi, A. (2023). Farm-level medicinal plants production and economic analysis in the Indian state of Punjab. *Journal of Applied Research on Medicinal and Aromatic Plants, 34*, 100486.
163. Singh, P. A., Bajwa, N., Chinnam, S., Chandan, A., & Baldi, A. (2022). An overview of some important deliberations to promote medicinal plants cultivation. *Journal of Applied Research on Medicinal and Aromatic Plants, 31*, 100400.

CHAPTER 4

Metabolic Pathways in Higher Plants and Their Determination

ARUN KUMAR,[1,*] MOHEMMED FARAZ KHAN,[1] KULDEEP SINGH,[1] MUHAMMAD ARIF,[1] MOHD. MURSAL,[1] SAHIL HUSSAIN,[1] and SYED KAYNAT FATIMA[2]

[1]*Department of Pharmaceutical Chemistry, Faculty of Pharmacy, Integral University, Lucknow, Uttar Pradesh, India*

[2]*Department of Molecular Biology, Staffordshire University, Stoke-on-Trent, UK*

*Corresponding author

ABSTRACT

In the realm of higher plants, metabolic pathways are the intricate roadmaps that guide the transformation of simple molecules into a diverse array of essential compounds. "Metabolic Pathways in Higher Plants and Their Determination" offers an in-depth exploration of these critical pathways and their role in shaping the production of secondary metabolites. This chapter embarks on a journey to unravel the secrets of plant metabolism, with a specific focus on the shikimic acid pathway, the acetate pathways, and the amino acid pathway. The foundation of our investigation begins with a concise overview of the fundamental metabolic pathways, highlighting their significance in synthesizing a wide array of secondary metabolites. We delve into the intriguing world of plant biochemistry, unveiling the intricate processes that give rise to compounds with vital ecological, medicinal, and industrial roles. A significant portion of our exploration is dedicated to three key metabolic pathways: the shikimic acid pathway, the acetate pathways, and the amino acid pathway.

The Essentials of Herbal Drugs. Varsha Tiwari, Abhishek Tiwari, and Ajay Sharma (Eds.)

DOI: 10.1201/9781998511778-4

Through detailed analysis and case studies, we shed light on the unique features of these pathways and their impact on the production of secondary metabolites in higher plants. Moreover, this chapter explores the innovative utilization of radioactive isotopes as powerful tools for biogenetic studies. We delve into the applications of these isotopes in tracing the biosynthetic routes of complex plant compounds, providing invaluable insights into their origin and metabolic pathways. "Metabolic Pathways in Higher Plants and Their Determination" is an essential resource for researchers, students, and enthusiasts of plant biochemistry, offering a comprehensive understanding of the metabolic pathways that govern secondary metabolite biosynthesis in higher plants. It invites readers to uncover the secrets of plant chemistry and the methodologies that enable us to decipher the mysteries of biogenetic studies.

4.1 INTRODUCTION

Plants generate an impressive assortment of chemical substances and stand out as highly proficient and graceful chemical synthesizers. A single plant has the capability to produce anywhere from 5 to 25,000 compounds simultaneously, and there are approximations suggesting that the plant kingdom may produce as many as 200,000 to 1,000,000 distinct metabolites. Metabolites are crucial for plants to complete their life cycles under typical growth conditions. In terms of quantity, they constitute the largest portion of the metabolome and generally consist of simpler compounds such as sugars, amino acids, and fatty acids. These compounds often serve as immediate building blocks for substances related to agricultural productivity, such as starch, protein, lipids, and cell walls. Approximately 10,000 years ago, human intervention, which resulted in the domestication of naturally occurring plant species, also brought about substantial changes in plant composition. In various crop plants, numerous secondary metabolites that once allowed plants to thrive in challenging natural environments have been reduced, while primary storage compounds have been deliberately promoted for maximal production through selective breeding and by providing ideal growth conditions [1].

The interaction between primary and secondary metabolites is of great importance for most plants, as they differ in distribution, chemical structure, and functional roles. Primary metabolites serve as crucial precursors for secondary metabolites, and two key metabolic pathways, the shikimic acid pathway and the Krebs cycle, provide essential building blocks for the biosynthesis of phenolic compounds, which are aromatic secondary metabolites. These phenolic molecules play diverse roles in plants, including involvement in electron transport, antioxidation, response to wounds, providing structural support, and serving as defense mechanisms. Aromatic amino acids like L-tryptophan, L-tyrosine, and L-phenylalanine act as precursors for secondary metabolites that are synthesized through the shikimate pathway. Chorismate, which is the final product of the shikimate pathway, becomes the starting point for the biosynthesis of various secondary metabolites as well as other important compounds like folate, phenylalanine, phylloquinone (vitamin K1), and tryptophan. In fungi, specific enzymes such as 3-dehydroquinate dehydratase (DHD) and shikimate dehydrogenase (SDH) play essential roles in key reactions within the shikimate pathway. These enzymes are involved in catalyzing important steps that lead to the production of chorismate, which is a critical branching point for the synthesis of secondary metabolites. In plants, SDH and DHD also have bifunctional roles, participating in these key reactions within the shikimate pathway, ensuring the production of chorismate, which subsequently supports the biosynthesis of various secondary metabolites and essential compounds [2, 3].

4.1.1 SHIKIMIC ACID PATHWAY

In bacteria, fungi, apicomplexan organisms, and plants, the shikimate biosynthesis pathway illustrated in Figure 4.1 serves as a reservoir of aromatic precursors. Notably, this pathway is absent in animals. The nomenclature of shikimic acid derives from its initial isolation from the exceedingly toxic Japanese shikimi flower (*Illicium anisatum*). This biochemical pathway plays a significant role in connecting primary and secondary metabolism, particularly in higher plants. In microorganisms, the shikimate pathway is responsible for generating essential aromatic amino acids, namely "L-tyrosine (L-Tyr), L-phenylalanine (L-Phe), and L-tryptophan (L-Trp)." They function as fundamental elements for constructing proteins. Within the plant kingdom, these aromatic amino acids play a dual role, serving as essential components for both protein synthesis and as precursors for a diverse array of secondary metabolites crucial for fostering plant growth. Plants produce phenolic compounds, referred to as secondary metabolites, in response to environmental demands, and these substances play a crucial role in facilitating the plant's adaptation to its surroundings. The exploration of these compounds contributes to the progress of biochemical techniques and molecular biology [4–6].

The primary aromatic phenolic compounds that originate from L-Phe and L-Tyr exhibit a wide variety, including but not limited to cinnamic acids and their esters, coumarins, phenylpropenes, chromones (composed of six carbon atoms and three carbon atoms), stilbenes, anthraquinones (formed by combining six carbon atoms, two carbon atoms, and another six carbon atoms), chalcones, flavonoids, isoflavonoids, neoflavonoids (comprising six carbon atoms, three carbon atoms, and another six carbon atoms), as well as their dimers and trimers (constructed from two or three sets of six carbon atoms and three carbon atoms). Additionally, there are lignans, neolignans (composed of sets of six carbon atoms and three carbon atoms repeated twice), lignans (consisting of sets of six carbon atoms and three carbon atoms repeated multiple times), aromatic polyketides, and diphenylheptanoids (composed of six carbon atoms, seven carbon atoms, and another six carbon atoms).

Furthermore, L-Trp serves as a precursor for alkaloids in the realm of secondary metabolism [4, 7]. The unique attributes of the shikimate pathway are indeed found exclusively in bacteria, fungi, and plants. This exclusivity underscores the potential importance of targeting the enzymes responsible for these reactions in the development of antibacterial agents and herbicides. One of the key enzymes in the shikimate pathway is "5-enolpyruvylshikimate 3-phosphate synthase (EPSP-synthase)." This enzyme plays a crucial role in catalyzing the transfer of the enolpyruvyl (carboxyvinyl) group from "phosphoenolpyruvate (PEP) to shikimic acid 3-phosphate (S3P)." This reaction is a critical step in the shikimate pathway, as it leads to the formation of 5-enolpyruvylshikimate 3-phosphate, which is subsequently converted into chorismate, a central intermediate in the biosynthesis of aromatic compounds and secondary metabolites. Because the shikimate pathway is unique to certain microorganisms and plants, targeting enzymes like EPSP-synthase in this pathway has been a strategy for developing selective herbicides that can effectively control weeds without harming other organisms. Additionally, disrupting the shikimate pathway in bacteria can be a target for the development of antibacterial agents, as it interferes with the synthesis of essential aromatic compounds required for bacterial growth and survival. This approach has been employed in the development of herbicides and antimicrobial compounds to combat various agricultural and health-related challenges [8]. Conversion of steps from substrate to product is shown in Table 4.1.

TABLE 4.1 Conversion Steps from Substrate to Product in the Shikimic Acid Pathway

Reaction Steps	Substrate	Product
1	Phosphoenolpyruvate (PEP), erythrose-4-phosphate 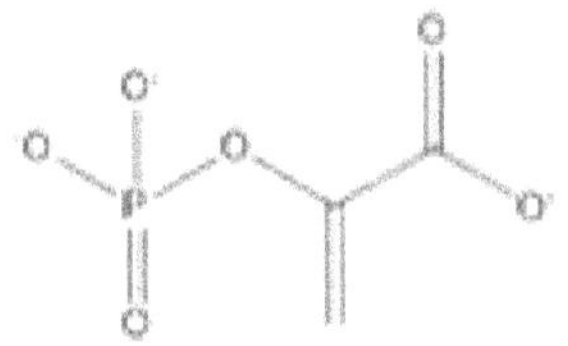	3-Deoxy-*D*-arabino-heptulosonic acid 7-phosphate (DAHP), Pi
2	3-Deoxy-*D*-arabino-heptulosonic acid 7-phosphate (DAHP) 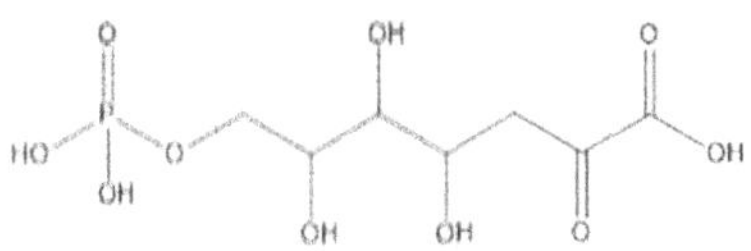	3-Dehydroquinic acid (DHQ), Pi
3	3-Dehydroquinic acid (DHQ) 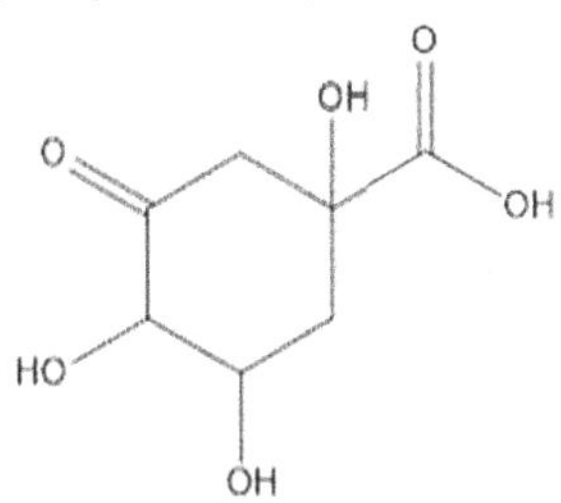	3-Dehydroshikimic acid (DHS), H_2O
4	3-Dehydroshikimic acid (DHS), NADPH + H^+ 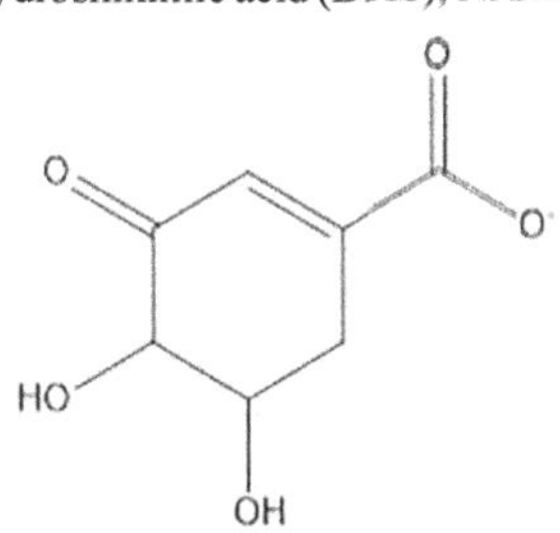	Shikimic acid, $NADP^+$

TABLE 4.1 *(Continued)*

Reaction Steps	Substrate	Product
5	Shikimic acid, ATP 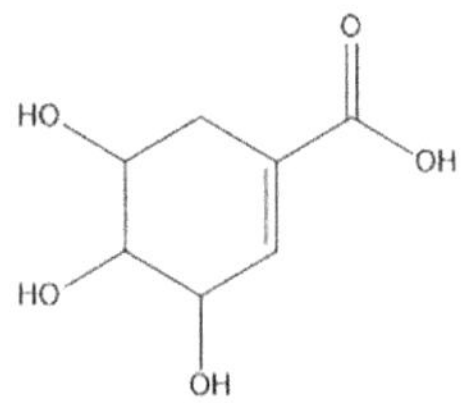	Shikimic acid 3-phosphate (S3P), ADP
6	Shikimic acid 3-phosphate (S3P), PEP 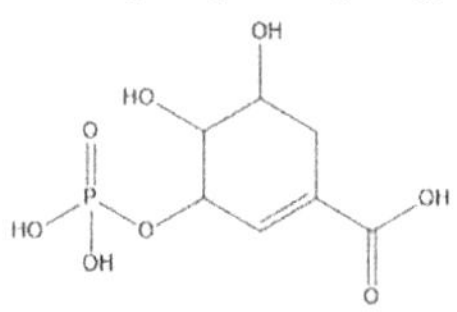	5-Enolpyruvylshikimate 3-phosphate (EPSP), Pi
7	5-Enolpyruvylshikimate 3-phosphate (EPSP) 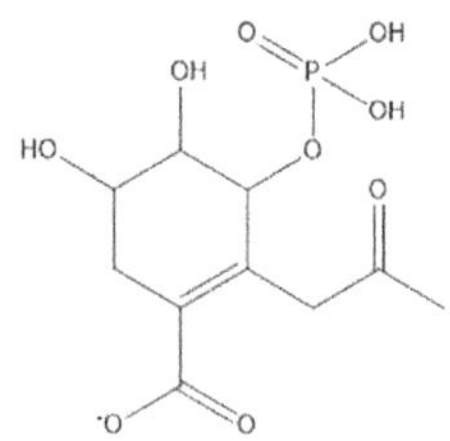	Chorismic acid, Pi

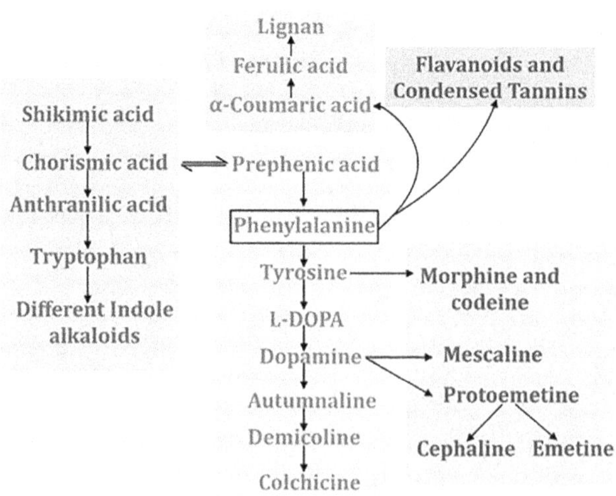

FIGURE 4.1 The shikimic acid pathway.

4.1.2 ACETATE PATHWAYS

The 3-hydroxy-3-methylglutaryl-CoA reductase (HMGCoAR) pathway, also known as the isoprenoid pipeline or the mevalonate pathway (Figure 4.2), is a metabolic system that provides molecules essential for several cellular activities in eukaryotes, archaea, and even some bacteria. This emphasizes how important it is to almost every living thing, including humans. Mevalonate, which HMGCoAR converts from acetoacetyl-CoA, goes through further changes to create sterol isoprenoids, such as cholesterol. Cholesterol serves as an essential precursor for lipoproteins, steroid hormones, and bile acids. Additionally, the pathway leads to the production of various hydrophobic compounds, including ubiquinone, heme-A, dolichol, isopentenyl tRNA, and nonsterol isoprenoids. Intermediates within this network also play pivotal roles in the posttranslational modification of numerous proteins involved in both inter- and intracellular signaling [9].

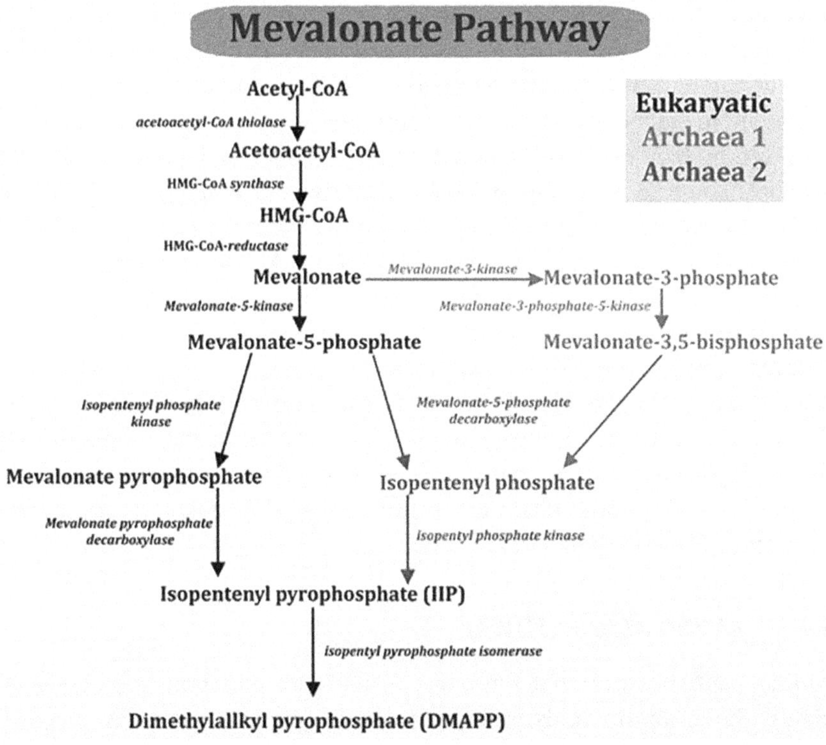

FIGURE 4.2 The mevalonate pathway.

The acetate-malonate pathway primarily yields fatty acids, encompassing both less common but widely distributed primary metabolites and more common ones. Furthermore, this pathway plays a significant role in the production of aliphatic and aromatic compounds in plants, accomplished through the synthesis of polyketides. In all living organisms, acetyl CoA, a versatile molecule, undergoes a continuous process of replenishment and depletion. Acetyl CoA is generated through various metabolic pathways, including glycolysis, as well as the breakdown of fatty acids and amino acids. Acetyl CoA is a crucial starting material for a wide range of primary and secondary metabolites, as shown in Figure 4.3 [10]. It is in charge of fatty acid biosynthesis. With an emphasis on spinach (*Spinacia oleracea*, Chenopodiaceae) chloroplasts, this route has been particularly well-studied in plants, and the enzymes involved have been fully defined. The first phase starts with the production of malonyl CoA, which is made possible by acetyl CoA carboxylase's carboxylation of acetyl CoA. Furthermore, malonate may be converted to malonyl CoA via a process similar to the one shown in Figure 4.3. Since oxaloacetate is produced in a variety of processes, malonate, a consequence of oxaloacetate catabolism, converts to malonyl CoA, a conversion that may be important in plants. In order to make butyrate, acetate is added to malonate, followed by the release of carbon dioxide (CO_2) and a decrease in the end product. The enzyme complex known as fatty acid synthetase is made up of the several enzymes involved in these different processes. This series of events repeats itself six more times until butyryl ACP is joined to six more malonyl units, resulting in the formation of C16 palmityl ACP. There is a termination response at this point. Plants have been shown to exhibit three different forms of termination reactions: the transfer of the palmityl radical to ACP, which is not connected to the *de novo* fatty acid synthase complex; the transfer to CoA; or the hydrolysis that results in the production of free acid. Because of this, palmitic acid is the main product of fatty acid synthesis, while shorter chain lengths might cause termination, producing acids with fewer carbon atoms [10].

4.1.3 AMINO ACID PATHWAY

Amino acids have crucial functions in the core metabolic processes of plants. Some amino acids, referred to as essential amino acids (EAAs), such as lysine and methionine, are not produced by humans or animals

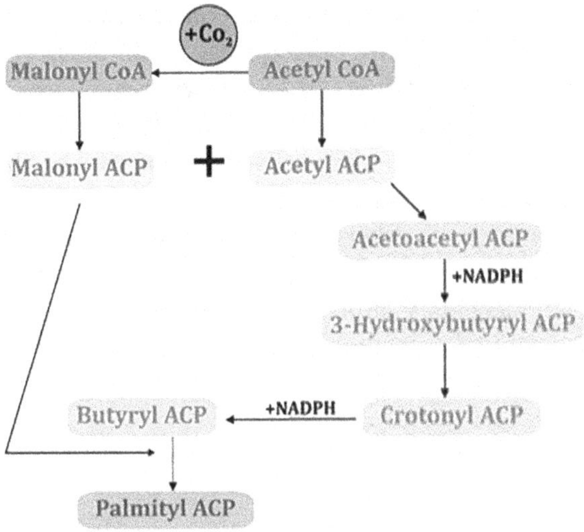

FIGURE 4.3 Formation of fatty acids by acetate-mevalonate pathway.

and must be obtained through dietary sources. Nevertheless, deficiencies in plant nutrition frequently arise due to a shortage of specific EAAs [11]. Amino acids also serve as intermediates in the synthesis of end-stage metabolites within specific metabolic pathways. Furthermore, they play a role in controlling various metabolic pathways, as well as other physiological and biochemical processes, thereby influencing a wide range of physiological processes in plants [12, 13]. Studies have shown that the regulation of a specific amino acid's metabolism may affect the concentrations of other amino acids. This phenomenon is mainly caused by the fact that amino acids that share a metabolic origin or are closely linked to different metabolic pathways often function as synthetic building blocks or intermediates, which alters the system's amino acid balance [14, 15]. Furthermore, amino acids function as precursors for a wide array of both primary and secondary metabolites. Amino acid consumption results in the production of many secondary metabolites. These pathways are typically distinct, and unlike isoprenes and polyketides, there are no regular patterns, except for the formation of peptides. Within this domain, as shown in "biomimetic synthesis," chemical syntheses conducted under moderate, "physiological" settings have become deeply entwined with theories of biosynthesis. Also, the shikimic acid route usually involves a different procedure for every particular product. There is no long history of conjecture about the function of shikimic acid in primary metabolism, since its significance was not completely recognized until 1951. Additionally, studies in this field have not kept pace with those conducted on the other three principal categories of secondary metabolites [16]. Additionally, they are essential for human nutrition, either as food components or as sources of nutraceutical chemicals. It is noteworthy that humans and other animals cannot generate 9 of the 21 proteinogenic amino acids, and that at least three of the others cannot be made in sufficient amounts to fulfill metabolic needs. As a result, eating is the only way to receive these physiologically necessary amino acids, with plants providing the bulk of these sources. Unlike animals and humans, plants are able to generate all 21 proteinogenic amino acids internally [11, 17] (Figure 4.4).

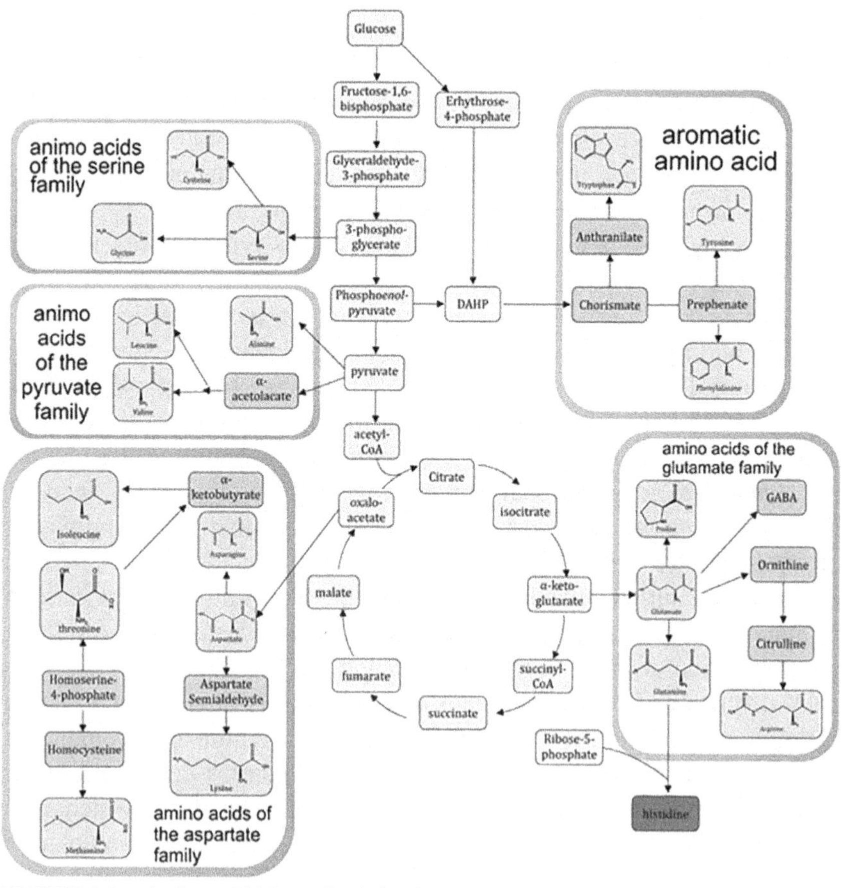

FIGURE 4.4 Amino acid biosynthesis in plants.

4.2 EXPLORING THE USE OF RADIOACTIVE ISOTOPES IN RESEARCHING BIOGENETICS

Researchers use five different approaches to investigate the biosynthetic pathway of primary and secondary metabolites. These methods encompass employing the tracer technique, utilizing isolated organs and tissues, implementing the grafting method, employing mutant strains, and conducting enzyme studies.

4.2.1 TRACER TECHNIQUES

Among the listed methods, the tracer technique stands out as the primary approach in investigating biogenetic studies. This method employs compounds labeled with radioactive isotopes to trace and identify various intermediates and steps within plant biosynthetic pathways, determining their progression at specific rates and times. These labeled compounds, upon administration to plants, integrate into the metabolic pool, collectively participating in the biological system's metabolic processes. Isotopes refer to elements sharing indistinguishable chemical properties or atomic numbers but differing in atomic mass numbers, meaning they are atoms of the same element characterized by identical proton numbers but varying neutron counts [18]. Isotopes exist in two main categories: stable isotopes, which do not change and do not release radiation (such as ^{13}C, ^{15}N, ^{18}O, and ^{2}H), and radioactive isotopes, which radiate and are unstable (like ^{3}H, ^{14}C, ^{13}N, ^{24}Na, ^{42}K, ^{32}S, ^{35}P, $^{13}1I$). The emission of radiation characterizes radioactive isotopes through a process known as radioactivity. Tracer techniques, which use these isotopes, prove valuable in assessing the creation of various metabolites within living organisms. A diverse array of isotopes is available to estimate metabolites, and these tracer techniques demonstrate high sensitivity, effectiveness, and simplicity in both administration and isolation. Accurate results are achievable with adequate metabolic time and techniques employed. For instance, the amount and location of a molecule, such as marked glucose, that contains the tracer isotope ^{14}C can be used to measure the amount of glucose present in a biological system. Various tracers can be employed for different studies; for instance, utilizing labeled nitrogen offers more precise insights into research related to alkaloids and amino acids compared to tracers based on carbon [19]. The process of tracing the biosynthetic route entails incorporating radioactive isotopes into the starting materials or precursors. For instance, by introducing ^{14}C into phenylalanine, it becomes possible to track the biosynthesis of cyanogenic glycosides and prunacin, enabling the determination of their location and quantity within a biological system. When studying proteins, alkaloids, and amino acids, the use of the nitrogen atom (^{13}N) provides more precise insights than employing carbon-based isotopes. Investigations concerning glycosidic linkage employ radioactive atoms like ^{14}C, ^{13}N, ^{32}S, and ^{15}O, while studies focusing on terpenoids involve the use of radioactive ^{1}H and ^{15}O atoms [20].

4.2.2 WORKFLOW IN TRACER TECHNIQUES

The process involves preparing a labeled compound, integrating this compound into the system under study, isolating it through separation techniques, and then analyzing the nature of the metabolites present in different biochemical fractions.

4.2.3 PREPARATION OF LABELLED COMPOUND

In biological research, employing bioactive isotopes allows for the monitoring of compound metabolism within living organisms, facilitating the detection and measurement of gentle, readily absorbed radiation emitted by labeled compounds. These compounds, whether using radioactive or stable isotopes, are synthesized for this purpose. Typically, radioactive carbon and hydrogen isotopes are preferred in biological investigations, particularly those with extended half-lives. The selection of tracer elements follows specific criteria: the initial concentration of the tracer element must be substantial enough to endure dilution during metabolism, knowledge of the compound's physical and chemical properties is necessary, and it should possess a sufficiently lengthy half-life. Additionally, it is important that the tracer does not harm the tissue system and emits low radiation energy. Instruments like scintillation chambers, GM counters, autoradiography, NMR, and MS utilizing ionization techniques are used to discern the properties of metabolites [21] (Table 4.2).

TABLE 4.2 Readily Available Radionuclides for Laboratory Synthesis

Nuclide	t1/2	Typical Chemical Form
^{3}H	12.5 yr	^{3}HHO, $^{3}H_2$
^{14}C	5730 yr	$^{14}CH_3OH$; $^{14}CH_3I$; $H^{14}CHO$
^{13}N	10 minutes	Amino acids
^{24}Na	15 hr	Himalayan pink salt
^{36}Cl	3×10^5 year	Aqueous $H^{36}Cl$
^{42}K	1.25 billion years	KCl
^{32}S	87 days	Sulfate in aqueous solution; $H_2{}^{32}SO_4$
^{35}P	14 days	Orthophosphate in dilute HCl
^{131}I	8 days	^{131}I in aqueous NaOH

4.2.4 INTEGRATING THE MARKED COMPOUND WITHIN THE TISSUE SYSTEM

The process of integrating labeled compounds into the tissue system involves various techniques such as spraying, infiltration, the floating technique, direct injection, root feeding, and stem feeding. Root feeding involves administering labeled compounds to the roots, which is particularly effective when roots serve as the biosynthetic sites of metabolites, as seen in Solanaceae plants. Stem feeding entails introducing labeled compounds through the cut ends of the stem immersed in a solution, although it might not be suitable for plants containing latex. Direct injection is employed in plants with hollow stems, such as Umbelliferae and capsule plants like opium poppy, using a microsyringe to inject the labeled compound solution directly. Infiltration, a wick-feeding method, involves drawing a thread through the stem dipped into a radioactive solution or, alternatively, cutting a flap in the stem and immersing it in the solution.

The floating method involves floating leaf discs or chopped leaves on a solution containing the labeled compound. Lastly, the spraying technique involves the absorption of radioactive compounds by leaves after being sprayed, which is suitable for substances like steroids.

4.2.5 THE PROCESS OF SEGREGATING AND EXTRACTING THE MARKED COMPOUND

The selection of methods for separating and isolating labeled compounds depends on the characteristics of the drug and its origin. Fresh soft tissues are typically subjected to infusion or maceration techniques. Hard tissues, on the other hand, are treated using methods such as decoction or hot percolation. Unorganized drugs undergo maceration utilizing both polar and non-polar solvents, while fat and oil components are isolated using non-polar solvents. Substances like alkaloids, glycosides, and flavonoids are extracted using slightly polar solvents, while plant phenols and flavonoids are separated using polar solvents.

4.2.6 IDENTIFYING AND MEASURING THE RADIOACTIVITY IN THE LABELED COMPOUND

In biogenetic investigations involving radioactive tracers, the importance of reliable approaches for detecting and quantifying the labeled substances becomes paramount. Liquid scintillation counters serve to detect soft, readily absorbed radiation emitted by ^{3}H and ^{14}C labeled compounds. Advanced instruments are utilized to handle mixed radiations like ^{3}H and ^{14}C. Various tools aid in determining metabolite characteristics: the GM Counter, scintillation or liquid scintillation counter, and ionization chamber. Stable isotope-containing compounds are analyzed via mass spectroscopy, yielding a molecular peak based on the mass/charge ratio, while NMR provides insight into carbon or proton composition. Autoradiography, an imaging method employing radioactive sources within the exposed sample, comes in two forms. In *in vitro* autoradiography, cellular components like DNA, RNA, proteins, or lipids are isolated and labeled with suitable radioisotopes. *In vivo* autoradiography involves the use of radioisotopes mixed with radioactive tracers, which are introduced into the body either through oral ingestion or injection. This method is used to evaluate the distribution of radiation in thin tissue sections or entire body cryosections, often employing laboratory animals. It is extensively applied in research for understanding metabolism, tracking disease progression, and conducting experiments for the development of new pharmaceuticals. Moreover, radioactivity on paper or thin layer chromatography can be identified, and the density measurement helps determine the quantity of radioactivity in different spots. Additionally, autoradiography allows viewing negative results of whole morphological parts like leaves or sections under a microscope [22].

4.3 IDENTIFYING THE CHARACTERISTICS OF METABOLITES WITHIN DIFFERENT BIOCHEMICAL FRACTIONS

Different instruments are employed to discern the chemical properties of intermediate and end products when utilizing various isotopes.

4.3.1 GEIGER-MULLER COUNTER

A Geiger counter, also known as a Geiger-Müller counter or G-M counter, is an electronic instrument designed to detect and quantify ionizing radiation. It finds usage in various fields such as radiation dosimetry, radiological safety, experimental physics, and the nuclear sector. This device functions by sensing ionizing radiation, such as alpha particles, beta particles, and gamma rays, through the process of ionization in a Geiger-Müller tube, which is the source of the device's name. Widely recognized as a portable radiation survey tool, it stands as one of the most globally familiar radiation detection devices. Comprising a Geiger-Müller tube as the sensing component responsible for radiation detection, coupled with processing electronics, it provides the displayed results [23]. Within the Geiger-Müller tube, an inert gas like helium, neon, or argon is maintained at low pressure and subjected to high voltage. When high-energy particles or gamma radiation ionize the gas, the tube briefly conducts electrical charge. The ionization effect undergoes significant amplification through the Townsend discharge effect within the tube, resulting in a detectable pulse. This amplified signal is then transmitted to the processing and display electronics for measurement and analysis [24].

4.3.2 SCINTILLATION OR LIQUID SCINTILLATION COUNTER

Utilizing the excitation effect of incoming radiation on a scintillating material and collecting the ensuing light pulses, a scintillation counter is a tool for the detection and measurement of ionizing radiation. It usually consists of a scintillator that releases photons when exposed to radiation and a sensitive photodetector that transforms this light into an electrical signal. Common photodetectors include photomultiplier tubes (PMTs), charge-coupled devices (CCDs), cameras, and photodiodes.

After that, this signal is processed and interpreted using electronics. These counters find extensive use in various fields such as radiation protection, assessing radioactive materials, and research in physics due to their cost-effectiveness, high quantum efficiency, and ability to gauge the energy and intensity of incoming radiation [25].

4.3.3 IONIZATION CHAMBER

Among gas-filled radiation detectors, the ionization chamber is the most basic and is often used to detect X-rays, gamma rays, and beta particles, among other forms of ionizing radiation. The phrase "ionization chamber" refers, in its conventional sense, only to detectors that collect all charges generated by the direct ionization of the gas through the application of an electric field. In order to provide a tiny direct current output, this detector makes use of discrete charges created by interactions between the gas and the incoming radiation. As a result, it is unable to quantify individual ionizing events and, thus, cannot distinguish between radiation types' intensities. However, it provides a comprehensive assessment of the collective ionizing effect. Its advantage lies in its uniform response across a broad spectrum of energies, making it well-suited for measuring high levels of gamma radiation, such as within radiation hot cells, enduring extended periods within high radiation fields without deterioration. Ionization chambers find widespread use across various domains, including the nuclear power industry, research laboratories, fire detection systems, radiation safety protocols, and environmental monitoring due to their reliability and versatility [26].

4.3.4 NMR SPECTROPHOTOMETER

The scientific technique known as nuclear magnetic resonance (NMR) spectroscopy uses the magnetic properties of individual atomic nuclei to determine the physical and chemical characteristics of the atoms or molecules that make them up. It revolves around NMR, offering intricate insights into the structure, dynamics, reactivity, and chemical surroundings of these molecules. Various biological fluids possess distinct physicochemical properties, influencing the selection of NMR experiments best suited to extract biochemical data from each fluid type effectively.

This technique unveils two types of information attainable from an NMR experiment on biological fluids: latent and patent biochemical details, each contributing to a comprehensive understanding of the fluid's composition and properties [27].

4.3.5 AUTORADIOGRAPHY

This method involves using photographic film or emulsion as an ionizing radiation detector to examine the distribution of radioactive materials within a plant item, such as histology tissue or a chromatography sheet. For a certain amount of time, referred to as the exposure duration, the specimen is maintained in close proximity to the emulsion. This technique involves immediately placing a sample containing a radioactively tagged metabolite onto an appropriate photosensitive medium, such as X-ray (photographic) film, and leaving it there for a predetermined amount of time. Understanding the distribution and movement of radioactive materials may be gained by analyzing the ensuing autoradiograph, or the captured pattern [28].

4.4 METHODS OF TRACER TECHNIQUES

The procedure entails injecting into the plant a labeled putative precursor of the investigated ingredient. The separated component is examined for radioactivity after a reasonable amount of time. However, merely detecting radioactivity in the isolated compound is not sufficient evidence that the fed compound directly contributed, as it could have entered broader metabolic pathways, randomly dispersing among various products. To strengthen the evidence, double and triple labeling experiments are conducted. These involve using different isotopes or placing labels at multiple positions within the molecule. For instance, distinct isotopes applied at two or more positions aid in tracking the compound's specific involvement in pathways. This methodology has been crucial in various applications, such as distinguishing the synthesis of hyoscine from hyoscyamine in *Datura stramonium*. It has also been useful in researching the biogenesis of ergot alkaloids and morphine. Notably, Leete utilized doubly labeled lysines to determine the specific nitrogen involvement in forming the piperidine ring of anabasine in *Nicotiana glauca*.

4.4.1 USE OF ISOLATED ORGANS AND TISSUES

The isolated organ perfusion technique is utilized to create an isolated circulation and perfusion for an organ, detached from the body's systemic circulation. This method serves multiple purposes, including organ-specific chemotherapy, targeted delivery of drugs or genetic material, organ transplants, and aiding organ injury recovery. Extensively studied in both animal models and humans over many years, the process involves selecting a suitable perfusion system, resembling an organ bath in some aspects.

However, it is important to note that the isolated organ perfusion technique is generally performed *in vivo*, meaning it is conducted within the living organism. It does not involve removing the entire organ from the body, but rather isolating its circulation and perfusion while it remains within the organism [29].

4.4.2 GRAFTING

The horticultural practice commonly referred to as grafting, or graftage, involves the fusion of plant tissues to stimulate their mutual growth and development. Grafting, also known as graftage, is a horticultural method that involves merging plant tissues to stimulate their coalescence and sustained growth. The combined plant is referred to as having a scion at the top and a rootstock at the bottom. The vascular tissues must unite, a spontaneous process that is similar to inosculation, for this procedure to be successful. Predominantly utilized in asexual propagation within the horticultural and agricultural sectors, the typical connection point for the scion to the rootstock is at the soil line. However, in top-work grafting, this union can occur at a higher point, forming an understock comprising the lower trunk and root system. Typically, the scion is chosen for its ideal branches, leaves, flowers, or fruits, conveying the appropriate genetic composition for future plant development, while the rootstock is chosen for its beneficial root features. Stem grafting is the process of attaching a shoot from a chosen plant variety onto the rootstock of another plant, while bud grafting involves attaching a dormant bud to the stem of a rootstock. After a successful graft, growth is promoted by cutting the rootstock's stem just above the new bud. For grafting to work, the vascular cambium tissues of both the rootstock and the scion must make contact, and they need to remain intact until the graft is fully integrated, typically over a span of weeks. Establishing a vascular connection between the grafted tissues is crucial for successful grafting. Studies on Arabidopsis thaliana hypocotyls have revealed that while the xylem connection might take up to seven days to establish post-grafting, the phloem connection can occur within three days [30].

4.4.3 USE OF MUTANT STRAINS

In biology, particularly in genetics, a mutant refers to an organism or a new genetic trait arising from a mutation, typically an alteration in the DNA sequence of an organism's genome or chromosome. This alteration leads to a characteristic that would not naturally occur in a specimen. Mutants are instrumental in exploring multiple pathways within a cell, often revealing parallel or interconnected routes. Each metabolic system exhibits distinctive features that aid in the selection of mutants. Moreover, each mutant chosen subsequently becomes a potential source for the discovery of new mutants. The use of appropriate mutants not only benefits metabolic studies but also aids in physiological investigations. These mutants help unravel the physiological roles of key metabolites like sterols, fatty acids, vitamins, and hemin. For instance, studying primary defects post-starvation or the effects of substituting one metabolite for another sheds light on the roles of these essential compounds. Furthermore, mutants unable to transform a specific metabolite provide an avenue to explore permeation mechanisms. By using such mutants, researchers can investigate the entry and quantity of a metabolite within a system independently of its utilization, offering insights into its pool size and transport mechanisms [31].

4.4.4 ENZYMATIC STUDIES

In drug metabolism studies, samples encompass enzymes, endogenous compounds, and varied concentrations of target drugs and their byproducts. Analyzing these metabolites within biological matrices typically involves a sample preparation step before introducing them into analytical instruments like high-performance liquid chromatography (HPLC). This sample preparation serves to purify, isolate, and concentrate the analytes, facilitating subsequent chromatographic analysis and the identification of drug structures and their metabolites. In patients with homocystinuria receiving high doses of pyridoxine, a range of biochemical responses occurs. Studies conducted before and after such treatment reveal diverse metabolic and enzymatic reactions. Interestingly, for patients showing a positive response, the impact of pyridoxine does not seem to affect the liver's cystathionine synthase [32].

4.5 CONCLUSION AND FUTURE DIRECTIONS

The plant cell serves as a hub for synthesizing diverse phytocomponents. Analyzing chemical bioactive compounds derived from medicinal plants begins with understanding plant physiology, metabolic processes, biosynthetic pathways, and metabolite degradation. This involves qualitative screening and *in vitro* analysis methods. Secondary metabolites in medicinal plants originate from glucose degradation through glycolysis in primary metabolism, yielding four major secondary metabolite categories through essential plant biosynthetic pathways. These phyto-components synthesized by plant cells accumulate in various plant parts like roots, bark, leaves, fruits, seeds, and wood. Extracting these plant materials yields biologically active phytocompounds, whose potential can be assessed based on biological activity. ADMET assessment and prediction help in confirming certain plant bioactive compounds as promising or unsuitable drug candidates. Determining potential drugs from plant secondary metabolites involves employing in silico molecular docking through bioinformatics. This computational approach utilizes tools and software to predict, visualize, and develop potential medicinal drugs derived from plants, providing a valuable method for advancing human health.

KEYWORDS

- **biochemistry**
- **isotopes**
- **metabolic pathway**
- **metabolite degradation**
- **phytocompounds**
- **plant cells**
- **plant secondary metabolites**
- **secondary metabolites**

REFERENCES

1. Beckles, D. M., & Roessner, U. (2012). Plant metabolomics: Applications and opportunities for agricultural biotechnology. In A. Altman & P. M. Hasegawa (Eds.), *Plant Biotechnology and Agriculture* (pp. 67–81). Academic Press. https://doi.org/10.1016/B978-0-12-381466-1.00005-5.
2. Eid, S. Y., El-Readi, M. Z., Fatani, S. H., Mohamed Nour Eldin, E. E., & Wink, M. (2015). Natural products modulate the multifactorial multidrug resistance of cancer. *Pharmacology & Pharmacy, 6*(3), 146–176. https://doi.org/10.4236/pp.2015.63017.
3. Reshi, Z. A., Ahmad, W., Lukatkin, A. S., & Javed, S. B. (2023). From nature to lab: A review of secondary metabolite biosynthetic pathways, environmental influences, and *in vitro* approaches. *Metabolites, 13*(8), 895. https://doi.org/10.3390/metabo13080895.
4. Dixon, R. A., & Strack, D. (2003). Phytochemistry meets genome analysis, and beyond. *Phytochemistry, 62*(6), 815–816. https://doi.org/10.1016/s0031-9422(02)00712-4.
5. Herrmann, K. M., & Weaver, L. M. (1999). The shikimate pathway. *Annual Review of Plant Physiology and Plant Molecular Biology, 50*, 473–503. https://doi.org/10.1146/annurev.arplant.50.1.473.
6. Tzin, V., & Galili, G. (2010). New insights into the shikimate and aromatic amino acids biosynthesis pathways in plants. *Molecular Plant, 3*(6), 956–972. https://doi.org/10.1093/mp/ssq048.
7. Cheynier, V., Comte, G., Davies, K. M., Lattanzio, V., & Martens, S. (2013). Plant phenolics: Recent advances on their biosynthesis, genetics, and ecophysiology. *Plant Physiology and Biochemistry, 72*, 1–20. https://doi.org/10.1016/j.plaphy.2013.05.009.
8. Macheroux, P., Schmid, J., Amrhein, N., & Schaller, A. (1999). A unique reaction in a common pathway: Mechanism and function of chorismate synthase in the shikimate pathway. *Planta, 207*(3), 325–334. https://doi.org/10.1007/s004250050489.
9. Karlic, H., & Varga, F. (2019). Mevalonate pathway. In P. Boffetta & P. Hainaut (Eds.), *Encyclopedia of Cancer* (3rd ed., pp. 445–457). Academic Press. https://doi.org/10.1016/B978-0-12-801238-3.65000-6.
10. Vickery, M. L., & Vickery, B. (1981). The acetate-malonate pathway. In M. L. Vickery & B. Vickery (Eds.), *Secondary Plant Metabolism* (pp. 56–87). Macmillan Education UK. https://doi.org/10.1007/978-1-349-86109-5_3.
11. Galili, G., Amir, R., & Fernie, A. R. (2016). The regulation of essential amino acid synthesis and accumulation in plants. *Annual Review of Plant Biology, 67*, 153–178. https://doi.org/10.1146/annurev-arplant-043015-112213.
12. Amir, R., Galili, G., & Cohen, H. (2018). The metabolic roles of free amino acids during seed development. *Plant Science: An International Journal of Experimental Plant Biology, 275*, 11–18. https://doi.org/10.1016/j.plantsci.2018.06.011.
13. Yang, Q. Q., Zhao, D. S., Zhang, C. Q., Wu, H. Y., Li, Q. F., Gu, M. H., Sun, S. S. M., & Liu, Q. Q. (2018). A connection between lysine and serotonin metabolism in rice endosperm. *Plant Physiology, 176*(3), 1965–1980. https://doi.org/10.1104/pp.17.01283.
14. Long, X., Liu, Q., Chan, M., Wang, Q., & Sun, S. S. M. (2013). Metabolic engineering and profiling of rice with increased lysine. *Plant Biotechnology Journal, 11*(4), 490–501. https://doi.org/10.1111/pbi.12037.

15. Song, S., Hou, W., Godo, I., Wu, C., Yu, Y., Matityahu, I., Hacham, Y., Sun, S., Han, T., & Amir, R. (2013). Soybean seeds expressing feedback-insensitive cystathionine γ-synthase exhibit a higher content of methionine. *Journal of Experimental Botany, 64*(7), 1917–1926. https://doi.org/10.1093/jxb/ert053.
16. Bentley, R. (1999). Secondary metabolite biosynthesis: The first century. *Critical Reviews in Biotechnology, 19*(1), 1–40. https://doi.org/10.1080/0738-859991229189.
17. Hou, Y., & Wu, G. (2018). Nutritionally essential amino acids. *Advances in Nutrition, 9*(6), 849–851. https://doi.org/10.1093/advances/nmy054.
18. Christian, J. E. (1948). The applications of radioactive tracer techniques to pharmacy and pharmaceutical research. *Journal of the American Pharmaceutical Association (Scientific ed.), 37*(6), 250–253.
19. Kumar, G. S., & Jayaveera, K. N. (2014). *A Textbook of Pharmacognosy and Phytochemistry*. S. Chand Publishing.
20. Evans, W. C. (1956). Advances in pharmacognosy. *Manufacturing Chemist and Aerosol News, 27*, 51–55.
21. Hu, S., Mao, X., Feng, W., Oy, H., Chai, Z., Wang, M., Xu, D., & Zhang, F. (2007). Study of the effect of a Chinese medicine on calcium absorption with isotopic tracer technique. *Journal of Radioanalytical & Nuclear Chemistry, 272*(3), 519–522.
22. Delgoda, R. (2016). *Pharmacognosy: Fundamentals, Applications and Strategies*. Academic Press.
23. Veall, N. (1948). A Geiger-Muller counter for measuring the beta-ray activity of liquids, and its application to medical tracer experiments. *The British Journal of Radiology, 21*(247), 347–351.
24. Grummitt, W. E., Brown, R. M., Cruikshank, A. J., & Fowler, I. L. (1956). Recent developments in low background Geiger–Müller counters. *Canadian Journal of Chemistry, 34*(3), 206–213.
25. Bray, G. A. (1960). A simple efficient liquid scintillator for counting aqueous solutions in a liquid scintillation counter. *Analytical Biochemistry, 1*(4, 5), 279–285.
26. Almond, P. R., & Svensson, H. (1977). Ionization chamber dosimetry for photon and electron beams. *Acta Radiologica: Therapy, Physics, Biology, 16*(2), 177–186.
27. Lindon, J. C., Nicholson, J. K., & Everett, J. R. (1999). NMR spectroscopy of biofluids. *Annual Reports on NMR Spectroscopy, 38*, 1–88.
28. Caro, L. G., & Van Tubergen, R. P. (1962). High-resolution autoradiography: I. Methods. *The Journal of Cell Biology, 15*(2), 173–188.
29. Vane, J. R. (1964). The use of isolated organs for detecting active substances in the circulating blood. *British Journal of Pharmacology and Chemotherapy, 23*(2), 360–373.
30. Melnyk, C. W., & Meyerowitz, E. M. (2015). Plant grafting. *Current Biology, 25*(5), R183–R188.
31. Lacroute, F. (1975). The use of mutants in metabolic studies. *Methods in Cell Biology, 11*, 235–245.
32. Elion, G. B. (1966). Enzymatic and metabolic studies with allopurinol. *Annals of the Rheumatic Diseases, 25*(Suppl 6), 608.

CHAPTER 5

Evolving Approaches in the Extraction and Assessment of Herbal Medicines: Progress in Methodologies and Utilization of Analytical Instruments

VED PAL,[1] ARCHITA KATROLIA,[2] and ROHIT SINGH[3]

[1]*Department of Pharmacognosy, College of Pharmacy, JSS Academy of Technical Education, Noida, Uttar Pradesh, India*

[2]*Department of Pharmaceutics, College of Pharmacy, JSS Academy of Technical Education, Noida, Uttar Pradesh, India*

[3]*Department of Pharmaceutical Chemistry, College of Pharmacy, JSS Academy of Technical Education, Noida, Uttar Pradesh, India*

*Corresponding author

ABSTRACT

The use of herbal drugs, deeply rooted in traditional medicine, remains vital in modern pharmaceutical and healthcare sectors. This book chapter delves into the multifaceted process of extracting and analyzing herbal drugs, emphasizing the selection of appropriate extraction methods and solvents, modern advancements in extraction techniques, and the integration of spectroscopy, chromatography, and electrophoresis for the isolation, purification, and characterization of crude drugs.

The extraction of active constituents from herbs using a suitable solvent is the cornerstone of herbal drug preparation. The choice of solvent and extraction method can vary depending on the specific herb and its intended use. The extraction process typically involves soaking the herbs in the

The Essentials of Herbal Drugs. Varsha Tiwari, Abhishek Tiwari, and Ajay Sharma (Eds.)

DOI: 10.1201/9781998511778-5

chosen solvent for a specified duration, allowing for the dissolution of active constituents. Subsequently, the mixture is strained to remove solid plant material, and the liquid extract is collected. This extract can be employed in various formulations, such as teas, tinctures, or topical applications. Furthermore, the chapter explores the cutting-edge techniques that have revolutionized herbal drug extraction. Modern methods, such as solid-phase microextraction, microwave-assisted extraction (MAE), and pressurized liquid extraction, are examined in detail, demonstrating their capacity to speed up processing and increase extraction efficiency.

The application of analytical tools, including spectroscopy, chromatography, and electrophoresis, is explored in the context of herbal drug analysis. Spectroscopic techniques such as UV-Vis, FTIR, and NMR spectroscopy are used to analyze herbal components both qualitatively and quantitatively, enabling the identification of active compounds and assessment of their purity. Gas chromatography, high-performance liquid chromatography, and thin-layer chromatography are discussed with a focus on their role in separating and quantifying herbal drug components. Additionally, electrophoresis methods, including capillary electrophoresis and gel electrophoresis, are examined for their potential in characterizing and purifying herbal drugs.

In conclusion, this book chapter provides a comprehensive overview of the extraction and analysis of herbal drugs, from the initial selection of extraction methods and solvents to the integration of modern techniques and analytical tools. By understanding these principles and embracing technological advancements, researchers and practitioners can advance the field of herbal medicine, ensuring the development of safe, effective, and standardized herbal drug products for the benefit of healthcare and pharmaceutical industries.

5.1 INTRODUCTION

The World Health Organization's (WHO) definition of herbal medicine includes herbs, herbal materials, herbal preparations, and finished herbal products that contain sections of plants or other plant materials that are active components, alone or in combination [1]. Phytochemicals or botanical medicine are other names for herbal medicine. Herbal medicines are used to prevent or treat illnesses and enhance health and well-being since they contain elements with therapeutic potential. Human illnesses have long been treated using herbal remedies made from terrestrial medicinal plants.

Most people view herbal medicine as an essential component of dietary supplements [2]. Herbal medicines result from a long history of traditional use of medicinal plants. These uses included extracts of various plant parts, such as seeds, roots, leaves, bark, flowers, or whole herbs; they also included fixed oils, gums, fresh juice, resins, and essential oils. These medicines were used to preserve health and to prevent, treat, or cure disease; their beneficial effects were attributed to the bioactive constituents of the plants [3, 4]. Due to their extensive use and the widespread perception that herbs are natural and inherently safe, herbal medicine is gaining popularity. Approximately 80% of the global population gets their primary medical treatment from traditional herbal medicine, according to the WHO [5]. Drugs derived from higher plants have garnered increasing interest during the past 20 years, particularly those known as phytotherapeutics. Approximately 25% of medications prescribed globally are sourced from plants. Around 11% of the 252 medications on the WHO's list of essential medicines is derived from plants [6]. According to estimates, a sizable portion of people in developed nations, including the USA (43%), Belgium (31%), Canada (71%), France (49%), and Australia (48%), have utilized complementary and alternative medicine (CAM) at least once for healthcare [7]. The growing trend of herbal medicine suggests that people in developed countries are not pleased with the conventional healthcare system (Figure 5.1).

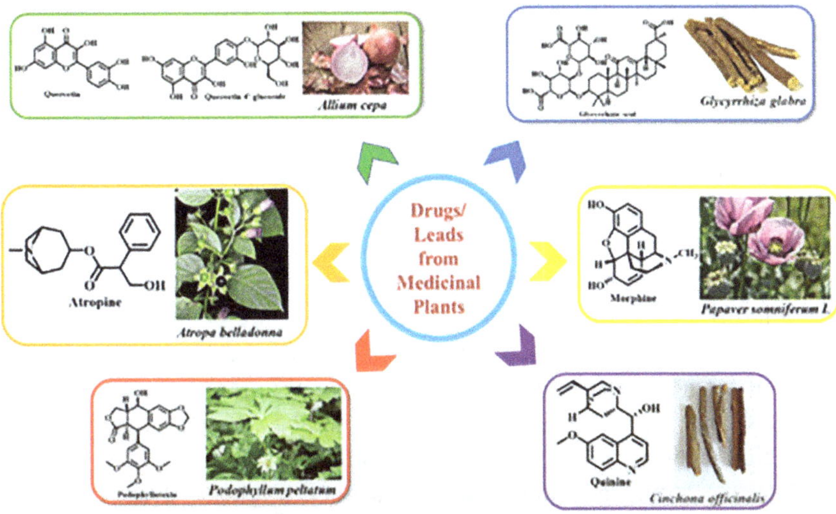

FIGURE 5.1 Structures of drugs/leads isolated from plant sources.

5.2 IMPORTANCE OF HERBS IN PHARMACEUTICALS

Humans have always depended on nature to provide their basic needs, which include the production of food, housing, clothes, tools for mobility, fertilizers, flavors, and aromas, and, last but not least, medications [8]. Plants are the cornerstone of sophisticated conventional medical systems that date back thousands of years. The earliest known written records, which date to 2600 BC and were discovered in Mesopotamia, contained references to almost 1000 compounds derived from plants [9]. The 19th century marked the beginning of the "modern" pharmaceutical era. In 1805, a young German chemist named Friedrich Sertürner isolated morphine—the first pharmacologically active substance—from the poppy plant [10]. Numerous active substances have since been extracted from natural goods. Natural ingredients have shown considerable promise in developing some medications, including antihypertensive, anticancer, and antimigraine drugs [11].

Owing to their unique chemical diversity that has evolved over millions of years, natural products (NPs) exhibit a broad spectrum of biological activity and characteristics found in drugs. These goods have developed into one of the main suppliers of innovative scaffolds and lead compounds. Natural goods will lead the way in the hunt for drugs that treat serious human ailments and will be employed consistently to meet the urgent need to develop effective treatments [12]. Many people believe that herbal medicine can provide an alternative treatment for a variety of illnesses, especially lifestyle disorders that create safety issues since they require long-term pharmaceutical medication. Traditional healthcare providers also believe that the phytoconstituents found in herbal medicine are more suited to the human system. Much research is being done on the phytochemicals found in herbs, both as potential medicinal agents and as lead molecules for developing novel synthetic or semisynthetic drugs [13]. The availability of high-throughput screening for target-based drug development and libraries containing several extremely pure phytochemicals has led to an increase in research interest in herbal medicine worldwide in the hunt for new medications. These lab animal models replicate human illnesses; they also serve as bioinformatics databases for long-term safety prediction and drug toxicity studies' profiling kits [14, 15].

A strong antimalarial medication, arteether, originates from a sesquiterpene lactone called artemisinin, separated from the plant *Artemisia annua* L. (Asteraceae), which is used in traditional Chinese medicine. Several artemisinin derivatives are undergoing clinical studies or are used at different phases as antimalarial medications [16]. Extracted from *Galanthus woronowii* Losinsk (Amaryllidaceae), galantamine is a naturally occurring substance that was initially identified via ethnobotanical research in Russia during the early 1950s [17]. Galantamine inhibits acetylcholinesterase (AChE), binds to and modifies the nicotinic acetylcholine receptor (nAChR), and slows the process of neurological degeneration. It is licensed for the treatment of Alzheimer's disease [18]. A natural dipyranocoumarin substance called calanolide A was extracted from the Malaysian rainforest tree *Calophyllum lanigerum* (Clusiaceae). Calanolide A is an anti-HIV medication that works against AZT-resistant strains of the virus and has a distinct and particular mode of action as a non-nucleoside reverse transcriptase inhibitor (NNRTI) of type-1 HIV [19, 20] (Figure 5.2).

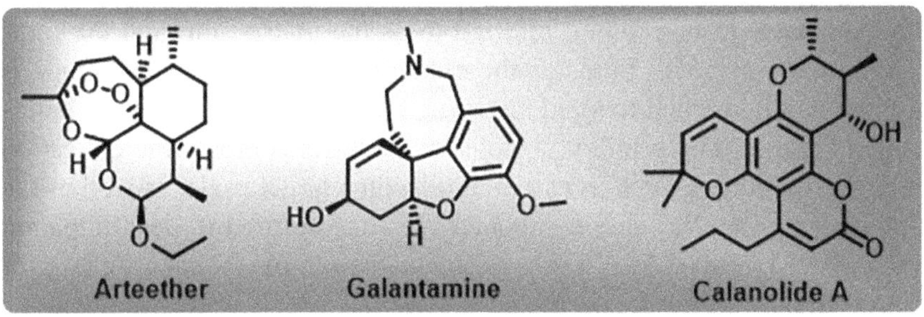

FIGURE 5.2 Chemical structures of active constituents.

In discovering new drugs from medicinal plants, existing chemicals with novel biological activities can yield significant therapeutic leads even in cases where novel chemical structures are not discovered. Since the human genome was sequenced, thousands of novel molecular targets have been identified as significant in various diseases [21]. It has already been demonstrated that several well-known substances derived from traditional medicinal plants function on recently established molecular targets. Indirubin, for example, explicitly inhibits cyclin-dependent kinases, and kamebakaurin inhibits NF-κB [22, 23].

In a nutshell, various therapeutically utilized medications have been made possible by natural compounds in medicinal plants (and their derivatives). Despite all the challenges facing drug discovery from these plants, it is reasonable to believe that natural compounds produced from medicinal plants will remain an important component of the search for innovative treatments.

5.3 MODERN TECHNIQUE OF EXTRACTION

5.3.1 SUPER CRITICAL FLUID EXTRACTION (SFE)

Because of $ScCO_2$'s (supercritical carbon dioxide) low polarity and strong infusibility, SFE can be used to extract highly efficient hydrophobic chemicals. Moreover, polar modifiers can be added to $ScCO_2$ to facilitate the extraction of polar molecules.

5.3.1.1 PRINCIPLE

SFE is a method employed for the separation of one component, termed the extractant, from another, referred to as the matrix, through the utilization of supercritical fluids as the extracting solvent. This technique is predominantly applied to solid matrices, although extraction from liquids is also feasible. The primary objectives of SFE encompass the collection of desired products, such as essential oils, on a larger scale, as well as the elimination of undesirable components, as exemplified in decaffeination processes. Moreover, SFE serves as a valuable sample preparation step for analytical purposes.

The essential oils obtained through SFE may comprise direct solvents, such as limonene, as integral constituents. The preeminent supercritical fluid employed in this process is carbon dioxide (CO_2), which can occasionally be modified with co-solvents like methanol or ethanol. The operative conditions for supercritical CO_2 extraction involve pressures surpassing the critical pressure of 74 bar and temperatures exceeding the critical temperature of 31°C.

5.3.1.2 ADVANTAGES

1. **Sensitivity:** Selective extraction is possible by adjusting the supercritical fluid's characteristics through temperature and pressure changes. For instance, modest pressures (100 bar) can be used to extract volatile oils from a plant, whereas liquid extraction would also remove lipids. Higher pressures of pure CO_2 can be

used to extract lipids; ethanol can then be added to the solvent to remove phospholipids [24]. Unsaturated fatty acids and polyphenols can be extracted independently from wine waste using the same methodology [25].

2. **Speed:** Both the extracted material and the solvent must diffuse into the matrix during the diffusion-based extraction procedure. An extraction using an organic liquid may take many hours, as opposed to supercritical fluid extraction, which can be completed in 10–60 minutes [26].

5.3.1.3 LIMITATIONS

Super critical fluid extraction (SFE) will only be utilized in situations where there are clear benefits because it is more expensive than conventional liquid extraction due to the need for high pressures. CO_2 is not usually an appropriate solvent on its own because it is non-polar and has a limited capacity to dissolve substances, particularly when working with polar solutes.

5.3.1.4 PROCEDURE

A comprehensive system for supercritical fluid extraction necessitates the integration of essential components, including a CO_2 pump, a pressure cell designed to securely contain the sample, mechanisms to uphold constant system pressure, and a collection vessel. The procedural sequence involves the elevation of CO_2 to supercritical temperatures through controlled pumping, directing the fluid to a designated heating zone. After this, the material targeted for extraction undergoes dissolution, facilitated by rapid diffusion into the solid matrix enclosed within the extraction vessel. Following the dissolution process, the extracted material undergoes a phase separation within the extraction cell. The dissolved components are expeditiously transported out of the extraction cell into a separator configured to operate at reduced pressure. Subsequently, the separated constituents settle out, completing the extraction process. The residual CO_2 may then undergo various disposition options, including release into the atmosphere, cooling, or recompression for subsequent utilization in the extraction cycle.

5.3.1.5 PUMPS

Carbon dioxide (CO_2) is typically delivered through the pumping process in its liquid state, maintaining a temperature of <5°C and a pressure of approximately 50 bar. The choice of utilizing the solvent in its liquid state is attributed to its near-incompressible nature at this phase; pumping it as a supercritical fluid would result in a substantial portion of the pump stroke being dedicated to the compression of the fluid rather than its effective conveyance. Syringe pumps or reciprocating CO_2 pumps are commonly used for smaller-scale extractions, up to a few grams per minute. Conversely, diaphragm pumps have become the preferred option for extractions carried out on a bigger scale.

The pump heads in operation typically necessitate cooling, and a parallel cooling procedure is implemented for the CO_2 prior to its introduction into the pump. This meticulous control over temperature conditions is imperative to optimize the efficiency of the pumping mechanism and the overall extraction process.

5.3.1.6 PRESSURE VESSELS

While most extractions are carried out at pressures lower than 350 bar, the minimum required pressure is 74 bar. However, occasionally, greater pressures will be necessary. For example, when extracting vegetable oils, 800 bar of pressure may be needed to ensure complete miscibility between the two phases [27].

5.3.1.7 PRESSURE MAINTENANCE

Sustaining consistent pressure levels throughout the system, from the pump to the pressure vessel, is imperative. In diminutive systems, typically those operating within the range of up to approximately 10 mL/min, a straightforward solution involves the incorporation of a basic restrictor for this purpose.

5.3.1.8 COLLECTION

A vessel that is not as pressurized as the extraction vessel receives the supercritical solvent. Supercritical fluids have a density that changes dramatically with pressure. As a result, the material precipitates for collection in the lower density CO_2, where its solubility is much lower. Fractionation of the dissolved material can be achieved by decreasing pressure in a series of vessels. Either recycle the CO_2 or depressurize it to atmospheric pressure before venting it. The pressure is usually reduced to air, and the now-gaseous CO_2 bubbles through a solvent to trap the precipitated components for analytical SFE.

5.3.1.9 COOLING AND HEATING

This is a crucial component. To maintain liquid conditions, the fluid is cooled prior to pumping and heated following pressurization. Heat must be applied to the fluid as it expands into the separator to avoid overcooling. For larger systems, the supercritical fluid's thermodynamic properties can be used to calculate the energy needed at each stage of the process [28].

5.3.1.10 OPTIMIZATION

When a plant is harvested for its essential oil, a large amount of CO_2 will be needed; however, a yield of 70–80% may be enough to yield a profit. "Complete" extraction is not necessary.

5.3.1.11 MAXIMUM DIFFUSION

This can be accomplished by lowering the particle size, expanding the matrix, or raising the temperature. There are instances when raising the solvent's pressure and adding modifiers will exacerbate matrix swelling. CO_2 causes significant swelling of certain polymers, especially elastomers, with diffusion sometimes increasing by several orders of magnitude [29].

5.3.1.12 MAXIMUM SOLUBILITY

In general, solubility will rise with increasing pressure. The impact of temperature is less certain because, in the vicinity of the critical point, rising temperatures result in drops in density and, consequently, in dissolving power. Solubility is expected to rise with temperature at pressures significantly above the critical pressure [30].

5.3.1.13 FLOW RATE OPTIMIZATION

The supercritical CO_2 density changes with temperature both before and during compression; hence, mass flow should be utilized to determine the flow rate rather than volume. Coriolis flow meters are the best choice for this kind of flow confirmation.

5.3.1.14 APPLICATION OF SFE IN PHARMACEUTICAL SCIENCES

SFE and CO_2 are used to extract desirable components from natural sources for application in the food, pharmaceutical, and nutraceutical sectors (Table 5.1).

TABLE 5.1 Application of SFE for Plant Drugs [31–33]

Solids	Extract and Component	Solvents	I Extraction Method	II Extraction Method
Dried ginger (*Zingiber officinale*)	Ginger aroma	Carbon dioxide	89 bars and 30°C	256 bar and 40°C
Coriandrum sativum (seeds)	Aroma	Carbon dioxide (sage-celery mixture)	350 bar and 40°C	90 bar and 20°C
Egg yolk	Phospholipids	Carbon dioxide with 5% ethanol	414 bar and 45°C	414 bar and 45°C

5.3.2 MICROWAVE EXTRACTION

The process known as MAE involves heating solvents that are in close contact with a sample using microwave energy. Analytes can be effectively extracted from the sample matrix into the solvent with the help of this technique. The main benefit of MAE is its intrinsic capacity to elevate the solvent-sample mixture's temperature quickly and evenly.

The use of a microwave extractor to extract bioactive compounds from plant samples has increased recently. This is because conventional extraction techniques require larger volumes of solvents, destroy heat-sensitive bioactive compounds, and take a long time to extract.

To get around the drawbacks of using traditional methods, it is crucial to investigate contemporary extraction techniques. MAE has drawn the most attention of all the modern extraction techniques because it uses less solvent, requires less time to operate, is repeatable, improves recovery yield, has good selectivity, and requires less sample manipulation [34, 35] (Table 5.2).

TABLE 5.2 Solvents, Accompanied by Their Respective Loss Tangents, Dielectric Losses, and Dielectric Constants

Sl. No.	Name of Solvent	Loss Tangent	Dielectric Loss	Dielectric Constant
1.	Hexane	0.200	0.038	0.020
2.	Toluene	0.040	0.096	0.040
3.	Water	9.899	12.30	9.889
4.	Ethanol	0.931	22.866	0.941
5.	Chloroform	0.081	0.437	0.091
6.	Ethylene glycol	1.250	37.00	1.350
7.	Dimethyl sulfoxide	0.725	37.125	0.825

Microwave irradiation operates within a specific frequency range of the electromagnetic field, closely resembling photochemically activated reactions. The frequencies utilized in this context fall within the spectrum of 300 MHz to 300 GHz. However, for applications in medical, scientific, and industrial domains, a more restricted frequency range of 0.915 to 2.45 GHz is globally sanctioned. In the context of MAE, dielectric heating emerges as a suitable mechanism for the treatment of heat-sensitive bioactive compounds [36].

When polar molecules or ionic species are used in the MAE framework, there is a sudden heating that causes collisions with molecules that are closer together without requiring an increase in pressure. The parameters governing microwave power and extraction duration typically span from 25 to 750 W and 30 to 10 minutes, respectively [37].

5.3.2.1 WORKING AND PRINCIPLE

The theory behind MAE is that when polarizable materials and polar solvent dipoles come into contact with microwave radiation, the forces between the magnetic and electric components quickly change direction. When polar solvent molecules align with the direction of the changing field, they heat up. The heating is inadequate for non-polar solvents without polarizable groups. This molecular-level thermal effect happens quickly, but it only affects a low percentage of the samples and the depths close to the surface. Conduction heats up the remaining portion of the samples. Since large samples or agglomerates of small samples cannot be heated uniformly, this is the main disadvantage of MAE. Although employing high-power sources to increase penetration depth is a possibility, once microwave radiation enters a solid that absorbs microwaves, it decays exponentially [38] (Table 5.3).

TABLE 5.3 Phytoconstituents Extracted Through MAE of Some Important Indian Traditional Medicinal Plants [34, 35, 39, 40]

Plant Name	Family	Phytoconstituents	Results (MAE)	Conclusion
Aloe (*Aloe barbadensis*)	Liliaceae	Aloe-emodin	Solvent = water/ethanol (20 mL, 20/80, v/v); Microwave power = 340 W; Solvent/feed ratio = 15; Time = 3 min	More yield as compared to alternative techniques.
Onion (*Allium cepa*)	Amaryllidaceae	Flavonoids and phenolic compounds	Microwave power = 500 W; Time = 23 minutes	Less time-consuming.
Green tea (*Camellia sinensis*)	Theaceae	Tea phenols, caffeine	Solvent = ethanol/water (50:50, v/v); Microwave power = 700 W; Solvent/feed ratio = 20; Temperature = 21°C; Time = 4 minutes	More yield compared to alternative extraction techniques.
Cardamom (*Elettaria cardamomum*)	Zingiberaceae	Linalool, cineole	Temperature = 100°C; Humidity = 67%; Microwave power = 390 W; Time = 75 min	Greater yields of bioactive compounds compared to other methods.
Fennel (*Foeniculum vulgare*)	Umbelliferae	Fenchone, ferulic acid – Global yield (1.14% db)	Temperature = 100°C; Solvent = water; Solvent/feed ratio = 2; Microwave power = 300 W; Time = 200 s	High yields compared to other extraction methods.

5.4 ISOLATION, PURIFICATION, AND CHARACTERIZATION OF DRUGS VIA SPECTROSCOPY, CHROMATOGRAPHY, AND ELECTROPHORESIS

In the realm of pharmaceutical development, the isolation, purification, and characterization of drugs are critical steps in ensuring the efficacy, safety, and quality of therapeutic agents. The journey of drug development often begins with the isolation of bioactive compounds from natural sources or synthesis in the laboratory. NPs, derived from plants, microorganisms, or marine organisms, often serve as the basis for drug discovery. The isolation process involves the extraction of these compounds from complex matrices, employing various techniques such as maceration, percolation, or supercritical fluid extraction. This initial step aims to obtain a crude extract containing a mixture of compounds, laying the groundwork for subsequent purification.

Purification is a crucial step to isolate the target drug compound from the myriads of co-extracted substances. Chromatographic techniques, such as high-performance liquid chromatography (HPLC) and column chromatography (CC), play a pivotal role in this phase. Upon obtaining a purified compound, spectroscopic techniques come into play for detailed structural elucidation. Mass Spectrometry (MS), Nuclear Magnetic Resonance (NMR) spectroscopy, and Infrared (IR) spectroscopy are commonly employed [41].

5.4.1 CHROMATOGRAPHIC TECHNIQUES

5.4.1.1 THIN LAYER CHROMATOGRAPHY (TLC)

Thin layer chromatography (TLC), as a chromatographic technique, plays a significant role in the initial stages of herbal drug analysis, offering rapid and cost-effective means for compound separation, identification, and isolation.

1. **Principle:** It is based on the principles of differential migration of components in a mixture over a thin layer of stationary phase on a flat support, commonly a glass or aluminum plate. The separation occurs due to the varying affinities of the compounds for the stationary and mobile phases. As the mobile phase (solvent) travels up the plate, compounds with different polarities move at different rates, leading to distinct bands or spots on the chromatogram.
2. **Isolation and Purification:** In the isolation of bioactive compounds from herbal extracts, TLC serves as a preliminary screening tool. The crude extract is first applied to the TLC plate, and as the solvent migrates, different compounds separate based

on their chemical properties. Visualizing the plate under ultraviolet (UV) light or by using specific detection reagents allows for the identification of spots corresponding to potential bioactive compounds. These spots can then be marked and targeted for further isolation [42].

Following the identification of target compounds, TLC can be employed for their purification. Preparative TLC involves using larger plates and higher quantities of the sample to obtain higher-purity fractions. Once the compound of interest is isolated, it can be eluted from the TLC plate, and the solvent can be evaporated to obtain a purified form of the bioactive compound. This technique is particularly advantageous for isolating compounds with similar polarities that might co-migrate in other chromatographic methods.

3. **Characterization:** It offers flexibility in terms of detection methods. While UV light is commonly used for visualizing all compounds, specific detection reagents can be employed for compounds with functional groups that might not be easily visible under UV light. For example, compounds containing phenolic or amino groups can be visualized using reagents like Dragendorff's reagent or ninhydrin, respectively.

5.4.1.2 GAS CHROMATOGRAPHY (GC)

Gas chromatography (GC) stands as a powerful analytical technique widely utilized in the isolation and purification of herbal drugs. Leveraging the principles of partition chromatography, GC enables the separation and identification of volatile and semi-volatile compounds present in complex mixtures, making it particularly well-suited for the analysis of essential oils and other volatile constituents commonly found in herbal extracts.

1. **Principle:** The differential partitioning of compounds between a stationary phase, usually a liquid coating on a solid substrate, and a mobile phase, usually an inert gas, is the basis for the GC concept. Compounds interact with the stationary phase as the sample is vaporized and injected into the GC column, resulting in separation depending on their volatility, polarity, and other physicochemical features. A chromatogram is then produced once the separated compounds are identified as they come out of the column.

2. **Isolation and Purification:** In the isolation of herbal drugs, particularly those rich in essential oils or volatile constituents, GC serves as an invaluable tool. The volatile components of the herbal extract are vaporized and injected into the GC system. The compounds travel through the column at different rates, resulting in their separation. The detector records the presence and abundance of each compound, producing a chromatogram that can be used for compound identification and quantification.
3. **Characterization:** One of the strengths of GC lies in its ability to offer selective detection for specific compounds. Different detectors, such as flame ionization detector (FID) or MS, can be coupled with GC for enhanced sensitivity and selectivity. MS provides mass spectra for each separated compound, aiding in the identification of individual components in complex herbal extracts.

5.4.1.3 COLUMN CHROMATOGRAPHY (CC)

Column chromatography (CC) is a powerful and widely employed separation technique in the isolation and purification of herbal drugs. Based on the principles of adsorption chromatography, CC facilitates the separation of complex mixtures by exploiting the differential affinities of compounds for a stationary phase within a column.

1. **Principle:** Column chromatography (CC) involves the packing of a vertical glass or plastic column with a stationary phase (commonly silica gel or alumina). The sample mixture is then introduced onto the top of the column, and elution is achieved by passing a solvent or a solvent mixture through the column.
2. **Isolation and Purification:** The crude extract, containing a complex mixture of compounds, is loaded onto the column. As the solvent system travels down the column, compounds with different polarities interact differently with the stationary phase, leading to their progressive separation. By selecting an appropriate solvent system, compounds can be eluted in order of increasing polarity, allowing for the targeted isolation of specific components.
3. **Characterization:** As fractions are collected during the elution process, monitoring the separation is essential. Various detection

methods, such as UV spectroscopy, refractive index measurement, or specific chemical tests, can be employed to identify the presence of compounds in each fraction. Combining CC with analytical techniques, such as thin-layer chromatography or GC, further aids in the characterization of isolated compounds.

5.4.1.4 HIGH-PERFORMANCE LIQUID CHROMATOGRAPHY (HPLC)

It is a robust and widely utilized chromatographic technique in the isolation and purification of bioactive compounds from herbal drugs. Renowned for its high resolution, sensitivity, and ability to handle a diverse range of compounds, HPLC plays a pivotal role in elucidating the complex chemical profiles of herbal extracts and obtaining purified fractions for further analysis.

1. **Principle:** HPLC employs a liquid mobile phase, often under high pressure, to pass through a column packed with a stationary phase. The sample is injected into the system, and as it traverses the column, compounds interact with the stationary phase based on factors such as polarity, size, and charge. The separation is achieved through differential affinities, and a detector monitors the eluting compounds, producing a chromatogram for analysis [43].
2. **Isolation and Purification:** The complex mixture obtained from the initial extraction is injected into the HPLC system. The chromatographic conditions, including the choice of column and mobile phase, can be tailored to target specific classes of compounds. The separated peaks in the chromatogram represent individual components, and fractions corresponding to the desired compounds can be collected for further analysis.
3. **Characterization:** HPLC provides various detection options, such as UV-Visible, fluorescence, or MS, allowing for selective identification of compounds based on their unique spectral characteristics. This selective detection enhances the specificity and accuracy of compound identification. Moreover, HPLC is inherently quantitative, enabling the determination of the concentration of each compound in the sample.

5.4.1.5 HIGH PERFORMANCE THIN LAYER CHROMATOGRAPHY (HPTLC)

HPTLC has become a valuable tool in the isolation, purification, and analysis of bioactive compounds from herbal drugs. Its combination of speed, efficiency, and versatility makes it an attractive option for researchers and pharmaceutical scientists aiming to unravel the complex chemical profiles of herbal extracts and identify potential therapeutic agents.

1. **Principle:** HPTLC shares the fundamental principles of traditional TLC but incorporates improvements in terms of plate quality, instrumentation, and detection capabilities. A thin layer of sorbent material, often silica gel or alternative stationary phases, is coated onto a glass or aluminum plate. The sample is applied as a spot, and the plate is developed in a suitable solvent system. Detection and quantification are achieved using specialized instruments equipped with high-resolution cameras or scanning densitometers.
2. **Isolation and Purification:** After applying the herbal sample onto the HPTLC plate, the plate is developed in a solvent system, separating the compounds based on their affinities. By visualizing and marking the bands corresponding to the compounds of interest, one can then cut and collect these portions of the plate. The compounds are subsequently eluted from the cut portion using a suitable solvent, and the eluted solution is concentrated. The isolated compounds can be further analyzed and characterized using complementary techniques.
3. **Characterization:** One of the strengths of HPTLC lies in its ability to provide selective detection of compounds. UV-Visible absorption spectra, fluorescence, or derivatization techniques can be utilized for enhanced sensitivity and specificity. Quantification can be achieved by comparing the intensity or area of the separated bands with those of standards.

5.4.2 SPECTROSCOPY TECHNIQUES

Various spectroscopy techniques play integral roles in elucidating the chemical composition and structural features of the extracted compounds, as mentioned in Table 5.4.

TABLE 5.4 Different Spectroscopy Techniques [44]

Sl. No.	Spectroscopy Technique	Description
1.	Nuclear magnetic resonance (NMR)	High-resolution NMR spectra unveil intricate details of the compounds' molecular structures, including the arrangement of atoms, bonding patterns, and stereochemistry. NMR also enables the identification of specific functional groups and allows researchers to monitor changes in chemical shifts, revealing diverse phytochemicals.
2.	Mass spectroscopy	Mass spectrometry (MS) is a pivotal technique in the isolation, purification, and characterization of herbal extracts, providing unparalleled insights into the composition and identity of bioactive compounds. During the isolation phase, MS aids in the rapid screening and identification of compounds based on their molecular weights. The characterization of herbal extracts relies heavily on MS for elucidating the chemical structure of individual constituents. Tandem MS (MS/MS) further enhances this process by providing fragmentation patterns, which facilitate the identification of functional groups and enable detailed determination of a compound's structure.
3.	Ultraviolet-visible (UV-Vis) spectroscopy	UV-Vis spectroscopy provides insights into the electronic transitions and overall composition of extracted compounds. During the isolation phase, it aids in the preliminary identification of compounds by analyzing their absorption spectra in the ultraviolet and visible regions. It also helps detect impurities or contaminants based on characteristic absorbance patterns. Additionally, UV-Vis spectroscopy allows for the quantitative analysis of specific compounds within herbal extracts, offering valuable information about their concentration and supporting the standardization of herbal formulations.
4.	Fourier transform infrared spectroscopy (FTIR)	FT-IR aids in the identification of functional groups present in extracted compounds, helping to discern and prioritize target molecules. It enables the detection of specific bonds, such as C=O, C–H, and O–H stretches, facilitating the elucidation of chemical composition and the identification of unique biomolecules within the herbal extract.
5.	Raman spectroscopy	Raman spectroscopy provides information about molecular vibrations and structural details.

By employing a combination of these techniques, one can comprehensively characterize isolated compounds, gaining a detailed understanding of their chemical, physical, and structural properties.

5.4.3 ELECTROPHORESIS

Electrophoresis, an influential separation methodology grounded in the displacement of charged particles within an electric field, has transformed into a multifaceted instrument for the scrutiny of biomolecules. Its utility extends to providing discernible advantages in terms of selectivity, sensitivity, and the capacity for high-resolution separation (Table 5.5).

TABLE 5.5 Electrophoretic Techniques [45, 46]

Sl. No.	Electrophoretic Technique	Description
1.	Gel electrophoresis	Gel electrophoresis is a widely utilized methodology for the separation and examination of biomolecules, specifically nucleic acids and proteins, based on their respective size and charge characteristics. The underlying principle of gel electrophoresis revolves around the directed migration of charged molecules through a gel matrix subjected to an electric field. This gel matrix, commonly composed of agarose or polyacrylamide, functions as a molecular sieve, retarding the migration velocity of molecules proportionally to their size.
2.	Agarose gel electrophoresis	This technique is particularly used for the separation and analysis of DNA molecules. The principle involves the migration of charged DNA fragments through a porous agarose gel matrix in response to an electric field. The gel's structure creates a sieve effect, allowing for the separation of DNA fragments based on their size.
3.	Capillary electrophoresis	This is a sophisticated separation technique that utilizes the principles of electrophoresis but is conducted in a narrow capillary tube. This technique allows for the separation of charged molecules, such as proteins, peptides, nucleic acids, and small ions, based on their size, charge, and shape. CE offers high resolution and rapid separations compared to traditional gel electrophoresis.
4.	Isoelectric focusing	IEF is a specialized electrophoresis technique where molecules are separated according to their isoelectric point (*pI*). The pH level at which a molecule has no net electric charge is known as the isoelectric point. In IEF, a pH gradient is established within a gel or capillary, and charged molecules migrate until they reach a pH equivalent to their *pI*, resulting in sharp bands of separation.

The isolation and purification of herbal extracts via electrophoresis represent a less conventional approach within the realm of phytochemical separation. Electrophoresis techniques, primarily designed for the separation of charged biomolecules based on their size and charge, are typically not employed for the isolation of entire herbal extracts due to their complex composition. However, in specific cases where a targeted compound within the herbal extract possesses distinct charge characteristics suitable for electrophoretic separation, techniques such as capillary electrophoresis might be considered. This would entail careful optimization of electrophoresis conditions, including buffer systems and pH gradients, to facilitate the migration and subsequent isolation of the desired compound. The process involves loading the herbal extract or a fraction enriched with the target compound, electrophoretic separation, and the collection of fractions based on migration positions. Subsequent concentration and analysis confirm the presence of the target compound. While not a conventional method, the application of electrophoresis for the isolation of specific charged compounds within herbal extracts highlights the adaptability of separation techniques in phytochemical research.

By subjecting isolated compounds to electrophoretic conditions, researchers can visualize the migration patterns and distinguish between different molecular species within a sample. This information is essential for confirming the identity of the isolated compounds, assessing their integrity, and providing insights into potential post-translational modifications or structural variations.

KEYWORDS

- **biomolecules**
- **chromatography**
- **electrophoresis**
- **electrophoretic conditions**
- **herbal drugs**
- **isoelectric point**
- **molecular vibrations**
- **Raman spectroscopy**

REFERENCES

1. Robinson, M. M., & Zhang, X. (2011). *Traditional Medicines: Global Situation, Issues and Challenges*. The World Medicines Situation 2011.
2. Woo, C. S., Lau, J. S., & El-Nezami, H. (2012). Herbal medicine: Toxicity and recent trends in assessing their potential toxic effects. In *Advances in Botanical Research, 62*, 365–384. Academic Press.
3. Kamboj, V. P. (2000). Herbal medicine. *Current Science, 78*(1), 35–39.
4. Yuan, H., Ma, Q., Ye, L., & Piao, G. (2016). The traditional medicine and modern medicine from natural products. *Molecules, 21*(5), 559.
5. Akerele, O. (1993). Nature's medicinal bounty: Don't throw it away. *World Health Forum, 14*(4), 390–395.
6. Sam, S. (2019). Importance and effectiveness of herbal medicines. *Journal of Pharmacognosy and Phytochemistry, 8*(2), 354–357.
7. World Health Organization. (2013). *WHO Traditional Medicine Strategy: 2014–2023*. World Health Organization.
8. Shi, Q., Li, L., Huo, C., Zhang, M., & Wang, Y. (2010). Study on natural medicinal chemistry and new drug development. *Zhongcaoyao = Chinese Traditional and Herbal Drugs, 41*(10), 1583–1589.
9. Fabricant, D. S., & Farnsworth, N. R. (2001). The value of plants used in traditional medicine for drug discovery. *Environmental Health Perspectives, 109*(Suppl 1), 69–75.
10. Hamilton, G. R., & Baskett, T. F. (2000). In the arms of Morpheus: The development of morphine for postoperative pain relief. *Canadian Journal of Anesthesia, 47*, 367–374.
11. Newman, D. J., Cragg, G. M., & Snader, K. M. (2003). Natural products as sources of new drugs over the period 1981–2002. *Journal of Natural Products, 66*(7), 1022–1037.
12. Galm, U., & Shen, B. (2007). Natural product drug discovery: The times have never been better. *Chemistry & Biology, 14*(10), 1098–1104.
13. Briskin, D. P. (2000). Medicinal plants and phytomedicines: Linking plant biochemistry and physiology to human health. *Plant Physiology, 124*(2), 507–514.
14. Ley, S. V., & Baxendale, I. R. (2002). New tools and concepts for modern organic synthesis. *Nature Reviews Drug Discovery, 1*(8), 573–586.
15. Geysen, H. M., Schoenen, F., Wagner, D., & Wagner, R. (2003). Combinatorial compound libraries for drug discovery: An ongoing challenge. *Nature Reviews Drug Discovery, 2*(3), 222–230.
16. Van Agtmael, M. A., Eggelte, T. A., & Van Boxtel, C. J. (1999). Artemisinin drugs in the treatment of malaria: From medicinal herb to registered medication. *Trends in Pharmacological Sciences, 20*(5), 199–205.
17. Heinrich, M., & Teoh, H. L. (2004). Galanthamine from snowdrop—The development of a modern drug against Alzheimer's disease from local Caucasian knowledge. *Journal of Ethnopharmacology, 92*(2–3), 147–162.
18. Pirttilä, T., Wilcock, G., Truyen, L., & Damaraju, C. V. (2004). Long-term efficacy and safety of galantamine in patients with mild-to-moderate Alzheimer's disease: Multicenter trial. *European Journal of Neurology, 11*(11), 734–741.

19. Kashman, Y., Gustafson, K. R., Fuller, R. W., Cardellina, J. H., McMahon, J. B., Currens, M. J., Buckheit, R. W., Hughes, S. H., Cragg, G. M., & Boyd, M. R. (1992). The calanolides, a novel HIV-inhibitory class of coumarin derivatives from the tropical rainforest tree *Calophyllum lanigerum*. *Journal of Medicinal Chemistry, 35*(15), 2735–2743.
20. Currens, M. J., Gulakowski, R. J., Mariner, J. M., Moran, R. A., Buckheit, R. W., Gustafson, K. R., McMahon, J. B., & Boyd, M. R. (1996). Antiviral activity and mechanism of action of calanolide A against the human immunodeficiency virus type-1. *Journal of Pharmacology and Experimental Therapeutics, 279*(2), 645–651.
21. Kramer, R., & Cohen, D. (2004). Functional genomics to new drug targets. *Nature Reviews Drug Discovery, 3*(11), 965–972.
22. Hoessel, R., Leclerc, S., Endicott, J. A., Nobel, M. E., Lawrie, A., Tunnah, P., Leost, M., Damiens, E., Marie, D., Marko, D., & Niederberger, E. (1999). Indirubin, the active constituent of a Chinese antileukemia medicine, inhibits cyclin-dependent kinases. *Nature Cell Biology, 1*(1), 60–67.
23. Hwang, B. Y., Lee, J. H., Koo, T. H., Kim, H. S., Hong, Y. S., Ro, J. S., Lee, K. S., & Lee, J. J. (2001). Kaurane diterpenes from *Isodon japonicus* inhibit nitric oxide and prostaglandin E_2 production and NF-κB activation in LPS-stimulated macrophage RAW264.7 cells. *Planta Medica, 67*(5), 406–410.
24. Tanaka, Y., & Takeshi, O. (2004). Extraction of phospholipids from salmon roe with supercritical carbon dioxide and an entrainer. *Journal of Oleo Science, 53*(9), 417–424. https://doi.org/10.5650/jos.53.417.
25. Aizpurua-Olaizola, O., Ormazabal, M., Vallejo, A., Olivares, M., Navarro, P., Etxebarria, N., & Usobiaga, A. (2015). Optimization of supercritical fluid consecutive extractions of fatty acids and polyphenols from *Vitis vinifera* grape wastes. *Journal of Food Science, 80*(1), E101–E107. https://doi.org/10.1111/1750-3841.12715.
26. Skoog, D. A., & Harris, D. C. (2007). *Principles of Instrumental Analysis* (6th ed., p. 863). Thomson Brooks/Cole.
27. King, J. W. (2002). Supercritical fluid technology for lipid extraction, fractionation, and reactions. In T. M. Kuo & H. Gardner (Eds.), *Lipid Biotechnology* (pp. 663–687). Marcel Dekker Inc.
28. Calculation of density, enthalpy and entropy for supercritical carbon dioxide with examples. (n.d.).
29. Clifford, T. (1999). *Fundamentals of Supercritical Fluids*. Oxford Science Publications.
30. Vandenburg, H. J., Clifford, A. A., et al. (1997). Analytical extraction of additives from polymers. *Analyst, 122*(9), 101R–115R. https://doi.org/10.1039/a704052k.
31. Supercritical fluid extraction, density considerations. (n.d.).
32. Yonei, Y., Ōhinata, H., Yoshida, R., Shimizu, Y., & Yokoyama, C. (1995). Extraction of ginger flavor with liquid or supercritical carbon dioxide. *The Journal of Supercritical Fluids, 8*(2), 156–161.
33. Durling, N. E., Catchpole, O. J., Grey, J. B., Webby, R. F., Mitchell, K. A., Foo, L. Y., & Perry, N. B. (2007). Extraction of phenolics and essential oil from dried sage (*Salvia officinalis*) using ethanol–water mixtures. *Food Chemistry, 101*(4), 1417–1424.

34. Wang, G., Su, P., Zhang, F., Hou, X., Yang, Y., & Guo, Z. (2011). Comparison of microwave-assisted extraction of aloe emodin in aloe with Soxhlet extraction and ultrasound-assisted extraction. *Science China Chemistry, 54*(1), 231–236.
35. Zill-e-Huma, Abert-Vian, M., Maingonnat, J. F., & Chemat, F. (2009). Clean recovery of antioxidant flavonoids from onions: Optimising solvent-free microwave extraction method. *Journal of Chromatography A, 1216*, 7700–7707.
36. Chee, K. K., Wong, M. K., & Lee, H. K. (1996). Microwave extraction of phthalate esters from marine sediment and soil. *Journal of Chromatography A, 42*, 378.
37. Kaufmann, B., & Christen, P. (2002). Recent extraction techniques for natural products: Microwave-assisted extraction and pressurized solvent extraction. *Phytochemical Analysis, 13*, 105–113.
38. Handa, S. S., Khanuja, S. P. S., Longo, G., & Rakesh, D. D. (2008). *Extraction Technologies for Medicinal and Aromatic Plants*. International Centre for Science and High Technology (ICS-UNIDO).
39. Pan, X., Niu, G., & Liu, H. (2003). Microwave-assisted extraction of tea polyphenols and tea caffeine from green tea leaves. *Chemical Engineering & Processing, 42*, 129.
40. Lucchesi, M. E., Smadja, J., Bradshaw, S., Louw, W., & Chemat, F. (2007). Solvent-free microwave extraction of *Elletaria cardamomum* L.: A multivariate study of a new technique for the extraction of essential oil. *Journal of Food Engineering, 79*(3), 1097–1086.
41. Brusotti, G., Cesari, I., Dentamaro, A., Caccialanza, G., & Massolini, G. (2014). Isolation and characterization of bioactive compounds from plant resources: The role of analysis in the ethnopharmacological approach. *Journal of Pharmaceutical and Biomedical Analysis, 87*, 218–228.
42. Liu, Y., Liu, H. Y., Li, S. H., Ma, W., Wu, D. T., Li, H. B., Xiao, A. P., Liu, L. L., Zhu, F., & Gan, R. Y. (2022). *Cannabis sativa* bioactive compounds and their extraction, separation, purification, and identification technologies: An updated review. *Trends in Analytical Chemistry, 149*, 116554.
43. Ramos-de-la-Peña, A. M., Renard, C. M., Montañez, J., de la Luz Reyes-Vega, M., & Contreras-Esquivel, J. C. (2016). A review through recovery, purification and identification of genipin. *Phytochemistry Reviews, 15*, 37–49.
44. Rasul, M. G. (2018). Extraction, isolation and characterization of natural products from medicinal plants. *International Journal of Basic Sciences and Applied Computing, 2*(6), F0076122618.
45. Cooke, R. J. (1995). Gel electrophoresis for the identification of plant varieties. *Journal of Chromatography A, 698*(1, 2), 281–299.
46. Pellati, F., & Benvenuti, S. (2007). Chromatographic and electrophoretic methods for the analysis of phenethylamine alkaloids in *Citrus aurantium*. *Journal of Chromatography A, 1161*(1, 2), 71–88.

CHAPTER 6

Isolation, Identification, and Analysis of Phytoconstituents

D. S. N. B. K. PRASANTH,[1] PRAVEEN KUMAR PASALA,[2] SUNEETHA ACHANTI,[3] JYOTI SHRIVASTAVA,[4] VIJENDER KUMAR PAREEKH,[5] and ARYA LAKSHMI MARISETTI[5,*]

[1]School of Pharmacy and Technology Management, SVKM's Narsee Monjee Institute of Management Studies (NMIMS), Polepally SEZ, TSIIC, Jadcherla, Mahbubnagar, Hyderabad, India

[2]Department of Pharmacology, Raghavendra Institute of Pharmaceutical Education and Research, Anantapuramu, Andhra Pradesh, India

[3]Department of Pharmaceutical Analysis, KVSR Siddhartha College of Pharmaceutical Sciences, Vijayawada, Andhra Pradesh, India

[4]Department of Pharmaceutical Chemistry, The Oxford College of Pharmacy, Hongasandra, Bangalore, India

[5]Department of Pharmacognosy and Phytochemistry, School of Pharmaceutical Sciences, Delhi Pharmaceutical Sciences and Research University, New Delhi, India

*Corresponding author

ABSTRACT

- **Terpenoids:** Menthol, citral and artemisinin.
- **Glycosides:** Glycyrrhetinic acid and rutin.
- **Alkaloids:** Atropine, quinine, reserpine and caffeine.

The Essentials of Herbal Drugs. Varsha Tiwari, Abhishek Tiwari, and Ajay Sharma (Eds.)

DOI: 10.1201/9781998511778-6

- **Resins:** Podophyllotoxin, curcumin.

Crude drugs are complex mixtures of thousands of phytoconstituents. Isolating, extracting, and identifying the pharmacologically active components of medicinal plants is one way to study their mechanisms of action. Different techniques have been adopted to extract phytoconstituents in suitable solvents. The phytoconstituent was isolated from the extract, and its purity was estimated. Extraction is a method of sifting the desired compounds from a mixture; isolation separates and purifies only pure compounds among those extracted. Because of the presence of other plant constituents (mainly proteins, fats, sugars, and tannins) in the crude extract, it is very difficult to isolate these active compounds. Therefore, the separation process uses powerful techniques with high efficiency and sensitivity. With the widespread application of plant products, there has been a demand for reliable techniques and standards to judge the quality, safety, and efficacy of these drugs or their concoctions. The current direction in which the herbal drug industry is trending is towards compounds with active phytoconstituents that have a more efficient therapeutic activity at and for specific sites. This chapter describes commercially important phytoconstituents of alkaloids, glycosides, terpenoids, and resins based on their isolation techniques [1, 2].

6.1 MENTHOL

Menthol is a monocyclic monoterpene alcohol found in various types of mint and peppermint oils. For this purpose, mint oil can be obtained from several species of the Lamiaceae family, including *Mentha piperita*, *M. arvensis*, *M. canadensis*, and other members of the genus (the name suggests what flowers must have been used here). Peppermint contains 1 to 3% volatile oil, and the latter must contain no less than 45% menthol. In addition to menthol, the oil contains (+)-neomenthol, (+)-isomenthol, menthone, menthofuran, menthyl acetate, and cineol. Menthol obtained from natural sources can be levorotatory (l-menthol) or racemic (dl-menthol). Menthol can also be artificially produced by hydrogenation of thymol. It is frequently found in the food industry, oral hygiene products, and preparations for treating mild throat pain or mouth irritation that arises when a canker sore occurs. Menthol is often used in various topical preparations because of its analgesic and counterirritant properties [3].

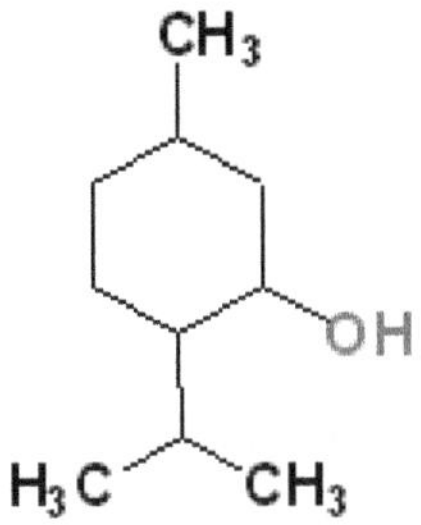

Menthol

6.1.1 ISOLATION OF MENTHOL

The first step in isolation is to obtain peppermint oil from the plant. This may be accomplished by hydrodistillation or steam distillation of the aboveground parts of the plant, which is performed before flowering. The resulting oil was desiccated using anhydrous sodium sulfate to remove moisture. The oil was then cooled to a temperature below –22 °C in a closed container for approximately 7 to 8 days, allowing menthol crystals to form. The crystals were filtered out of the oil and then squeezed between filter papers to remove any residual oil. Finally, the crystals were recovered via recrystallization. Even after the removal of crystals, there was still some menthol in the filtrate, as well as menthone and other terpenes. The filtrate was treated with boric acid and boiled for 3 hours to eliminate menthone. Menthone was removed by distillation. The filtrate was then washed with alcoholic potassium hydroxide under reflux for approximately an hour to saponify the menthol borate. The solution was then set aside to cool, and the menthol crystals remained separate. The two types of crystals were mixed and dried thoroughly [4].

6.1.2 IDENTIFICATION TESTS

1. The melting point of menthol was found to be 41–44°C.
2. A small amount of menthol was added to an equal volume of thymol or camphor in the test tube. If liquefied, then it is menthol.
3. Ten milligrams of menthol crystals were mixed with four drops of concentrated sulfuric acid. A few drops of vanillin sulfuric acid were added to this solution. A small amount of water was added, and the orange-yellow color turned violet.

4. A few crystals of menthol were dissolved in glacial acetic acid, and 4 ml of a mixture (three parts sulfuric acid to 1-part nitric acid) was added. The mixture resulted in neither green nor bluish-green coloration, which is indicative of menthol.

6.1.3 ANALYSIS/ESTIMATION OF MENTHOL

6.1.3.1 TITRIMETRIC METHOD

Menthol (2 g) was accurately weighed and added to a flask containing 20 mL of a mixture of dehydrated pyridine and acetic anhydride in an 8:1 ratio. A reflux condenser was attached, and the mixture was heated in a water bath for two hours. After the solution cooled, the condenser was removed and rinsed with 20 mL of water. Thereafter, the flask contents were titrated with a 1 M alcoholic sodium hydroxide solution, using phenolphthalein as an indicator. Reading = "a" mL. Perform a blank determination and record the reading as "b" mL. The difference between "b" milliliters and "a" milliliters gives the volume of titrant equivalent to one gram-atom of the acetylic radical eliminated with respect to menthol. The equivalent factor of 1 M alcoholic sodium hydroxide, which is 156.27 milligrams, determines the percentage of free menthol.

6.1.3.2 THIN LAYER CHROMATOGRAPHY OF MENTHOL

For thin-layer chromatography (TLC) of menthol, approximately 1 mg was dissolved in approximately 1 ml of methanol. The solution was then applied to a silica gel GF254 plate. The plates were then eluted with pure chloroform. Thereafter, the dried plate was sprayed with 1% vanillin sulfuric acid reagent and heated at 110°C for 10 minutes. At normal chamber saturation and 24°C, the *Rf* value of menthol should fall between 0.48 and 0.62.

6.2 CITRAL

Two geometric isomers have been reported, that is, Geranial and Neral. They can be derived from the essential oil obtained by steam distillation of either *Cymbopogon citratus* or *Cymbopogon flexuosus*, which belong to the Graminae family. They have also been discovered to some degree in the oils of verbena, lemon, lime, orange, ginger roots, and various citrus plants [5].

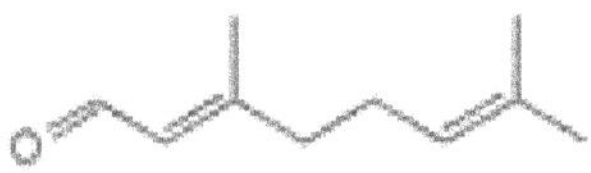

Geranial

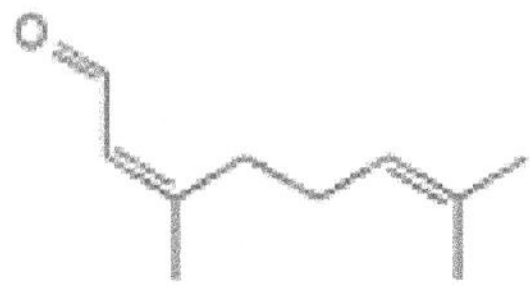

Neral

6.2.1 *ISOLATION OF CITRAL*

To isolate citral from lemongrass oil, the oil was shaken with a 5% (w/v) solution of sodium bisulfite for about half an hour. The adduct was washed in a Buchner funnel with solvent ether or ethanol to obtain pure crystals. The sodium bisulfite adduct was dissolved in a dilute sodium hydroxide solution to give crude citral. Finally, under reduced pressure, the crude citral was dissolved to obtain pure citral.

Separation of Geranial and Neral—because they are insoluble in water, the sodium bisulfate complex of Geranial is sparingly soluble, whereas that of Neral is readily soluble. This property can be used to separate Geranial and Neral. In addition, if citral (a mixture of Geranial and Neral) is shaken for a short time with alkaline cyanoacetic acid solution, the more reactive component in the mix, Geranial, reacts faster to produce anhydride.

6.2.2 *TESTS FOR IDENTIFYING CITRAL*

1. Citral, having two ethylenic and one aldehydic bond, is reactive with oxidizing agents. In particular, it can be attacked by excess air to form linalool, which has a strong yellow color.
2. When treated with Tollen's reagent, geranial becomes geranic acid.
3. In a slightly acidic solution, geranial was hydrogenated with sodium amalgam to form citronellal or citronellol.
4. When it is treated with potassium bisulfite, geranial is converted into para-cymene.

6.2.3 ESTIMATION OF CITRAL

6.2.3.1 BY COLORIMETRY

The citral content of lemongrass oil can be estimated by the colorimetric method using Ehrlich-Miller as a chromophore. This technique ensures accurate results. Color development is rapid and stable over a long period of time. According to the Ehrlich–Miller procedure, 5% p-dimethylaminobenzaldehyde was dissolved in acetic acid (carrying out this operation first) and mixed with a solution of 10% phosphoric acid, as previously described. During the coloring tests, 1 ml of each solution was added to different amounts of dissolved citral. An Ethan A colorimeter was used to determine both the percentage absorbance and extinction of colored citral as it changed from blue to pink. Calibration graphs were plotted, and the citral in solution was compared to a known strength, allowing us to determine the proportion of citral present.

6.2.3.2 HPTLC METHOD

1. **Stationary Phase:** Aluminum foil-backed plates (20 cm × 10 cm) coated with a layer of silica gel (silica gel 60F254) with a thickness of approximately 20 μm were used for the HPTLC tests.
2. **Mobile Phase:** The common method of plate development is linear ascent. Toluene and ethyl acetate mixed in a ratio of 8.5:1.5 (v/v) were used as binary mobile phases for developing plates.
3. **Visualization:** The plates were sprayed with vanillin sulfuric acid reagent for visualization. The reagent consisted of 0.5 grams of vanillin dissolved in a solution of 85 parts methanol, 10 parts glacial acetic acid, and five (v/v) parts sulfuric acid. The spots were well defined when the chamber was saturated with the mobile phase for 30 minutes at 25 ± 2°C. *Rf* values for trans and cis-citral were 0.55 ± 0.03 and 0.34 ± 0.05, respectively.
4. **Densitometric Method:** The densitometric method involves scanning the absorbance at 595 nm with the CAMAG TLC Scanner III. Trans- and cis-citral samples of varying concentrations were spotted onto a plate. The use of toluene and ethyl acetate at a ratio

of 8.5:1.5 (v/v) results in well-defined peaks for both compounds, with trans-citral showing an *Rf* value of 0.55 ± 0.03 and cis-citral showing an *Rf* value of 0.34 ± 0.05.

6.3 ARTEMISININ

Malaria is a parasitic disease caused by *Plasmodium falciparum*, and one of its treatments is artemisinin. It comes from the Chinese herb *Artemisia annua* and is more effective than older treatments, such as quinine or its derivatives, because the parasite has developed resistance to these drugs. Artemisinin, which contains a unique peroxide linkage essential for its activity, was discovered by Chinese scientist Tu Youyou in 1972. For cancer treatment, artemisinin has shown promise in preclinical studies. It dissolves in organic solvents but not in water [6, 7].

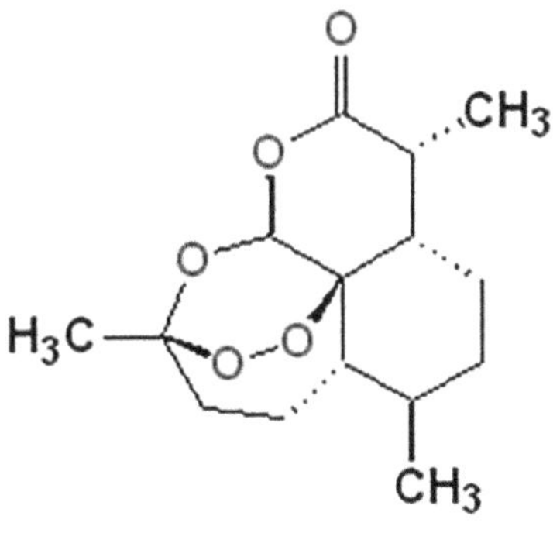

Artemisinin

6.3.1 *ISOLATION OF ARTEMISININ*

1. The leaves were dried from *Artemisia annua* and ground into a powder. A kinetic maceration technique using methanol was employed to extract the compound. This process was repeated several times until the methanol became colorless.
2. The methanol extract was mixed, and its volume was reduced to 100 ml under vacuum at 40°C.

3. The methanol extract was separated using hexane until it was colorless.
4. Two fractions are currently available: methanolic and hexane fractions.
5. To make it hydroalcoholic, a small amount of water was added to the methanol extract. The hydroalcoholic extract was partitioned with ethyl acetate several times until the ethyl acetate layer was colorless.
6. This gives rise to two semi-polar and polar fractions.
7. Each fraction was separated under vacuum at 40°C.
8 Artemisinin, the most viscous extract, was further separated using column chromatography (CC), where a mixture of ethyl acetate and hexane was used.
9. The fractions containing artemisinin were then available for preparative TLC to isolate pure artemisinin.

6.3.2 IDENTIFICATION TEST FOR ARTEMISININ

The TLC method was used to test for the presence of artemisinin by employing a mobile phase consisting of n-hexane and ethyl acetate in a 75:25 ratio, along with anisaldehyde sulfuric acid reagent derivatization. Through this process, artemisinin was separated at an *Rf* value of 0.28 [8].

6.3.3 ESTIMATION/ANALYSIS OF ARTEMISININ

6.3.3.1 ESTIMATION BY HPLC

Artemisinin analysis in plant extracts was conducted using reverse-phase HPLC with a mobile phase of formic acid (50%) and acetonitrile (50%). A calibration curve was constructed for the Artemisia samples to quantify artemisinin content. The average quantity of artemisinin was determined from three separate determinations.

6.3.3.2 ESTIMATION BY HPTLC

The concentration of hexane extract from A. annua is determined by HPTLC, with standard artemisinin dissolved in methanol serving as a reference solution. The TLC plate is developed using a mobile phase of n-hexane: ethyl acetate (75:25 v/v), derivatization with anisaldehyde-sulfuric acid, and heating at 110°C for 10 minutes. The presence of artemisinin was also confirmed by a pink spot at *Rf* = 0.28. The amount of artemisinin in the sample was determined using a calibration curve versus standards (i.e., resolution and density were measured with an HPTLC densitometer at 540 nm).

6.4 GLYCOSIDES

A substance that yields one or more sugar molecules when hydrolyzed is termed a glycoside. They are organic compounds chemically bound to sugars and are found in natural products derived from plants or animals. Its sugar portion is called the glycone, while its non-sugar portion is called the aglycone. The link between the glycone and aglycone is the glycosidic linkage [9].

Glycosides possess a range of properties, including:

1. They can be crystalline or amorphous.
2. Glycosides can be easily separated into water, mineral acids, and enzymes.
3. They are optically active; normally, they show levorotation.
4. Glycosides only reduce Fehling's solution after hydrolysis.
5. Although they contain sugar, the physical and chemical properties of glycosides are ascribed mainly to their aglycone portion. The glycone part allows the glycoside to be absorbed and helps in transporting the aglycone to its place of action.
6. Some glycosides dissolve in water and dilute alcohol, whereas resin-based glycosides do not. In contrast, aglycones are soluble in organic solvents.

6.5 GLYCYRRHETINIC ACID

It is a pentacyclic triterpenoid derived from the roots and rhizomes of the licorice plant *Glycyrrhiza glabra* (family Leguminosae). This compound is also known as glycyrrhetic acid or enoxolone. This compound is formed by the hydrolysis of glycyrrhizin, the principal glycoside in licorice. Glycyrrhetinic acid has many applications. It is used as an expectorant and to treat peptic ulcers. It is also used in pharmaceuticals as a flavoring agent and to mask the bitterness of aloe and quinine. In addition, glycyrrhetinic acid possesses mineralocorticoidal properties. Its clinical application includes the treatment of inflammatory diseases, rheumatism, and Addison's disease [10, 11].

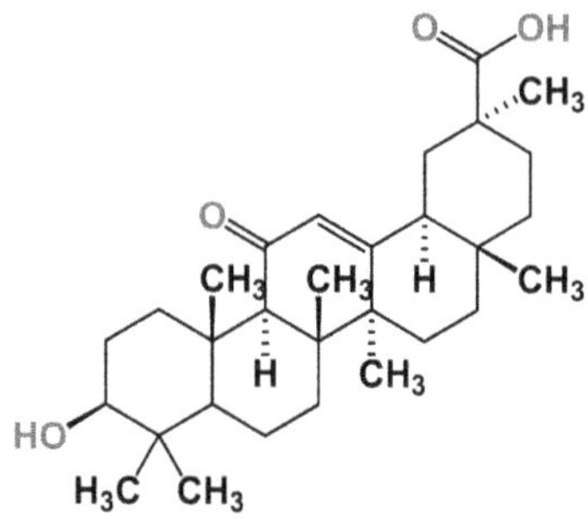

Glycyrrhetinic Acid

6.5.1 ISOLATION OF GLYCYRRHETINIC ACID

Glycyrrhetinic acid was obtained using the following method:

1. **Method I:**
   - i. About 20 g of powdered drug was added to a mixture of acetone and dilute nitric acid, taking two milliliters. All the ingredients were mixed well. Shake occasionally and let macerate for approximately 2 hours.
   - ii. The resulting mixture was filtered and extracted again with a small amount of acetone by heating in a boiling water bath. The extract was filtered, and the filtrates were combined before concentrating under vacuum.
   - iii. An appropriate amount of dilute ammonia solution was added to the acetone extract to precipitate ammonium glycyrrhizinate.
   - iv. The precipitate was filtered and washed with 5–10 mL of acetone.
   - v. The product was dried and weighed to determine the yield (usually 4–5% w/w).
2. **Method II:**
   - i. An accurate weight of liquid powder was obtained by extracting chloroform through Soxhlet extraction.

ii. The contents of the flask were filtered. Discard the filtrate.
iii. The marc was treated with 0.5 M H_2SO_4 for two to three hours.
iv. After passing the contents of the flask through a filter, the filtrate was removed.
v. The filtrate was extracted three times using a separating funnel with chloroform (25 mL of chloroform three times).
vi. The chloroform extracts were pooled and concentrated to dryness, yielding glycyrrhetinic acid residue.

6.5.2 *IDENTIFICATION TESTS*

- **Libermann Test:** 2 ml of the test solution and 2 ml of acetic anhydride were added to a container. Heat was applied, and 0.5 ml of sulfuric acid was added and mixed well. A blue color indicates the presence of glycyrrhetinic acid.

6.5.3 *ESTIMATION OF GLYCYRRHETINIC ACID BY USING TLC–DENSITOMETRY*

1. The stationary phase used was Kieselghur 60 HF coated onto a TLC plate.
2. The mobile phase comprises n-butanol, acetic acid, and water (7:1:2).
3. After using a visualizing agent in 1% ceric sulfate with 10% sulfuric acid, the section was heated to dryness for 5 minutes and boiled for another five.
4. A stock solution was prepared by dissolving a known quantity (0.5 to 2 mg/ml) of glycyrrhetinic acid in ethanol.
5. The sample solution was prepared by letting 1 g of the sample sit at reflux with 50 ml of cold ethanol (containing both water and alcohol) until tired, filtering while warm, and refluxing again with additional hot alcohol. The residue was solubilized in 50% ethanol (1.0 m).
6. The chromatograms are run out to around 13–14 cm.
7. The spots are typically observed and measured in the densitometer; then, this part is integrated to form a percentage of the total sample area.

6.6 RUTIN

Rutin is found in the dried ripe fruits of *Fagopyrum esculentum* (also known as buckwheat), a member of the Polygonaceae family. Other sources of rutin are the leaves of the tobacco plant *Nicotiana tabacum* and the family Solanaceae. The proportion of glycosides is highest in buckwheat leaves and flowers during the blossom stage; however, after maturation, it begins to deplete. It is insoluble in water, ether, petroleum ether, or chloroform. Rutin dissolves well in ethanol and acetone, is used to reduce the fragility and permeability of capillaries, and is applied in therapy for retinal hemorrhages [12, 13].

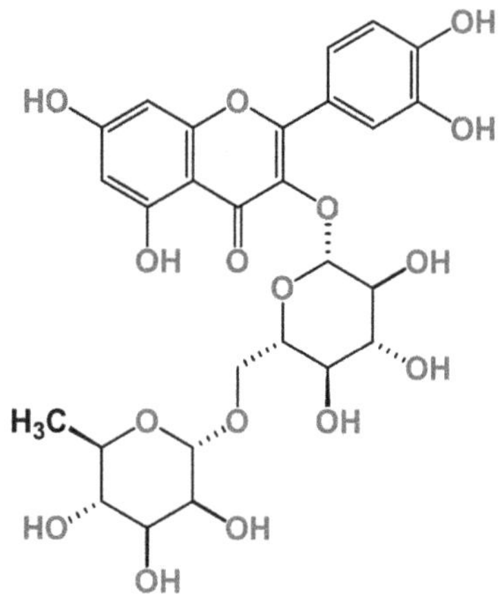

6.6.1 ISOLATION OF RUTIN

1. Dried ground plant material (150 g) was extracted with two separate portions of 80% ethanol, each containing 200 ml.
2. The resulting hydroalcoholic extract was filtered and reduced to 50–60 ml.
3. The extract was then divided into separate layers by using ether in a separating funnel.
4. After this process was repeated, the ether layer was discarded.
5. The remaining aqueous extract was reduced to a volume of 10 ml.
6. The solution was cooled overnight to below 5°C, during which the rutin crystals were allowed to separate.

7. The resulting crude rutin was subjected to CC for further purification.

6.6.2 *IDENTIFICATION TESTS*

1. When combined with basic lead acetate, rutin produces a vibrant yellow color.
2. After treatment with a ferric chloride solution, rutin was greenish-brown.

6.6.3 *ESTIMATION OF RUTIN BY SPECTROPHOTOMETRY*

1. **Prepare the Sample Solution:** Dissolve a 0.5 mg sample in 50 ml of methanol, and pass the solution through a filter. Mix 2 ml of ammonium molybdate and double-distilled water to make up a volume of 50 ml in a volumetric flask. The volume was adjusted to the mark using water.

2. **Prepare the Standard Solution:** Dissolve the standard (0.5 mg) in methanol and filter it. Proceed as for sample solution preparation.

The absorbance of both the standard and sample solutions was measured at 360 nm. The rutin percentage was calculated using the following formula:

$$\%\text{ of Rutin} = \frac{A_{\text{sample}} \times C \times 50 \times 100}{A_{\text{standard}} \times W \times 2}$$

where; A_{sample} is the absorbance of sample at 360 nm; $A_{standard}$ is the absorbance of standard at 360 nm; C is the concentration of standard solution (g/ml); and W is the weight of the sample.

6.7 ALKALOIDS

Alkaloids are organic substances that are either naturally occurring or synthetic in nature. Their basic character is due to the presence of one or more heterocyclic nitrogen atoms in their structure. Even when used in small amounts, they can have certain physiological effects on humans or animals. Alkaloids are classified based on their origin and nitrogen position as follows:

1. **True Alkaloids:** These are derived from amino acids and contain nitrogen in the heterocyclic ring. Example: Atropine.
2. **Protoalkaloids:** Derived from amino acids but without nitrogen in the heterocyclic ring. Example: Ephedrine.
3. **Pseudoalkaloids:** Not from amino acids but contain nitrogen in the heterocyclic ring. However, they may lack the characteristics of a typical alkaloid yet still test positive in standard qualitative tests for an alkaloid. Example: Conesine.

6.7.1 PROPERTIES OF THE ALKALOIDS

1. Generally, alkaloids are colorless crystalline solids with sharp melting points.
2. Some alkaloids are amorphous in nature, whereas others, such as nicotine and anabasine, are liquids.
3. Most alkaloids are chiral molecules, resulting in isomers with different chemical properties. For instance, one isomer may have a physiological function, whereas the other does not.
4. Alkaloid free bases dissolve in organic solvents but do not dissolve in water, while most alkaloid salts readily dissolve in water.
5. In nature, alkaloids can exist in various forms, including as a free base, amine, or salt with an acid or alkaloid N-oxide.

6.7.2 GENERAL CHEMICAL TESTS FOR ALKALOIDS

1. **Mayer's Test:** When Mayer's reagent (potassium mercuric iodide) is added to a solution of the drug, it turns creamy white.
2. **Wagner's Test:** When a few drops of Wagner's reagent (diluted iodine solution) are added to a drug solution, a reddish-brown precipitation occurs.
3. **Dragendorff's Test:** Dragendorff's reagent (potassium bismuth iodide) with the drug solution turns orange-red.
4. **Hager's Test:** A few drops of picric acid led to the formation of yellow crystals.
5. **Tannic Acid Test:** When drops of tannic acid solution are added to a drug solution, the latter turns buff-colored.

6.7.3 GENERAL EXTRACTION TECHNIQUE

1. **Method A:** The powdered material containing alkaloidal salts is moistened with alkaline substances like sodium bicarbonate, ammonia, or calcium hydroxide. These substances react with acids, tannins, and other phenolic compounds, releasing the alkaloid bases. Extraction is then carried out using organic solvents such as ether or petroleum spirits. The concentrated organic liquid is then shaken with an aqueous acid and allowed to separate. Alkaloid salts are present in the aqueous liquid, while many impurities remain in the organic liquid.
2. **Method B:** The powdered material was initially extracted with water or aqueous alcohol containing dilute acid. To remove pigments and other unwanted substances, chloroform and other organic solvents were added and shaken. The free alkaloids were then precipitated by the addition of excess alkalis, such as sodium bicarbonate or ammonia, and separated via filtration or extraction with organic solvents. Volatile liquid alkaloids such as nicotine and coniine were isolated through distillation. Alternatively, the powdered material containing alkaloids was extracted with water, and the resulting aqueous extract was rendered alkaline using sodium carbonate or ammonia. Subsequently, the alkaloid was distilled off with steam, collected, and purified.

6.8 ATROPINE

Atropine, a tropane alkaloid, is sourced from the dried leaves of either Atropa belladonna (European belladonna) or Atropa acuminata (Indian belladonna), both belonging to the Solanaceae family. Commonly referred to as belladonna or deadly nightshade leaf, it acts as a mydriatic, dilating the pupil of the eye, and reduces secretions such as saliva, tears, perspiration, and acidic gastric juices. It is also administered intravenously as an antidote for pilocarpine poisoning and for treating bradycardia. Atropine exhibits high solubility in ethanol [9, 14].

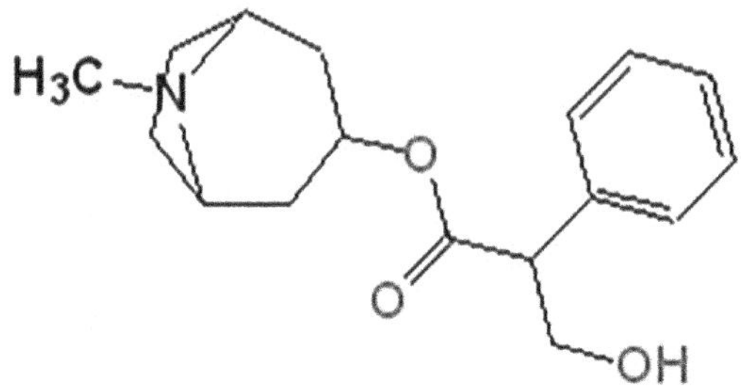

Atropine

6.8.1 ISOLATION OF ATROPINE

1. The powdered drug material was extracted with ethanol.
2. The solvent was filtered and evaporated to yield the syrupy extract. The extract was treated with dilute hydrochloric acid to form an alkaloidal salt, and resinous matter precipitated out.
3. The solution was filtered, and the resinous matter was retained on the filter paper.
4. The acidic solution was partitioned using petroleum ether and chloroform in a separating funnel.
5. The chloroform/petroleum ether layer was collected and removed by distillation to obtain a crude alkaloid mixture, which was further treated with oxalic acid.
6. Atropine and hyoscyamine oxalates are separated by fractional crystallization from acetone and ether, yielding crystals of atropine oxalate.

6.8.2 IDENTIFICATION TEST

The Vitali Morin Test involves adding fuming nitric acid to an extract and then evaporating it in a water bath until it is dry. A methanolic solution of potassium hydroxide is then added to the resulting nitrated residue. The appearance of a deep purple color indicates the presence of a tropane alkaloid.

6.8.3 ESTIMATION OF ATROPINE

6.8.3.1 TITRIMETRIC DETERMINATION OF ATROPINE SULFATE CONTENTS

Atropine content, expressed as atropine sulfate, is determined by the titrimetric method. An accurately weighed quantity of the test solution (i.e., sulfate salt dissolved in 50 mL of glacial acetic acid and titrated with 0.1 N perchloric acid, with the endpoint determined by potentiometry) is used. The factor obtained from the blank determination is then applied to calculate the amount of atropine sulfate present. About 1 mL of 0.1 N perchloric acid is equivalent to 0.677 mg of atropine sulfate.

6.8.3.2 BY TLC

- Standard Solution: A 1% solution of atropine is added to 2N acetic acid.
- Stationary Phase: Silica gel G.
- Mobile Phase: Strong ammonia solution: methanol (1.5:100).
- Derivatizing Agent: Dragendorff's reagent.
- Rf Value: 0.18.

6.9 QUININE

Quinine is obtained from the bark of different species of cinchona, viz. *Cinchona officinalis*, *C. calisaya*, *C. ledgeriana*, and *C. succirubra* (Rubiaceae). It is a quinoline-type alkaloid. Quinine, quinidine, cinchonine, and cinchonidine make up cinchona. Quinine and quinidine are stereoisomers of one another. They form many salts, but therapeutically, the sulfates alone figure most commonly.

With different species, the total alkaloid content ranges from 5% to 10%. The amount of total alkaloids in *C. ledgeriana* is approximately 610%, with 75% quinine. Quinine serves as an antimalarial.

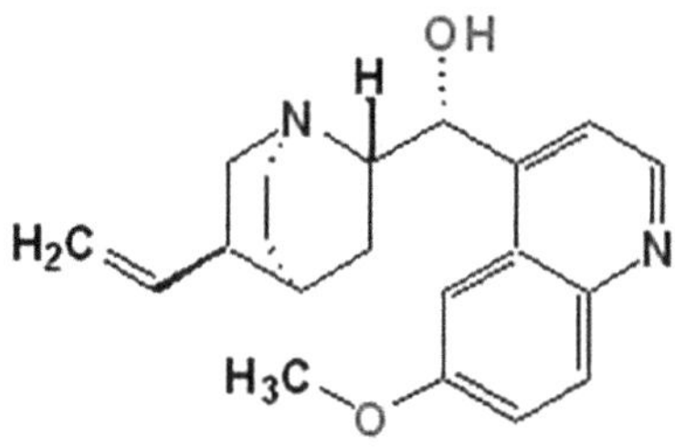

Quinine

6.9.1 *ISOLATION OF QUININE*

1. Thoroughly mix finely powdered cinchona bark with a sufficient quantity of calcium hydroxide solution and convert it to a paste by mixing in 5% sodium hydroxide solution.
2. Extract the paste with benzene in a Soxhlet extractor for 6 hours.
3. Transfer the resultant extract into a separating funnel and extract several times with warm dilute sulfuric acid for complete extraction of alkaloids.
4. Adjust the pH of the acid layer to about 6.5 by the addition of sodium hydroxide solution.
5. Allow the resultant mixture to cool and then centrifuge it for the separation of crystals of quinine sulfate.
6. Purify the quinine sulfate obtained by recrystallization from hot water.
7. Dissolve quinine sulfate crystals in warm dilute sulfuric acid; to this, add dilute ammonia solution until the solution becomes alkaline.
8. Quinine precipitates out as amorphous crystals; filter it and wash with water to remove sodium and ammonium salts.

6.9.2 *IDENTIFICATION TESTS FOR QUININE*

- **Thalleioquin Test:** To a small quantity of dilute acidic solution of quinine in a test tube, add a few milliliters of bromine water with gentle shaking. After the addition of dilute ammonia solution, the formation of an emerald green color, which turns blue after neutralization, indicates the presence of quinine.

- **Acetic Acid Test:** To a small quantity of quinine in a test tube, add a small quantity of glacial acetic acid. After heating the mixture in the test tube, the formation of purple vapors at the upper part indicates the presence of quinine.

6.9.3 ESTIMATION OF QUININE BY TLC

1. **Stationary Phase:** Silica gel G coated TLC plates
2. **Mobile Phase:** Chloroform: Methanol: Ammonia (60:10:1)
3. **Preparation of Standard Quinine Solution:** A 1 mg/ml solution of standard quinine is prepared by dissolving 1 mg of quinine in 1 ml of chloroform.
4. **Preparation of Sample Solution:** A 1 mg/ml solution of cinchona extract is prepared in chloroform.

Both the sample and standard solutions are applied on the TLC plate and allowed to develop in a previously saturated development chamber. The *Rf* value of quinine is 0.6.

KEYWORDS

- **alkaloids**
- **chloroform**
- **isolation**
- **menthol**
- **phytoconstituents**
- **quinine**
- **recrystallization**
- **thalleioquin test**
- **thin layer chromatography**

REFERENCES

1. Kinghorn, A. D. (2001). Pharmacognosy in the 21st century. *Journal of Pharmacy and Pharmacology, 53*(2), 135–148.
2. McCreath, S. B., & Clement, Y. N. (2023). *Pharmacognosy: Fundamentals, Applications, and Strategies*. Elsevier.
3. Lawrence, B. M. (2006). *Mint: The Genus Mentha*. CRC Press.
4. Abascal, K. (2002). A handbook of medicinal herbs. *Alternative & Complementary Therapies, 8*(5), 300–304.
5. Lawrence, B. M. (2011). Progress in essential oils. *Perfumer & Flavorist, 36*(11), 52–58.
6. Elfawal, M. A., Towler, M. J., Reich, N. G., Golenbock, D., Weathers, P. J., & Rich, S. M. (2012). Dried whole plant *Artemisia annua* as an antimalarial therapy. *PLOS ONE, 7*(12), e52746.
7. Tu, Y. (2016). Artemisinin—A gift from traditional Chinese medicine to the world (Nobel lecture). *Angewandte Chemie International Edition, 55*(35), 10210–10226.
8. Konstat-Korzenny, E., Ascencio-Aragón, J. A., Niezen-Lugo, S., & Vázquez-López, R. (2018). Artemisinin and its synthetic derivatives as a possible therapy for cancer. *Medical Sciences, 6*(1), 19.
9. Shah, B. N. (2009). *Textbook of Pharmacognosy and Phytochemistry*. Elsevier India.
10. Yano, S., Harada, M., Watanabe, K., Nakamaru, K., Hatakeyama, Y., Shibata, S., et al. (1989). Antiulcer activities of glycyrrhetinic acid derivatives in experimental gastric lesion models. *Chemical and Pharmaceutical Bulletin, 37*(9), 2500–2504.
11. Graebin, C. S. (2018). The pharmacological activities of glycyrrhizinic acid ("glycyrrhizin") and glycyrrhetinic acid. In *Sweeteners* (pp. 245–263).
12. Koja, E., Ohata, S., Maruyama, Y., Suzuki, H., Shimosaka, M., & Taguchi, G. (2018). Identification and characterization of a rhamnosyltransferase involved in rutin biosynthesis in *Fagopyrum esculentum* (common buckwheat). *Bioscience, Biotechnology, and Biochemistry, 82*(10), 1790–1802.
13. Ganeshpurkar, A., & Saluja, A. K. (2017). The pharmacological potential of rutin. *Saudi Pharmaceutical Journal, 25*(2), 149–164.
14. Shah, V. V., Shah, N. D., & Patrekar, P. V. (2013). Medicinal plants from Solanaceae family. *Research Journal of Pharmacy and Technology, 6*(2), 143–151.

CHAPTER 7

Advancements in Plant Tissue Culture: A Historical Perspective

MOHD. MUJEEB* and PRERNA SAXENA

Department of Pharmacognosy and Phytochemistry, School of Pharmaceutical Education and Research, Jamia Hamdard, New Delhi, India

*Corresponding author

ABSTRACT

The practice of maintaining or expanding plant cells, tissues, or organs on a nutrient culture medium under sterile circumstances is known as plant tissue culture. It is frequently used in a process called micropropagation to create clones of plants. Many plant components have the capacity to regenerate into a complete plant, and these totipotent cells, which can differentiate into a variety of specialized cells, are the basis for plant tissue culture. Given the necessary nutrients and plant hormones, it is frequently possible to create a new plant on culture media using single cells, plant cells without cell walls (protoplasts), or fragments of leaves, stems, or roots. Plant tissue culture has emerged as a versatile platform for the sustainable production of pharmaceuticals and secondary metabolites, offering advantages such as rapid propagation, controlled growth conditions, and enhanced biosynthetic capacity. Various aspects of plant tissue culture relevant to pharmaceutical applications, including the selection of elite plant species, optimization of tissue culture protocols, and manipulation of culture conditions to enhance secondary metabolite biosynthesis, are discussed. Plant tissue culture techniques play an important role in the production of pharmaceuticals and secondary metabolites. It is also

The Essentials of Herbal Drugs. Varsha Tiwari, Abhishek Tiwari, and Ajay Sharma (Eds.)

DOI: 10.1201/9781998511778-7

used for the development of new improved crops and edible vaccines. Historical developments and advancements in plant tissue culture, types of cultures, nutritional requirements, growth, maintenance, and applications of plant tissue in pharmaceuticals and secondary metabolite production are summarized in this chapter.

7.1 INTRODUCTION

Our exploration into the historical perspective of advancements in plant tissue culture takes us on a captivating journey through the latter half of the 20th century and into the 21st century. This period witnessed unprecedented breakthroughs in the field, shaping the landscape of agriculture, horticulture, and biotechnology. The advancements discussed in this chapter represent a pivotal phase where plant tissue culture transcended the confines of laboratory experimentation, finding widespread application in commercial agriculture and becoming an indispensable tool for precision breeding [1].

The late 20th century marked a paradigm shift as researchers seamlessly integrated genetic engineering techniques into plant tissue culture, ushering in a new era of biotechnological possibilities. The discovery and utilization of plant hormones in the 1920s and 1930s set the stage for subsequent breakthroughs, including the callus culture era of the 1940s and 1950s, organogenesis and somatic embryogenesis in the 1960s and 1970s, and the advent of genetic engineering in the 1980s. These advancements paved the way for commercial applications, transforming the way we propagate plants, combat diseases, and enhance agricultural productivity [2].

The chapter unfolds with a detailed exploration of the early experiments and discoveries in the late 19th to early 20th century, laying the groundwork for plant tissue culture. We delve into the origins of nutrient solutions, the identification of auxins and cytokinins, and the development of standardized nutrient media. The narrative then transitions to the callus culture era, discussing the intriguing phenomenon of dedifferentiation, the emergence of callus as a mass of undifferentiated cells, and the subsequent refinement of tissue culture techniques [3].

Moving into the 1960s and 1970s, we explore the era of organogenesis and somatic embryogenesis. The controlled development of shoots, roots, and embryos from cultured tissues revolutionized the practical applications of tissue culture. The elucidation of hormonal influences and the standardization of protocols set the stage for widespread adoption in commercial agriculture.

The narrative takes a ground breaking turn as we delve into the 1980s and beyond, witnessing the integration of genetic engineering and transformation techniques. Agrobacterium-mediated transformation and particle bombardment became instrumental tools for introducing foreign genes into plant cells, leading to the creation of transgenic plants with novel traits. This era saw the commercial release of genetically modified crops, marking a transformative period in modern agriculture [4].

The chapter gives an exploration of the commercial applications and biotechnological innovations that ensued in the 1990s and persisted into the present day. Tissue culture became synonymous with clonal propagation, disease-free plant production, and precision breeding. Specialty crops, forestry applications, and ecosystem restoration projects flourished through the strategic application of tissue culture methods. Genetic engineering further diversified the biotechnological landscape, addressing global challenges and sparking debates over societal impacts and regulatory frameworks [5].

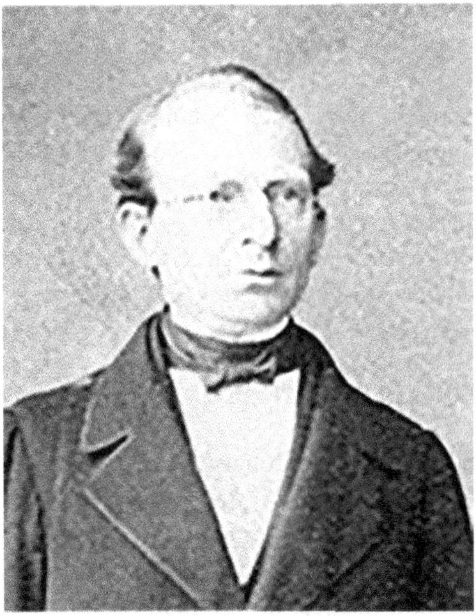

Wilhelm Knop

7.2 EARLY EXPERIMENTS AND DISCOVERY

The roots of plant tissue culture can be traced back to a period of scientific curiosity and experimentation in the late 19th century. At this time, botanists and researchers were driven by a desire to understand the fundamental processes governing plant growth and development. The pioneering work of Wilhelm Knop, a German botanist, played a pivotal role in setting the stage for the subsequent evolution of plant tissue culture [6].

In 1865, Wilhelm Knop conducted groundbreaking experiments that involved growing plant cells in a liquid nutrient medium. Knop's work laid the foundation for the concept of *in vitro* plant growth, demonstrating that plants could be sustained without being anchored in soil. His nutrient solutions, containing essential minerals and nutrients, provided the necessary elements for plant cells to proliferate and thrive outside their natural environment. Building upon Knop's findings, Austrian botanist Gottlieb Haberlandt (1902) furthered the exploration of *in vitro* plant cell culture. Haberlandt introduced the term "totipotency" to describe the remarkable ability of plant cells to differentiate into complete organisms. His experiments involved isolating individual cells and observing their potential to give rise to callus—a mass of undifferentiated cells. This phenomenon of dedifferentiation marked a crucial step in the understanding of plant cell behavior [7].

Around the same time, French botanist Georges Nobécourt made significant contributions to the field. Nobécourt (1894) experimented with liquid media, demonstrating that plants could be cultured in a more fluid environment than previously believed. His work emphasized the adaptability of plant cells to different growth conditions, further expanding the possibilities for *in vitro* cultivation [8].

7.3 CONCEPT OF CELL CULTURE

In the early 20th century, researchers such as Raoul Francé and Ernst Steward began working with tissue slices and fragments, demonstrating the potential for cultivating plant tissues outside the intact organism. This marked a shift from whole-plant experiments to a focus on specific plant tissues, laying the groundwork for the concept of "cell culture" [9].

Collectively, the late 19th to early 20th century represents a period of foundational discoveries and experimental groundwork that paved the way for the formalization of plant tissue culture techniques. The early experiments of Knop, Haberlandt, Nobécourt, and others laid a solid foundation for subsequent researchers to build upon, eventually leading to the sophisticated science of plant tissue culture we know today [10].

7.3.1 PLANT HORMONES (1920s–1930s)

The 1920s and 1930s marked a significant turning point in the history of plant tissue culture, as researchers delved deeper into understanding the role of plant hormones in regulating growth and development. This period witnessed the identification and isolation of key hormones, specifically auxins and cytokinins, which played instrumental roles in advancing the field [11].

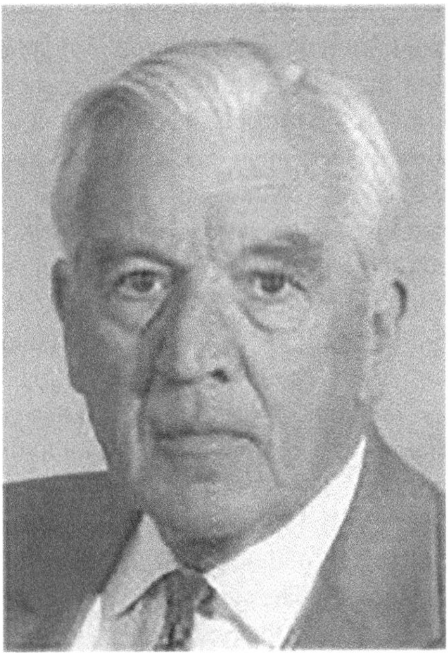

Frits Warmolt Went

Dutch scientist Frits Warmolt Went (1962) conducted pioneering experiments that led to the identification of auxins—a class of plant hormones crucial for promoting cell elongation and differentiation. Went's work involved studying the effects of coleoptile tips on oat seedlings. He discovered that the substance responsible for promoting growth in the seedlings was a hormone later named auxin. This discovery laid the foundation for understanding how plant hormones could be manipulated to control cell behavior in tissue culture [12].

The term "cytokinin" was coined by German plant physiologist Carl Miller in the early 20th century, but it was not until the 1950s that the first cytokinin, kinetin, was isolated by Miller and his colleagues. However, in the 1930s, the idea of plant hormones promoting cell division gained traction. F.C. Steward's work with coconut milk as a nutrient source demonstrated the presence of substances that stimulated cell division. Later identified as cytokinins, these hormones became pivotal in tissue culture for inducing shoot and root formation. The collaboration between Went and Miller in the 1930s led to the formulation of the Cholodny-Went theory, which highlighted the synergistic action of auxins and cytokinins in controlling plant growth. This theory provided a conceptual framework for manipulating plant tissues *in vitro*. Researchers realized that by carefully balancing the concentrations of auxins and cytokinins in the nutrient media, they could induce specific responses in cultured tissues, such as callus formation, organogenesis, and somatic embryogenesis [13].

Plant physiologists Toshio Murashige and Folke Skoog, in 1957, introduced a groundbreaking nutrient medium that became widely adopted in plant tissue culture laboratories. The Murashige and Skoog (MS) medium contained optimal concentrations of auxins and cytokinins, providing a standardized and reliable formula for promoting plant cell growth and development. This medium revolutionized tissue culture practices, making experiments more reproducible and facilitating the systematic study of plant physiology. The identification and understanding of plant hormones in the 1920s and 1930s not only revolutionized plant tissue culture but also laid the groundwork for advancements in plant physiology and molecular biology. The synergy between auxins and cytokinins became a cornerstone for researchers seeking to manipulate plant growth and development *in vitro*. Subsequent chapters will explore how these hormone-driven discoveries paved the way for the induction of specific developmental pathways and the emergence of biotechnological applications in plant tissue culture [14].

7.3.2 THE CALLUS CULTURE ERA (1940s–1950s)

The period spanning the 1940s to the 1950s witnessed a pivotal phase in the history of plant tissue culture—the advent of callus culture. Building upon earlier discoveries related to plant hormones, researchers began to explore the unique characteristics of callus, an undifferentiated mass of cells, and its implications for tissue culture techniques [15].

The discovery of callus formation was a result of experiments conducted by researchers such as Gautheret and White in the 1940s. They observed that when plant tissues were cultured *in vitro*, they often exhibited the intriguing phenomenon of forming a mass of unorganized, dedifferentiated cells—commonly referred to as callus. This discovery marked a significant departure from traditional plant tissue culture practices, where the emphasis was on cultivating whole plants or specific organs. Callus culture provided researchers with a unique insight into the dedifferentiation potential of plant cells. The ability of specialized cells to revert to a pluripotent state, where they could potentially differentiate into various cell types, opened new possibilities for manipulating plant tissues. The callus culture era highlighted the plasticity of plant cells and their capacity to undergo developmental changes in response to environmental cues provided in the *in vitro* culture setting [16].

The study of callus culture paved the way for the induction of organogenesis—the development of roots and shoots from callus tissues. Researchers, including Skoog and Miller, began to experiment with the addition of specific combinations of auxins and cytokinins to the nutrient medium, manipulating these conditions to prompt the formation of shoot buds and roots. The controlled induction of organogenesis represented a significant advancement in plant tissue culture, enabling the regeneration of entire plants from callus tissues. In addition to organogenesis, the 1950s saw the emergence of somatic embryogenesis—a process where embryos are formed from somatic cells. Researchers like Steward and colleagues observed that under certain conditions, callus cells could undergo a developmental pathway resembling embryogenesis. This discovery held immense promise for clonal propagation, as it provided an alternative route to regenerate plants from somatic cells, bypassing the need for traditional seeds [17].

The 1950s also witnessed efforts to standardize tissue culture techniques. Researchers sought to develop reproducible methods for inducing callus formation, organogenesis, and somatic embryogenesis. The establishment of standardized protocols, often building upon the MS medium, marked a critical step in making tissue culture a reliable and widely applicable tool for plant scientists and horticulturists. The callus culture era of the 1940s and 1950s laid the foundation for subsequent advancements in plant tissue culture. The discovery and understanding of callus formation, dedifferentiation, and the induction of specific developmental pathways marked a transformative period. This era not only expanded the theoretical understanding of plant growth but also introduced practical applications for clonal propagation and the manipulation of plant traits. As the historical narrative unfolds, subsequent chapters will delve into further developments, including the commercial applications and biotechnological implications of plant tissue culture [18].

7.3.3 ORGANOGENESIS AND SOMATIC EMBRYOGENESIS (1960s–1970s)

The 1960s and 1970s witnessed a significant leap forward in plant tissue culture with the exploration and refinement of organogenesis and somatic embryogenesis. Researchers, building on the foundation laid during the callus culture era, focused on inducing the development of distinct plant organs and embryos from cultured tissues, opening new avenues for clonal propagation and genetic manipulation. During this period, researchers like Toshio Murashige and Folke Skoog made crucial contributions by elucidating the roles of plant hormones, particularly auxins and cytokinins, in the regulation of organ development. Their groundbreaking research led to the formulation of the MS medium in 1962, a nutrient-rich solution optimized for promoting the growth of plant tissues and the induction of specific organs [19].

Organogenesis, the controlled formation of shoot and root structures from cultured tissues, became a focal point in tissue culture research. By manipulating the concentrations of auxins and cytokinins in the nutrient medium, researchers were able to guide the differentiation of callus tissues into specific organ types. This marked a significant advancement in the practical application of tissue culture for clonal propagation, allowing for the regeneration of entire plants with predetermined traits [20].

Somatic embryogenesis emerged as a revolutionary concept in plant tissue culture during the 1970s. Researchers like Peter R. White demonstrated that under specific conditions, somatic cells could undergo a developmental pathway that resembled embryogenesis. This process allowed for the regeneration of embryos directly from non-reproductive, somatic cells, bypassing the need for traditional seeds. Somatic embryogenesis provided a powerful tool for clonal propagation, allowing for the production of large numbers of genetically identical plants. The advancements in organogenesis and somatic embryogenesis during the 1960s and 1970s laid the groundwork for the application of plant tissue culture in various fields. The ability to induce the development of specific organs and embryos not only facilitated large-scale propagation of elite plant varieties but also opened doors for genetic engineering applications. Researchers could now manipulate specific tissues to express desired traits, paving the way to produce genetically modified plants with enhanced characteristics [21].

The practical applications of organogenesis and somatic embryogenesis fueled the commercialization of tissue culture techniques. Nurseries and agricultural industries adopted these methods for the mass production of disease-free and genetically uniform plants. Ornamental crops, fruits, and forestry species became prime candidates for large-scale clonal propagation, contributing to increased agricultural productivity and the conservation of valuable plant varieties. The 1960s and 1970s marked a dynamic period in the history of plant tissue culture, characterized by profound advancements in the controlled development of organs and embryos. The elucidation of hormonal influences and the refinement of tissue culture techniques paved the way for widespread applications in agriculture, horticulture, and biotechnology. As we move forward in this historical narrative, subsequent chapters will explore the continued evolution of plant tissue culture, including the rise of genetic engineering and the commercialization of genetically modified crops [22].

7.3.4 GENETIC ENGINEERING AND TRANSFORMATION (1980s–PRESENT)

The 1980s marked a revolutionary phase in plant tissue culture with the integration of genetic engineering techniques, allowing researchers to manipulate and engineer plant genomes. This era witnessed a transformative shift from traditional clonal propagation to the targeted modification of plant DNA, ushering in new possibilities for crop improvement, pest resistance, and enhanced agricultural productivity. One of the breakthroughs in genetic engineering applied to plant tissue culture was the utilization of Agrobacterium tumefaciens as a vector for gene transfer. The bacterium, naturally capable of transferring genetic material into plants, was harnessed as a tool for introducing foreign genes into plant cells. This technique enabled scientists to selectively introduce desired traits, such as resistance to pests, pathogens, or herbicides, into the plant genome [23].

In the early 1980s, researchers achieved a monumental milestone by creating the first transgenic plants. A team led by Mary-Dell Chilton and colleagues successfully introduced a bacterial gene into tobacco plants using agrobacterium-mediated transformation. The transgenic plants exhibited resistance to the antibiotic kanamycin, demonstrating the feasibility of incorporating novel traits into plants through genetic engineering.

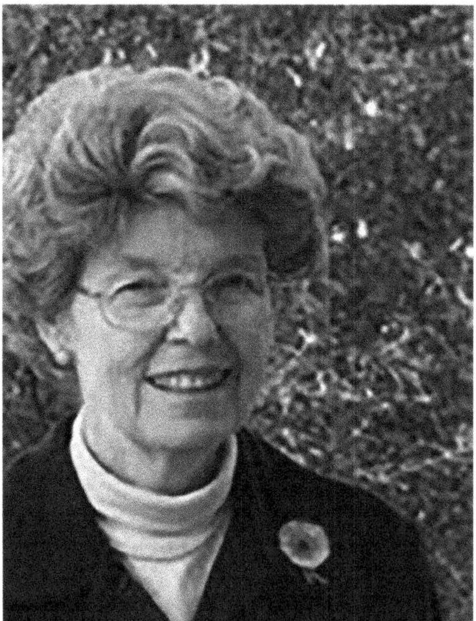

Mary-Dell Chilton

Parallel to agrobacterium-mediated transformation, another technique emerged known as particle bombardment or biolistic. This method involved propelling small particles coated with foreign DNA into plant cells. The "gene gun," developed by John Sanford and colleagues, became a valuable tool for introducing genes into plant tissues that were resistant to agrobacterium infection, broadening the scope of plant species amenable to genetic transformation. The application of genetic engineering in plant tissue culture led to the development of crops with enhanced traits. In the 1990s, the commercial release of the first genetically modified crops took place. Herbicide-resistant crops, engineered to withstand specific herbicides, allowed for more effective weed control. Simultaneously, insect-resistant crops, incorporating genes from *Bacillus thuringiensis* (Bt), provided built-in protection against specific pests. The advent of genetic engineering in plant tissue culture opened new avenues for biotechnological applications. The production of crops with improved nutritional content, enhanced tolerance to environmental stresses, and increased yields became realistic goals. Researchers explored the manipulation of metabolic pathways to enhance the synthesis of valuable compounds, turning plants into biofactories for pharmaceuticals, enzymes, and other high-value products [24].

While genetic engineering in plant tissue culture brought about unprecedented possibilities, it also sparked debates and controversies. Concerns over environmental impact, food safety, and ethical considerations led to increased scrutiny and regulatory measures. Public discourse on the acceptance and regulation of genetically modified organisms (GMOs) became a defining aspect of the biotechnological era. The incorporation of genetic engineering techniques in plant tissue culture during the 1980s fundamentally altered the landscape of agriculture and biotechnology. The ability to precisely manipulate plant genomes opened doors to innovative solutions for global challenges in food security, sustainability, and resource conservation. Subsequent chapters will delve into the commercial applications, societal impacts, and ongoing developments in the realm of genetically modified crops and plant biotechnology [25].

7.3.5 COMMERCIAL APPLICATIONS AND BIOTECHNOLOGY (1990S–PRESENT)

The 1990s ushered in an era of widespread commercialization of plant tissue culture techniques, as the field transitioned from academic research to practical applications in agriculture, horticulture, and biotechnology. This period saw the integration of genetically modified crops into commercial agriculture, the development of disease-resistant plants, and the emergence of tissue culture as a cornerstone of modern plant breeding. One of the immediate and tangible outcomes of advancements in plant tissue culture during the 1990s was the commercial-scale production of clonally propagated plants. Elite plant varieties, including fruits, ornamental crops, and forestry species, could be efficiently and consistently propagated in large quantities. Commercial nurseries adopted tissue culture techniques, offering disease-free and genetically uniform planting materials to meet the demands of the global market.

Plant tissue culture played a pivotal role in the production of disease-free planting materials. Through meticulous sterilization techniques and controlled culture conditions, researchers and nurseries could eliminate pathogens, viruses, and other contaminants from plant tissues. This ensured the production of healthy, disease-resistant plants, reducing the need for chemical treatments and enhancing overall crop quality. The integration of tissue culture with emerging molecular biology techniques in the late 20th century paved the way for precision breeding strategies. Researchers utilized genetic markers to identify desirable traits and selectively propagate plants with specific genomic compositions. Marker-assisted selection became a powerful tool for accelerating the breeding process, allowing for the development of crops with improved yield, quality, and resilience.

Plant tissue culture also contributed to the development of specialty crops with unique characteristics. Ornamental plants with novel flower colors, shapes, and sizes became popular in the horticultural industry. Additionally, the production of exotic fruits, high-value medicinal plants, and plants with enhanced nutritional profiles became feasible through tissue culture methods. The 1990s witnessed the expansion of plant tissue culture into forestry and ecosystem restoration projects. Researchers and conservationists explored the propagation of tree species for reforestation, habitat restoration, and the conservation of endangered plant species. Tissue culture became a valuable tool in efforts to preserve biodiversity and restore ecosystems impacted by deforestation and other environmental challenges [26].

Plant tissue culture became an integral component of the broader biotechnological landscape. The development of genetically modified crops with traits such as drought tolerance, enhanced nutrient content, and resistance to specific environmental stresses further highlighted the potential of plant biotechnology. These innovations aimed to address global challenges related to climate change, population growth, and sustainable agriculture. The commercialization of genetically modified crops and widespread adoption of plant tissue culture techniques raised societal concerns and regulatory challenges. Debates over food safety, environmental impact, and intellectual property rights became central to discussions surrounding biotechnology in agriculture. Governments and international organizations developed regulatory frameworks to address these concerns and ensure the responsible deployment of GMOs.

The historical evolution of plant tissue culture from the 1990s to the present underscores its profound impact on agriculture, horticulture, and biotechnology. The commercial applications of tissue culture techniques have transformed plant breeding and propagation, offering innovative solutions to global challenges. As we delve into subsequent chapters, we will explore the ongoing developments, ethical considerations, and prospects of plant tissue culture in the ever-evolving landscape of plant science and biotechnology (Table 7.1; Figure 7.1).

TABLE 7.1 Summary of Historical Prospective of Plant Tissue Culture

Year	Scientist Name	Remark
1980	Mary Dell Chilton	Using agrobacterium mediated transformation, in tobacco plants introduced a bacterial gene.
1970	Peter R. White	Somatic cells undergo a pathway resembling embryogenesis.
1962	Frits Warmolt Went	Pioneering experiments leading to identification of auxins.
1962	Toshio Murashige and Folke Skoog	Optimized the growth of plant tissues and induction of specific organs.
1957	Toshio Murashige and Folke Skoog	Introduced a nutrient medium in plant tissue culture.
1940	Gautheret and White	Conducted experiment resulting in discovery of callus formation.
1902	Gottlieb Haberlandt	Introduced term "totipotency," observed the potential of plants by isolating cells.
1894	Georges Nobecourt	Expanded the possibilities for *in vitro* cultivation.
1865	Wilhelm Knop	Experimented or Worked on growth of plant cells in liquid nutrient medium.

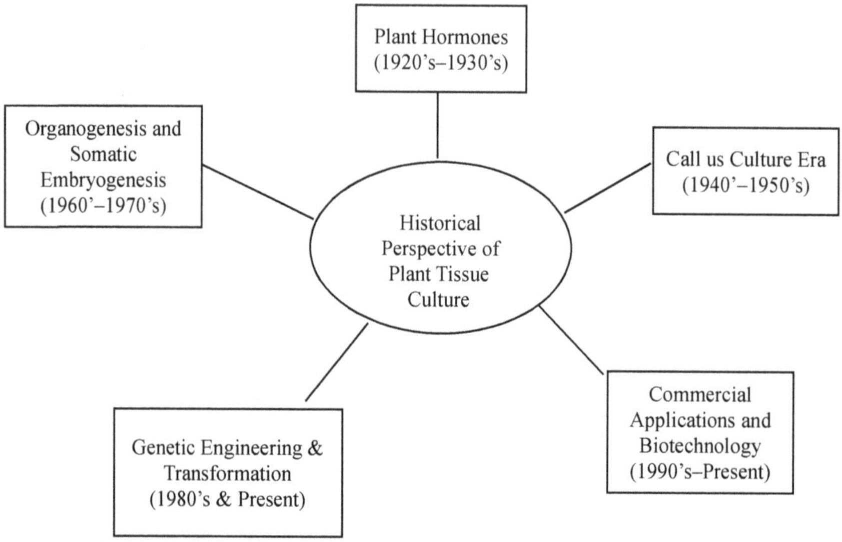

FIGURE 7.1 Historic perspective of plant tissue culture.

7.4 ADVANCES IN PLANT TISSUE CULTURE

7.4.1 INTERVENTIONS AGAINST EXPLANT RECALCITRANCE UNDER IN VITRO CULTURE SYSTEMS

Explant recalcitrance poses a significant challenge in *in vitro* plant tissue culture, hindering the successful propagation and manipulation of certain plant species. Overcoming this recalcitrance requires a comprehensive understanding of the physiological and biochemical factors influencing tissue response to culture conditions. These strategies encompass optimizing culture media composition, employing pre-culture treatments, implementing rigorous surface sterilization protocols, employing controlled wounding techniques, selecting appropriate explant sources and ages, manipulating phytohormone ratios, exploring additives, utilizing co-culture techniques, and employing genetic approaches. By integrating these strategies and continually refining culture protocols through empirical testing and optimization, researchers can improve the success rate of *in vitro* propagation and manipulation of recalcitrant plant species. Such advancements hold promise for accelerating breeding programs, conservation efforts, and biotechnological applications in agriculture and horticulture [27].

7.4.2 EMBRYO SALVAGE: A PROMISING TECHNIQUE FOR IMPROVEMENT OF ECONOMICALLY VIABLE CROPS

Embryo rescue has emerged as a powerful technique for the improvement of economically important crops, offering solutions to challenges such as wide hybridization, embryo abortion, and seed sterility. By rescuing embryos from incompatible crosses or stressed maternal environments, researchers can circumvent barriers to seed development and unlock genetic diversity for trait improvement. The technique involves excising immature embryos from seeds or ovules and culturing them under controlled *in vitro* conditions to promote germination and plantlet development. Embryo rescue enables the recovery of valuable hybrids, introgressions, and genetic variants that may otherwise be lost, facilitating the introgression of desirable traits such as disease resistance, stress tolerance, and agronomic performance. Additionally, embryo rescue has proven instrumental in facilitating distant hybridization, somatic embryogenesis, and haploid induction, thereby accelerating breeding programs and germplasm enhancement efforts. By leveraging embryo rescue as a versatile tool in plant breeding, researchers can enhance the resilience, productivity, and sustainability of crop production systems, addressing global food security challenges and fostering agricultural innovation [27].

7.4.3 GENETIC TRANSFORMATION VIA PLANT TISSUE CULTURE METHODOLOGIES: PRESENT AND FUTURE STRATEGIES

Genetic transformation via plant tissue culture techniques has revolutionized plant biotechnology by enabling the introduction of desired traits into economically important crops. The advent of tissue culture-based transformation methods, such as Agrobacterium-mediated gene transfer and direct DNA uptake, has facilitated the development of transgenic plants with enhanced agronomic traits, including pest resistance, herbicide tolerance, and improved nutritional profiles. Recent advancements in transformation protocols, such as the optimization of culture conditions, selection systems, and marker-free technologies, have contributed to increased efficiency and precision in transgene integration and expression. Additionally, emerging techniques such as genome editing tools (e.g., CRISPR/Cas9) and synthetic biology platforms offer novel avenues for targeted gene manipulation and trait engineering. Furthermore, it examines the ethical, environmental, and regulatory considerations surrounding the deployment of genetically modified crops and highlights the importance of biosafety measures and public engagement in shaping the future of plant biotechnology. By harnessing the power of genetic transformation techniques, researchers can accelerate crop improvement efforts, address global agricultural challenges, and contribute to sustainable food production systems in the face of climate change and population growth [28].

7.4.4 PLANT TISSUE CULTURE: SOMATIC EMBRYOGENESIS AND ORGANOGENESIS

Plant tissue culture techniques, including somatic embryogenesis and organogenesis, have revolutionized plant propagation, breeding, and biotechnology. Somatic embryogenesis involves the regeneration of embryos from somatic cells, bypassing the sexual reproduction process, while organogenesis entails the induction of shoots, roots, or other organs from explants under controlled *in vitro* conditions. These techniques offer efficient means of clonal propagation, germplasm conservation, and genetic transformation in various plant species, including crops, ornamentals, and woody plants. Somatic embryogenesis and organogenesis have been harnessed to produce elite varieties, the multiplication of disease-free planting materials, and the enhancement of secondary metabolite production. Recent progress in understanding the molecular and physiological mechanisms underlying somatic embryogenesis and organogenesis has led to the development of improved protocols and biotechnological tools for enhancing regeneration efficiency and genetic stability. Furthermore, advancements in omics technologies, such as transcriptomics, proteomics, and metabolomics, offer insights into the regulatory networks and metabolic pathways governing regeneration processes, facilitating targeted manipulation and trait improvement. By harnessing the potential of somatic embryogenesis and organogenesis, researchers can accelerate crop improvement efforts, conserve endangered species, and contribute to sustainable agriculture and biotechnology.

7.4.5 HISTORICAL DEVELOPMENTS AND ADVANCEMENTS OF PLANT GROWTH REGULATORS IN TISSUE CULTURE

The application of plant growth regulators (PGRs) in tissue culture has revolutionized the field, enabling the manipulation of plant growth and development for various applications. Initially employed for callus induction and organogenesis, PGRs such as auxins and cytokinins have been instrumental in regulating cellular differentiation and morphogenesis *in vitro*. Subsequent advancements in PGR formulations, delivery methods, and synergistic interactions have enhanced the efficiency and versatility of tissue culture techniques, enabling precise control over plant regeneration pathways and genotype-independent propagation. Recent breakthroughs include the discovery of novel PGR analogs, the elucidation of signaling pathways governing PGR responses, and the integration of omics technologies for systems-level characterization of PGR-mediated processes. Moreover, innovative strategies such as micropropagation, somatic embryogenesis, and synthetic biology approaches have expanded the scope of PGR applications in crop improvement, conservation biology, and biopharmaceutical production. By leveraging the diverse properties and applications of PGRs, researchers can harness the full potential of tissue culture for advancing agriculture, horticulture, and biotechnology, addressing global challenges, and contributing to sustainable development goals [29].

7.4.6 ORIENTATION TO AND LINEAGE OF PLANT TISSUE CULTURE: PAST, PRESENT, AND FUTURE ASPECTS

Plant tissue culture, a cornerstone of modern plant biotechnology, has evolved significantly since its inception, offering unprecedented opportunities for the manipulation, propagation, and improvement of plant species. In the early 20th century, for understanding plant development, tissue culture techniques have since become indispensable tools in various fields, including agriculture, horticulture, forestry, and pharmaceuticals. The historical journey of plant tissue culture encompasses key milestones such as the discovery of totipotency, the establishment of culture media formulations, and the development of regeneration protocols for diverse plant species [18, 19].

In the current era, tissue culture techniques have been refined and optimized to address contemporary challenges in crop improvement, germplasm conservation, and biopharmaceutical production. Advancements in culture media composition, hormonal manipulation, and culture vessel design have led to enhanced efficiency, reproducibility, and scalability of tissue culture systems. Moreover, emerging technologies such as genetic engineering, omics approaches, and synthetic biology are reshaping the landscape of plant tissue culture, enabling precise trait manipulation and accelerating breeding programs [20–24].

Looking ahead, the future of plant tissue culture holds immense promise for addressing pressing global issues such as food security, climate change resilience, and ecosystem restoration. Continued research efforts are focused on overcoming remaining challenges, including explant recalcitrance, genotype dependence, and regulatory constraints associated with genetically modified organisms (GMOs). Additionally, the integration of tissue culture with novel biotechnological tools and interdisciplinary collaborations is poised to unlock new avenues for sustainable agriculture, biodiversity conservation, and bioproduct innovation.

By embracing the rich legacy and advancing the frontiers of plant tissue culture, researchers can harness the transformative potential of this technology to address the evolving needs of society, foster economic development, and safeguard the planet's botanical wealth for future generations [27].

7.4.7 APPLICATIONS OF PLANT TISSUE CULTURE MEDIUM INGREDIENTS

Plant tissue culture medium components play a pivotal role in regulating the growth, development, and differentiation of plant cells *in vitro*. This provides an overview of the essential components of tissue culture media and their functions in supporting plant growth and morphogenesis. The composition of tissue culture media typically includes inorganic salts, organic supplements, vitamins, amino acids, sugars, and PGRs. Inorganic salts provide essential nutrients such as nitrogen, phosphorus, potassium, and micronutrients necessary for cellular metabolism and growth. Organic supplements, including carbon sources such as sugars and complex organic compounds, serve as energy sources and precursors for biosynthesis. Vitamins and amino acids play critical roles as cofactors and building blocks in various metabolic pathways, while PGRs such as auxins, cytokinins, and gibberellins regulate cell division, differentiation, and organogenesis.

Recent advancements in medium optimization, such as the utilization of alternative carbon sources, organic supplements, and hormone combinations, are highlighted for their potential to improve culture performance and overcome species-specific challenges. Additionally, the importance of understanding the physiological requirements and responses of target plant species to tissue culture media components is emphasized to tailor culture protocols for specific applications and genetic backgrounds.

By elucidating the roles and dynamics of tissue culture medium components, researchers can refine tissue culture protocols, expand the range of amenable species, and accelerate the application of tissue culture techniques in agriculture, horticulture, forestry, and biotechnology. This comprehensive understanding of medium composition and its effects on plant development lays the foundation for advancing plant tissue culture as a versatile tool for plant propagation, genetic transformation, and germplasm conservation [24–29].

7.4.8 SOMATIC EMBRYOGENESIS IN MEDICINAL PLANTS

Somatic embryogenesis, a remarkable phenomenon in plant tissue culture, holds immense promise for the propagation and production of valuable secondary metabolites in medicinal plants. It explores the principles, methodologies, and applications of somatic embryogenesis in the context of medicinal plant species. Somatic embryogenesis offers a reproducible and scalable approach for mass propagation of elite germplasm, circumventing limitations associated with conventional propagation methods such as seed germination and vegetative propagation. Moreover, somatic embryogenesis provides a controlled environment to produce bioactive compounds, including pharmaceuticals, nutraceuticals, and phytochemicals, with consistent quality and yield.

By harnessing the potential of somatic embryogenesis, researchers can accelerate the development of elite cultivars, optimize production systems for high-value secondary metabolites, and contribute to the conservation and sustainable utilization of medicinal plant resources. This underscores the significance of somatic embryogenesis as a transformative tool in medicinal plant biotechnology, offering opportunities for innovation, economic development, and public health enhancement [24–29].

7.4.9 REFINING CROPS VIA TRANSGENIC BREEDING: TECHNOLOGICAL ADVANCES AND PROSPECTS

Transgenic breeding stands at the forefront of modern agricultural innovation, offering a potent toolkit for enhancing crop traits to meet the challenges of global food security, climate change, and sustainability. This provides an overview of the technological advances and prospects in transgenic breeding for crop improvement. By harnessing genetic engineering techniques, such as gene editing, RNA interference, and synthetic biology, researchers can precisely manipulate the genetic makeup of crops to confer desired traits, including resistance to pests and diseases, tolerance to abiotic stresses, and improved nutritional content [20–29].

7.4.10 APPLICATION OF PLANT TISSUE CULTURE IN PHARMACEUTICALS AND SECONDARY METABOLITES PRODUCTION

Plant tissue culture has emerged as a versatile platform for the sustainable production of pharmaceuticals and secondary metabolites, offering advantages such as rapid propagation, controlled growth conditions, and enhanced biosynthetic capacity. Various aspects of plant tissue culture relevant to pharmaceutical applications include the selection of elite plant species, optimization of tissue culture protocols, and manipulation of culture conditions to enhance secondary metabolite biosynthesis. Key factors influencing metabolite production in tissue culture systems include culture media composition, hormonal regulation, elicitation techniques, and bioreactor design.

In addition to pharmaceuticals, plant tissue culture holds promise for producing high-value secondary metabolites used in nutraceuticals, cosmetics, and flavoring agents. The scalability, reproducibility, and sustainability of tissue culture systems make them attractive alternatives to traditional methods of secondary metabolite extraction from wild or cultivated plant sources.

Overall, plant tissue culture represents a valuable tool for pharmaceutical and secondary metabolite production, offering opportunities for innovation, cost-effectiveness, and environmental sustainability in the pharmaceutical industry. By leveraging advances in tissue culture techniques, biotechnology, and metabolic engineering, researchers can unlock the full potential of plant-derived compounds for therapeutic and commercial applications, addressing global health challenges and improving human well-being [18–30].

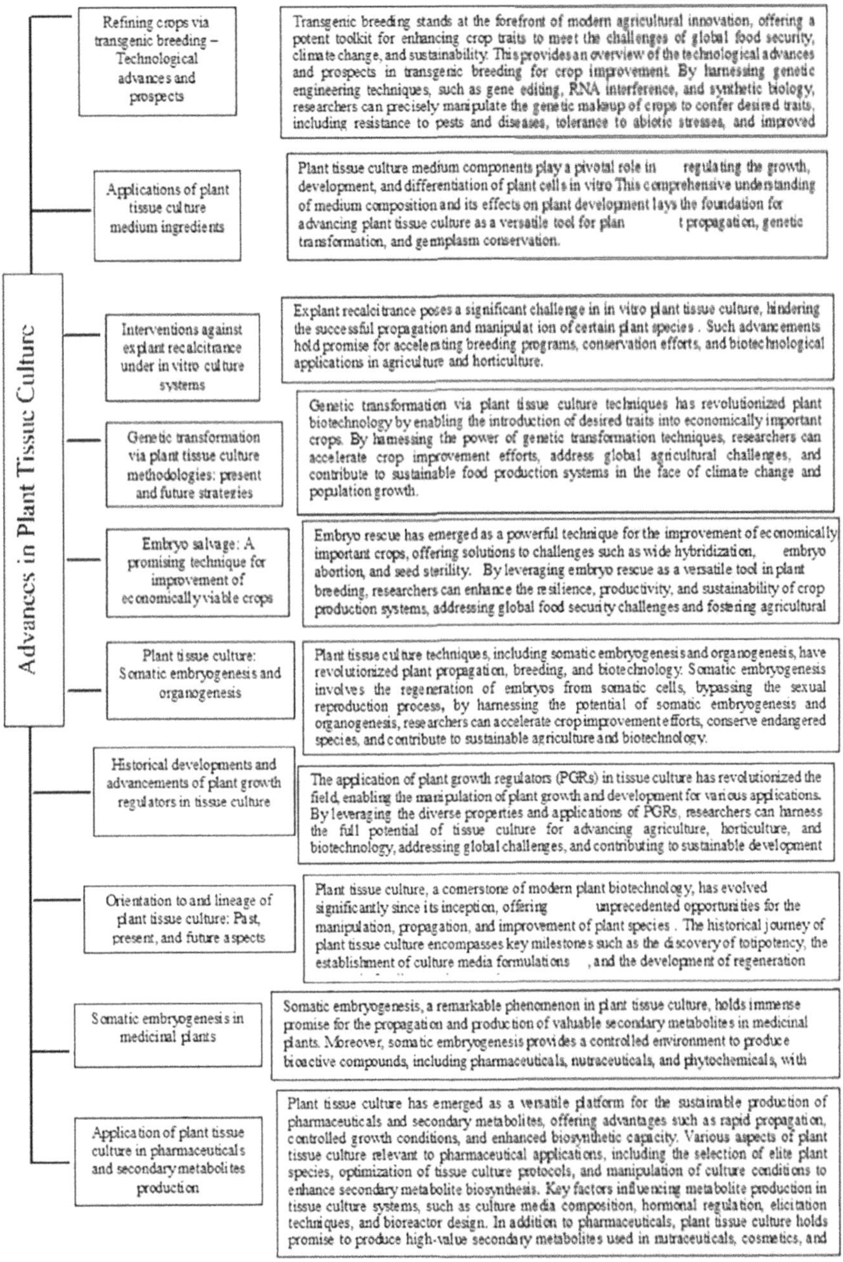
Advances in Plant Tissue Culture
Refining crops via transgenic breeding – Technological advances and prospects
Transgenic breeding stands at the forefront of modern agricultural innovation, offering a potent toolkit for enhancing crop traits to meet the challenges of global food security, climate change, and sustainability. This provides an overview of the technological advances and prospects in transgenic breeding for crop improvement. By harnessing genetic engineering techniques, such as gene editing, RNA interference, and synthetic biology, researchers can precisely manipulate the genetic makeup of crops to confer desired traits, including resistance to pests and diseases, tolerance to abiotic stresses, and improved
Applications of plant tissue culture medium ingredients
Plant tissue culture medium components play a pivotal role in regulating the growth, development, and differentiation of plant cells in vitro This comprehensive understanding of medium composition and its effects on plant development lays the foundation for advancing plant tissue culture as a versatile tool for plan t propagation, genetic transformation, and germplasm conservation.
Interventions against explant recalcitrance under in vitro culture systems
Explant recalcitrance poses a significant challenge in in vitro plant tissue culture, hindering the successful propagation and manipulation of certain plant species . Such advancements hold promise for accelerating breeding programs, conservation efforts, and biotechnological applications in agriculture and horticulture.
Genetic transformation via plant tissue culture methodologies: present and future strategies
Genetic transformation via plant tissue culture techniques has revolutionized plant biotechnology by enabling the introduction of desired traits into economically important crops. By harnessing the power of genetic transformation techniques, researchers can accelerate crop improvement efforts, address global agricultural challenges, and contribute to sustainable food production systems in the face of climate change and population growth.
Embryo salvage: A promising technique for improvement of economically viable crops
Embryo rescue has emerged as a powerful technique for the improvement of economically important crops, offering solutions to challenges such as wide hybridization, embryo abortion, and seed sterility. By leveraging embryo rescue as a versatile tool in plant breeding, researchers can enhance the resilience, productivity, and sustainability of crop production systems, addressing global food security challenges and fostering agricultural
Plant tissue culture: Somatic embryogenesis and organogenesis
Plant tissue culture techniques, including somatic embryogenesis and organogenesis, have revolutionized plant propagation, breeding, and biotechnology. Somatic embryogenesis involves the regeneration of embryos from somatic cells, bypassing the sexual reproduction process, by harnessing the potential of somatic embryogenesis and organogenesis, researchers can accelerate crop improvement efforts, conserve endangered species, and contribute to sustainable agriculture and biotechnology.
Historical developments and advancements of plant growth regulators in tissue culture
The application of plant growth regulators (PGRs) in tissue culture has revolutionized the field, enabling the manipulation of plant growth and development for various applications. By leveraging the diverse properties and applications of PGRs, researchers can harness the full potential of tissue culture for advancing agriculture, horticulture, and biotechnology, addressing global challenges, and contributing to sustainable development
Orientation to and lineage of plant tissue culture: Past, present, and future aspects
Plant tissue culture, a cornerstone of modern plant biotechnology, has evolved significantly since its inception, offering unprecedented opportunities for the manipulation, propagation, and improvement of plant species . The historical journey of plant tissue culture encompasses key milestones such as the discovery of totipotency, the establishment of culture media formulations , and the development of regeneration
Somatic embryogenesis in medicinal plants
Somatic embryogenesis, a remarkable phenomenon in plant tissue culture, holds immense promise for the propagation and production of valuable secondary metabolites in medicinal plants. Moreover, somatic embryogenesis provides a controlled environment to produce bioactive compounds, including pharmaceuticals, nutraceuticals, and phytochemicals, with
Application of plant tissue culture in pharmaceuticals and secondary metabolites production
Plant tissue culture has emerged as a versatile platform for the sustainable production of pharmaceuticals and secondary metabolites, offering advantages such as rapid propagation, controlled growth conditions, and enhanced biosynthetic capacity. Various aspects of plant tissue culture relevant to pharmaceutical applications, including the selection of elite plant species, optimization of tissue culture protocols, and manipulation of culture conditions to enhance secondary metabolite biosynthesis. Key factors influencing metabolite production in tissue culture systems, such as culture media composition, hormonal regulation, elicitation techniques, and bioreactor design. In addition to pharmaceuticals, plant tissue culture holds promise to produce high-value secondary metabolites used in nutraceuticals, cosmetics, and

7.5 CONCLUSION

The history of plant tissue culture is a testament to the perseverance and ingenuity of scientists who have continuously pushed the boundaries of knowledge. From the early experiments in nutrient media to the sophisticated genetic engineering techniques of today, plant tissue culture has evolved into a powerful tool for plant biologists, breeders, and biotechnologists. As we look to the future, ongoing research promises even more exciting possibilities for the manipulation and improvement of plants through tissue culture techniques.

KEYWORDS

- **callus culture**
- **genetic engineering**
- **micropropagation**
- **plant tissue culture**
- **secondary metabolites**
- **totipotent cells**

REFERENCES

1. Thorpe, T. A. (2007). History of plant tissue culture. *Molecular Biotechnology, 37*, 169–180.
2. Phillips, G. C., & Garda, M. (2019). Plant tissue culture media and practices: An overview. *In Vitro Cellular & Developmental Biology-Plant, 55*, 242–257.
3. Gamborg, O. L., Murashige, T., Thorpe, T. A., & Vasil, I. K. (1976). Plant tissue culture media. *In Vitro, 12*(7), 473–478.
4. Smith, R. H. (2012). *Plant Tissue Culture: Techniques and Experiments*. Academic Press.
5. García-Gonzáles, R., Quiroz, K., Carrasco, B., & Caligari, P. (2010). Plant tissue culture: Status, opportunities, and challenges. *International Journal of Agriculture and Natural Resources, 37*(3), 5–30.
6. Ahloowalia, B. S., Prakash, J., Savangikar, V. A., & Savangikar, C. (2004). Plant tissue culture. *Low-Cost Options for Tissue Culture Technology in Developing Countries, 1*, 3.

7. Mineo, L. (1990). Plant tissue culture techniques. *Tested Studies for Laboratory Teaching, 11*, 151–174.
8. Saad, A. I., & Elshahed, A. M. (2012). Plant tissue culture media. *Recent Advances in Plant In Vitro Culture*, 30–40.
9. Gaspar, T., Kevers, C., Penel, C., Greppin, H., Reid, D. M., & Thorpe, T. A. (1996). Plant hormones and plant growth regulators in plant tissue culture. *In Vitro Cellular & Developmental Biology-Plant, 32*, 272–289.
10. Bhojwani, S. S., & Dantu, P. K. (2013). *Plant Tissue Culture: An Introductory Text.* Springer.
11. Loyola-Vargas, V. M., & Ochoa-Alejo, N. (2018). An introduction to plant tissue culture: Advances and perspectives. *Plant Cell Culture Protocols, 1815*, 3–13.
12. Bhojwani, S. S., & Razdan, M. K. (1986). *Plant Tissue Culture: Theory and Practice*. Elsevier.
13. Trigiano, R. N., & Gray, D. J. (1999). *Plant Tissue Culture Concepts and Laboratory Exercises*. CRC Press.
14. Gaba, V. P. (2005). Plant growth regulators in plant tissue culture and development. In *Plant Development and Biotechnology* (pp. 87–99).
15. Aitken-Christie, J., Kozai, T., & Takayama, S. (1995). Automation in plant tissue culture—General introduction and overview. In *Automation and Environmental Control in Plant Tissue Culture* (pp. 1–8).
16. Espinosa-Leal, C. A., Puente-Garza, C. A., & García-Lara, S. (2018). *In vitro* plant tissue culture: Means for production of biological active compounds. *Planta, 248*, 1–8.
17. Kozai, T., & Smith, M. A. (1995). Environmental control in plant tissue culture—General introduction and overview. In *Automation and Environmental Control in Plant Tissue Culture* (pp. 301–318).
18. Cloutier, S., & Landry, B. S. (1994). Molecular markers applied to plant tissue culture. *In Vitro Cellular & Developmental Biology-Plant, 30*, 32–39.
19. Sathyanarayana, B. N., & Varghese, D. B. (2007). *Plant Tissue Culture: Practices and New Experimental Protocols*. IK International Pvt Ltd.
20. Smulders, M. J., & De Klerk, G. J. (2011). Epigenetics in plant tissue culture. *Plant Growth Regulation, 63*, 137–146.
21. Gamborg, O. L. (2002). Plant tissue culture: Biotechnology milestones. *In Vitro Cellular & Developmental Biology-Plant, 38*, 84–92.
22. Gamborg, O. L., & Wetter, L. R. (1975). *Plant Tissue Culture Methods.* Saskatoon: National Research Council of Canada, Prairie Regional Laboratory.
23. Aremu, A. O., Bairu, M. W., Doležal, K., Finnie, J. F., & Van Staden, J. (2012). Topolins: A panacea to plant tissue culture challenges. *Plant Cell, Tissue, and Organ Culture (PCTOC, 108*, 1–6.
24. Kumar, P. P., & Loh, C. S. (2012). Plant tissue culture for biotechnology. In *Plant Biotechnology and Agriculture* (pp. 131–138). Academic Press.
25. Bhatia, S., & Dahiya, R. (2015). Concepts and techniques of plant tissue culture science. In *Modern Applications of Plant Biotechnology in Pharmaceutical Sciences* (pp. 121–156).

26. Dias, M. I., Sousa, M. J., Alves, R. C., & Ferreira, I. C. (2016). Exploring plant tissue culture to improve the production of phenolic compounds: A review. *Industrial Crops and Products, 82*, 9–22.
27. George, E. F., Hall, M. A., & De Klerk, G. J. (2008). Plant tissue culture procedure—Background. In *Plant Propagation by Tissue Culture: The Background* (Vol. 1, pp. 1–28). Dordrecht: Springer Netherlands.
28. George, E. F., Hall, M. A., & De Klerk, G. J. (2007). *Plant Propagation by Tissue Culture: Volume 1. The Background.* Springer Science & Business Media.
29. Rai, A. C., Kumar, A., Modi, A., & Singh, M. (2022). In *Advances in Plant Tissue Culture.* Academic Press.
30. Smith, R. H. (2005). In *Plant Tissue Culture: Techniques and Experiments* (2nd ed.). Elsevier, Academic Press.

CHAPTER 8

Nutraceuticals

POPAT MOHITE,[1] ABHIJEET PURI,[1] SHUBHAM MUNDE,[1] RAMDAS PANDHARE,[2] DESHRAJ CHUMBALE,[3] and SUDARSHAN SINGH,[4,5,*]

[1]*AET's St. John Institute of Pharmacy and Research, Palghar, Maharashtra, India*

[2]*MES's College of Pharmacy, Sonai, Ahmednagar, Maharashtra, India*

[3]*Amrutwahini College of Pharmacy, Sangamner, Ahmednagar, Maharashtra, India*

[4]*Office of Research Administration, Chiang Mai University, Chiang Mai, Thailand*

[5]*Faculty of Pharmacy, Chiang Mai University, Chiang Mai, Thailand*

*Corresponding author

ABSTRACT

The chapter explores the multifaceted role of antioxidants, polyunsaturated fatty acids (PUFAs), and herbs as functional foods in promoting health and preventing chronic diseases. Beginning with an introduction to the significance of functional foods, the focus shifts to antioxidants and PUFAs, elucidating their importance in combating oxidative stress, preventing chronic diseases, and supporting cardiovascular health. The chapter further delves into the classification of herbs as functional

The Essentials of Herbal Drugs. Varsha Tiwari, Abhishek Tiwari, and Ajay Sharma (Eds.)

DOI: 10.1201/9781998511778-8

foods, highlighting their medicinal properties and health benefits. We go into great length about certain herbs, including spirulina, broccoli, ginseng, garlic, soybean, black cohosh, green and herbal tea, flaxseeds, and turmeric, discussing their origins, signature compounds, chemical makeup, and variety of health uses. The discussion extends to the formulation and standardization of nutraceuticals, addressing challenges and considerations in their development. Regulatory aspects and adherence to FSSAI guidelines are explored to ensure the safety and efficacy of functional foods. The chapter concludes with a comprehensive overview of the selected herbs, emphasizing their culinary and therapeutic applications. Future trends and research directions in nutraceutical development, including personalized nutrition, advanced formulations, and the integration of traditional and modern medicine, are also discussed.

8.1 INTRODUCTION

The categories of regular food (including drinks) and food supplements (such as energy bars, teas, and liquids) are becoming increasingly overlapping. When we consider nutraceuticals and functional foods, this overlap increases even further. In certain contexts, a product labeled as a functional food may also be referred to as a dietary supplement, medical food, food for special dietary use, or nutraceutical, depending on its ingredients (active components) and the claims made about it [1]. Although the definition of a dietary supplement is very straightforward and comprehensible, the line separating food, food supplements, and medications is still blurred when it comes to what constitutes a nutraceutical. "Food or a portion of a food that delivers medical or health benefits, including the prevention and/or treatment of a disease" is how Stephen DeFelice first coined the phrase nutraceutical. The term "nutraceuticals" is a neologism that combines the terms "pharmaceutical" and "nutrient" [2]. This idea has been proposed as a contemporary method of studying food science, with the definition of its potential application being outside of the diet but prior to medication. Despite this idea, there are currently conflicting definitions of nutraceuticals and a valid evaluation of their medical potential that is far from being shared and acknowledged globally [3].

8.2 FOOD SUPPLEMENT

Food products that are marketed in dosed formulations, like capsules, tablets, or pills, and that are meant to be taken in small, measured amounts individually, are concentrated sources of nutrients or other substances that, either alone or in combination, have physiological or nutritional effects. These products can be used as a supplement to a regular diet. The phytochemicals that are found in edible fruits and vegetables that people can eat daily (measured in grams) and that have the potential to positively modify human metabolism to prevent cancer and other diseases include isoflavones, resveratrol, garlic allyl sulfides, tomato lycopene, onion quercetin, and others. Nutraceuticals are food or food components that have health or medical benefits, such as aiding in the treatment or prevention of an illness [2].

Food additives are one or more of the following nutritional substances that can be found in a product: vitamins, minerals, amino acids, or other botanical or dietary elements. Goods (not including tobacco) that come in the form of powder, gel caps, soft gels, or capsules are meant to be added to food to improve health [4]. Nutraceuticals are food items that, in addition to their basic nutritional value, offer health advantages (either as a dietary supplement or fortified food) [5]. Nutritional goods have therapeutic and health effects, such as those for illness treatment and prevention [6]. Functional foods are nutrients that are ingested normally but that, within the food matrix, contain one or more active chemicals (that have physiological effects and may improve health) [7]. Foods that are functional products satisfactorily prove that, in addition to providing sufficient nutritional benefits, they positively affect one or more target functions of the organism, significantly improving welfare and health status or reducing the risk of disease [8]. Foods are any meal or substance that, in addition to being nutritious, has a favorable effect on a person's physical or mental well-being [9].

Food for medical use, full nutritional food that is formulated according to criteria; for the recipient, it may be their only source of nutrition. Alternatively, full nutritious food that has been specially formulated to meet the needs of a particular disease, disorder, or medical condition; this meal may be the only source of nutrition for the person receiving it. Alternatively put, nutritionally deficient food that has been modified to meet the needs of a particular illness, condition, or disease but is still not a sufficient source of nutrition on its own.

There is often overlap between the recognized definition of food supplements and the nutraceutical concept [10, 11], and the justification for using these goods is increasingly crucial to their uniqueness. Nutraceuticals are constantly in development and are expanding rapidly across the globe. Conflicting information currently accessible in the sector is creating uncertainty regarding the potential usefulness of these medications, which are sold and distributed by pharmacies. Supplemental foods can help those in need of better health based on their micronutrient content. Generally speaking, there may not be enough scientific evidence to support the many health claims made about food supplements, pro- and prebiotics, herbal items, and functional foods regarding their safety, effectiveness, and impact on pathological or general health issues [12]. Most of the claims are unsupported because there are insufficient investigations on potential mechanisms of action and *in vivo* studies that validate the positive health effects on clinical diseases. The data reported in the literature, which primarily originates from *in vitro* studies focused on individual food constituents (micronutrients), is another important factor to consider. These studies are predicated on the idea that because micronutrients are derived from commonly used foods or food components, they can be regarded as safe or recognized as such. Safety is crucial since these goods may contain pollutants with both organic and inorganic origins [13]. Furthermore, the substances themselves can have negative health consequences, and the label ought to include accurate information about any potential adverse effects. From our perspective, it is critical to obtain a deeper comprehension of the mechanism of action and bioavailability of these drugs, as well as additional data on safety and efficacy based on clinical trials rather than only *in vitro* investigations. Nutraceuticals must first be distinguished from other food-derived products, particularly food supplements, which should not always be included in a regular diet unless there is a specific need, in order to assess their efficacy [14].

In order to assess the efficacy of nutraceuticals, it is necessary to first distinguish them from other food-derived products, particularly food supplements, which should not always be included in a regular diet unless there is a specific need. The differences in the accepted definitions of nutraceuticals and the regulatory issues that follow will be very challenging to resolve. An overview of the absence of common rules pertaining to pharma-foods, or nutraceuticals, is required. Nutraceuticals are viewed as falling into the gray area, following nutrition but preceding medication.

Given their potential application and utility in the pharmaceutical industry, it is crucial to ascertain their specificity [15].

8.3 INORGANIC MINERAL SUPPLEMENTS

Minerals are inorganic compounds that are found in nature and are not produced by plants or animals. While mammals ingest minerals through their diet, plants absorb them from the nearby rocks, soil, and water. Minerals can be divided into two categories: major minerals, which require more than 100 milligrams per day, and trace minerals, which require less than 100 milligrams per day. Although they are required in smaller quantities, trace minerals are equally as vital to overall health as major minerals [16, 17].

8.3.1 MINERALS IN FOOD

Foods made from plants have a higher mineral content than the soils in which the plants were raised. The Great Lakes and the Appalachians were part of the "goiter belt," which encompassed the central and northwest parts of the United States, where goiter was common in the early 1900s. These regions of the country had low iodine soil, which affected the local foods that people consumed. Iodine was added to table salt to address this health issue, and the frequency of goiter decreased [18].

The quantity of a mineral in meals and how well your body absorbs it affect its availability. For instance, the body absorbs and uses only roughly 10–30% of the calcium that is present in meals. Numerous factors, including the composition of the meal and the method of preparation, might affect the absorption of minerals. Foods are intricate concoctions of numerous distinct substances, some of which cause absorption problems. For instance, oxalic acid, a binding agent found in spinach, might decrease the availability of calcium from other foods eaten at the same time. This effect is negligible in a diet rich in variety, though. On the other hand, absorption is boosted when specific vitamins, including vitamins C and D, are present. Similar-sized and ionic-charged minerals frequently compete with one another for absorption during digestion. One unforeseen consequence of over-supplementing a diet with one mineral is that it may reduce the absorption of another. The best defense against these issues and to guarantee proper mineral absorption is to eat a variety of meals [19].

8.3.2 MINERALS WITH ELECTROLYTE PROPERTIES

8.3.2.1 ELECTROLYTES

Electrolytes are minerals with an electrical charge that assist your body in controlling fluids and preserving the acid-base balance. Some examples of dietary-important electrolytes that must be found in food are potassium, sodium, chloride, and phosphorus (as phosphate) [20].

8.3.2.2 SODIUM

In the modern food supply, sodium is extensively dispersed, and Americans have little trouble getting enough of it. It is used in the production of food to produce desired textures and tastes, as well as to stop microbiological growth and prevent food spoilage [21]. The diets of ancient hunter-gatherers were low in sodium and high in potassium. This link has been reversed by the easy access to table salt and contemporary methods of food processing, leading to a diet heavy in sodium and low in potassium [22].

Extracellular spaces, or fluids outside of cells, contain sodium ions. These ions are used by the body to control how much water enters and leaves cells. The kidneys control the amount of sodium in urine, so when consumption is high, more sodium is excreted in the urine, helping to maintain appropriate salt levels. The body's sodium reserves can be reduced by prolonged vomiting or diarrhea, but eating salty meals usually suffices to make up for the loss. Low in potassium and high in sodium [23].

Sodium is present in all food sources, including tap water! Although grazing animals like deer and cattle may experience insufficient food, omnivores like humans rarely experience this issue. Additionally, because salt is a common ingredient in flavorings and preservatives, our highly processed, modern meals are rich in sodium. When food is cooked or served, sodium is also added to it along with salt. Some, but not all, individuals have a link between hypertension and excessive salt intake [24]. This phenomenon is referred to as salt sensitivity, or salt-sensitive blood pressure. Eating foods heavy in salt raises your risk of hypertension, or elevated blood pressure, if you have salt sensitivity. Keep your daily sodium consumption to less than 2300 milligrams to reduce this effect. Following the Dietary Reference Intake requirements requires conscious effort; this includes paying attention to nutrition facts labels and reducing salt intake at mealtimes [25].

8.3.2.3 POTASSIUM

Similar to sodium, potassium is also utilized to keep fluid equilibrium; however, it is found intracellularly, not extracellularly, in body cells. During digestion, the majority of the potassium in the food you eat is absorbed. Once the body's reserves are replenished, any excess is eliminated via the kidneys. As dietary potassium is linked to a drop in blood pressure, as opposed to salt, eating a banana a day is a well-known suggestion. However, those who have kidney disease need to watch what they eat and stay away from excesses that the kidneys cannot eliminate. Because of worries about inadequate intake, nutrition facts label purposefully indicate the amount of potassium in a serving of food, along with a percent daily value. Individuals on drugs that deplete reserves—such as diuretics, which remove extra fluid from the body—should concentrate on eating meals high in these reserves and talk to their doctors about supplements. Among many other foods, foods high in potassium include kidney beans, bananas, apricots, lentils, prunes, squash, milk, yogurt, chicken, and beef. A well-rounded diet that includes whole grains, unprocessed fruits and vegetables, meats, dairy products, and vegetable oils is an excellent method of obtaining enough potassium [25].

8.3.2.4 CHLORIDE

Fluids that are extracellular, or outside of cells, contain the necessary mineral chloride. It is essential to gastric (stomach) juices and aids in the preservation of electrolyte and fluid balance. What is the main source of the chloride found in food? Salt! The saltshaker on the table and processed foods both contain sodium chloride, or salt. Although water contains some chloride, it is negligible compared to the quantity added to our food by salting it. Chloride is present in human milk in somewhat greater amounts than sodium. Both salt and chloride levels are decreased by extreme perspiration, prolonged vomiting or diarrhea, trauma, and renal (kidney) illness [26].

8.3.2.5 CALCIUM

The bones and teeth contain 99% of the calcium in your body. Throughout life, bone remodeling, a metabolic process that involves the reabsorption and subsequent reconstitution of bone tissue, requires calcium from food. While calcium is best known for its role in maintaining healthy bones, it also plays a key part in blood clotting, muscular contraction, and neuron function. Less than 1% of the body's total calcium is found in the blood, where levels are kept within an extremely small range by the small intestine (absorption) and kidneys (excretion). Because bones can move calcium into and out of bone tissue as needed, they also aid in maintaining blood levels [26].

Food's nutrients affect the amount of calcium that is retained after a meal. Calcium absorption from the small intestine is facilitated by vitamin D. Vitamin C-containing beverages, like orange juice, can aid in absorption. Phytic and oxalic acid-rich foods bind to calcium and decrease absorption. This group of foods includes beans, sweet potatoes, and spinach. Carbonated drinks and other high-phosphate beverages enhance the excretion of calcium in the urine and its secretion into the intestines.

One cannot stress how important it is to maximize bone mineralization during the first 30 years of life. A persistently low calcium intake causes osteopenia, which is characterized by a decline in bone mineral density (BMD) and eventually leads to osteoporosis, or porous, weak bones. For women, the first 17 years of life and the first 21 years of life account for the majority (95%) of adult bone mass. After reaching the third decade, there is a slow loss of bone mineral that lasts the rest of a person's life. Exercises involving weight-bearing, as well as sufficient consumption of calcium and vitamin D, can lower the rate of bone mass loss. Although fortified orange juice, breads, cereals, tofu, green vegetables, and legumes are rich sources of calcium, few Americans consume enough of these items to meet their needs. Less than ideal levels are obtained from a diet deficient in rich sources, such as milk and dairy products, calcium-enhanced tofu, and enriched cereals [26].

8.3.2.6 IRON

Sufficient iron intake is essential for muscle contraction and workout efficiency. Compounds containing iron help the body produce energy, support the immune system, and assist the liver in detoxifying drugs. Iron is a component of myoglobin, a protein in muscle tissue that stores oxygen; hemoglobin, a blood protein molecule that carries oxygen throughout the body; and ferritin, a form of iron storage found in the liver, spleen, and bone marrow [27].

Low iron levels can put a surprising number of people at risk for chronic fatigue, appetite loss, and apathy. If iron deficiency is not addressed, iron deficiency erythropoiesis, or the manufacture of red blood cells, progresses from depleted stores to low hemoglobin levels in the blood and a decrease in hematocrit, or the proportion of red blood cells in the blood.

Meats have higher bioavailability (the amount of iron that is absorbed and used) than plant-based diets. In comparison to a mixed diet, where the presence of heme iron (an animal source) improves the absorption of non-heme iron (a plant source), a strict vegetarian diet has reduced iron bioavailability. Therefore, vegetarians should focus especially on maintaining a balanced diet that includes foods rich in vitamin C, which improves absorption, and foods rich in iron. Around the world, where access to meat and fish is restricted and intestinal parasites cause blood losses that deplete storage, iron deficiency is frequent [28]. Athletes who engage in prolonged training, such as distance running, may lose more iron. These individuals may be undernourished and have a higher rate of erythrocyte (blood cell) turnover. Athletes who regularly engage in intensive exercise have an Estimated Average Requirement (EAR) that is 30% higher than those who do not [29].

8.3.2.7 MAGNESIUM

All of the body's cells require magnesium. It contributes to the preservation of ideal bone and cardiovascular health, as well as proper nerve and muscle function. Magnesium is an essential component for several enzyme systems that control biological processes. Chronic alcoholism, certain drugs, type 2 diabetes, and gastrointestinal disorders can all increase a person's chance of developing a magnesium deficit. Deficiency symptoms include weakness, weariness, nausea, and vomiting. Severe shortages cause problems with nerve and cardiac function, as well as the balance of calcium and potassium.

There is a lot of magnesium in food and drink. Legumes, seeds, and unprocessed whole grains are examples of sources. Foods high in magnesium includes cashew nuts, baked beans, soybeans, and pumpkin seeds.

Spinach and other dark green, leafy plants are excellent providers of magnesium because chlorophyll contains it. Dried beans and legumes are sources, as are milk and yogurt. In comparison to a mixed diet, where the presence of heme iron (an animal source) improves the absorption of non-heme iron (a plant source), a strict vegetarian diet has reduced iron bioavailability. A diet heavy in meats, dairy products, and refined carbohydrates is low in magnesium [30].

8.3.2.8 ZINC

In addition to supporting immunological response and helping with wound healing, DNA synthesis, cell division, and protein synthesis, zinc is an enzyme cofactor. Adequate zinc is necessary for normal taste and smell; however, the body cannot retain zinc; therefore, it needs to be regularly supplemented. Normal growth and development from infancy through adolescence depend on zinc [31].

Zinc can be found in foods high in quality protein, such as chicken and red meat. Whole cereals, legumes, and grains are good sources of zinc; however, they also contain phytates, which are phosphorus compounds stored in plants that bind zinc and hinder its absorption. This characteristic explains the term "antinutritional factors" for phytates. Deficiencies are present in populations where the main supply of zinc is phytate-containing cereals (wheat, rice, and maize) [31].

Throat lozenges and syrups containing zinc lessen the symptoms of the common cold by preventing rhinovirus attachment in the sinuses and nose. It is easy to overindulge in zinc supplements, and doing so increases the risk of negative health outcomes, such as heart disease (which is caused by a decrease in HDL production) and immune system dysfunction [32].

8.3.3 DIGESTIVE ENZYMES

Digestive enzymes, once relegated to the realm of physiological processes within the human body, have now found a prominent role in the domain of nutraceuticals. Emerging as valuable supplements, digestive enzymes play a pivotal role in supporting the efficient breakdown of macronutrients, facilitating their absorption and utilization. These nutraceuticals encompass a spectrum of enzymes such as amylases, proteases, and lipases, each tailored to target specific components of the diet. Amylases aid in the digestion of carbohydrates, proteases tackle proteins, and lipases break down fats. Incorporating digestive enzymes as nutraceuticals is particularly relevant in modern dietary contexts, where processed foods and lifestyle factors can challenge the body's natural digestive processes. By supplementing with these enzymes, individuals aim to optimize digestion, alleviate digestive discomfort, and potentially enhance nutrient absorption. As the understanding of the intricate interplay between nutrition and digestive function deepens, digestive enzymes stand as versatile allies in promoting gastrointestinal health and overall well-being.

8.3.4 DIETARY FIBERS

Dietary fibers derived from cereals and grains have emerged as valuable sources of nutraceuticals, contributing significantly to overall health and well-being. These fibrous components, often found in the outer layers of grains, play a crucial role in promoting digestive health, managing weight, and regulating blood sugar levels. Soluble fibers, such as beta-glucans in oats and barley, have been associated with cholesterol reduction and cardiovascular health. Insoluble fibers, prevalent in wheat bran and whole grains, support bowel regularity and aid in preventing constipation. Cereals like quinoa and amaranth are not only rich in fibers but also provide essential amino acids (EAAs), making them wholesome sources of plant-based nutrition. The consumption of these nutraceutical-rich grains has been linked to a range of health benefits, including improved gut microbiota and reduced risk of chronic diseases. As the interest in functional foods grows, cereals and grains continue to be at the forefront of the nutraceutical landscape, offering a natural and sustainable approach to enhancing health through dietary choices.

8.4 HERBS AS FUNCTIONAL FOODS, POLYUNSATURATED FATTY ACIDS (PUFA), AND ANTIOXIDANTS

Food items that provide health advantages beyond their fundamental nutritional worth are referred to as functional foods. They contain bioactive compounds that can positively impact physiological functions and contribute to overall well-being. The significance of functional foods lies in their potential to promote health, prevent diseases, and improve the quality of life. This chapter explores the integral components of functional foods, focusing on antioxidants, polyunsaturated fatty acids (PUFAs), and herbs [4, 33, 34].

8.5 SIGNIFICANCE OF FUNCTIONAL FOODS

Foods that include bioactive substances and offer health advantages above and beyond basic nourishment are referred to as functional foods. These compounds may include vitamins, minerals, phytochemicals, probiotics, and other essential nutrients. The significance of functional foods lies in their ability to enhance various physiological functions and contribute to the prevention or management of diseases. Unlike traditional foods, functional foods are intentionally designed to have positive effects on health [35–37]. Functional foods can play a crucial role in promoting wellness, supporting specific health conditions, and addressing nutritional deficiencies. Examples include foods fortified with vitamins, minerals, omega-3 fatty acids, and those containing probiotics or antioxidants. The growing interest in functional foods reflects a shift toward proactive health management and a recognition of the strong connection between diet and well-being.

8.6 ROLE OF ANTIOXIDANTS AND POLYUNSATURATED FATTY ACIDS (PUFA) IN HEALTH

Antioxidants and PUFAs are key components of functional foods known for their profound impact on health.

8.6.1 ANTIOXIDANTS

Compounds known as antioxidants aid in the body's defense against dangerous free radicals. Free radicals are produced by both environmental and regular metabolic activities. They can harm cells and play a role in aging and several diseases, such as cancer and cardiovascular conditions. Fruits, vegetables, and other plant-based diets are rich in antioxidants, which are essential for reducing inflammation and oxidative stress [38].

8.6.2 POLYUNSATURATED FATTY ACIDS (PUFAS)

The body is unable to generate PUFAs, which include omega-3 and omega-6 fatty acids, on its own. These facts are essential for controlling inflammation, preserving brain function, and maintaining cell integrity. Omega-6 fatty acids are present in vegetable oils, but omega-3 fatty acids are prevalent in walnuts, flaxseeds, and fatty fish. For general health, a balanced ratio of omega-3 to omega-6 must be achieved [39].

8.7 HERBS AS POTENTIAL SOURCES OF FUNCTIONAL COMPOUNDS

Herbs, with their rich array of phytochemicals and bioactive compounds, are increasingly recognized as valuable contributors to functional foods. These plant-derived substances often exhibit antioxidant, anti-inflammatory, and other health-promoting properties.

8.7.1 MEDICINAL PROPERTIES

Herbs such as ginseng, garlic, turmeric, and others have been traditionally used for their medicinal properties. These include anti-inflammatory, antimicrobial, and immune-boosting effects.

8.7.2 HEALTH BENEFITS

Herbs are beneficial to the immune system, the cardiovascular system, and cognitive function. Furthermore, herbs are frequently rich in vitamins, minerals, and antioxidants that support general health [38–40].

8.7.3 ANTIOXIDANTS

A broad class of substances known as antioxidants is essential to preserving the delicate equilibrium of oxidative reactions in the body. These compounds neutralize the damaging effects of unstable molecules called free radicals that lack paired electrons. Normal metabolic processes, exposure to environmental contaminants, and other stressors can all produce free radicals. As scavengers, antioxidants neutralize free radicals and stop them from harming tissues and cells [40].

8.7.3.1 TYPES OF ANTIOXIDANTS

Comprising a wide range of molecules, antioxidants are essential for preserving the delicate equilibrium of oxidative reactions in the body. The negative effects of free radicals, which are unstable molecules with unpaired electrons, are mitigated by these compounds. In addition to exposure to environmental contaminants, regular metabolic processes can also produce free radicals. By neutralizing free radicals and stopping them from damaging cells and tissues, antioxidants function as scavengers (Figure 8.1) [41].

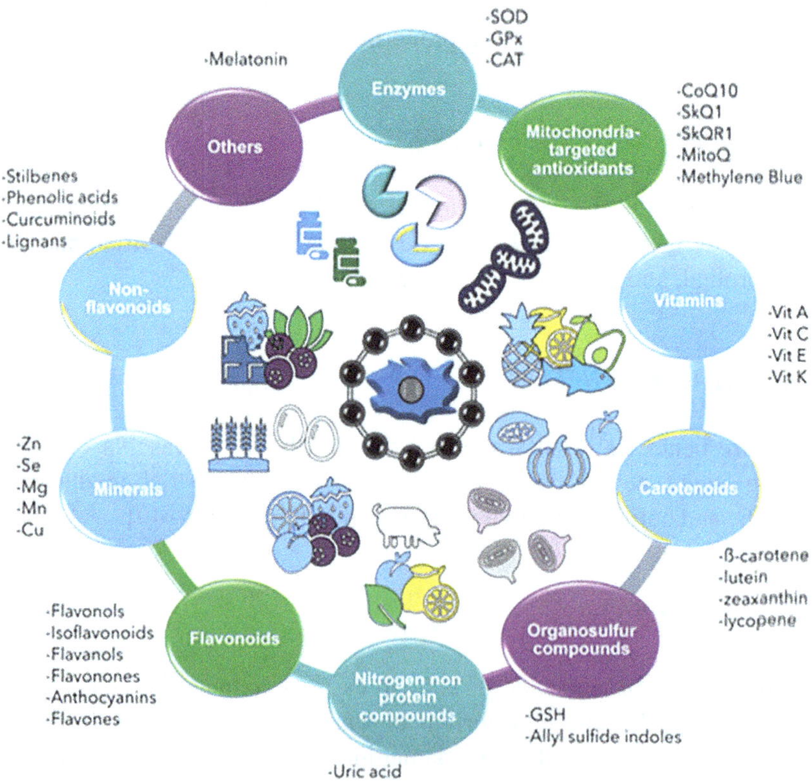

FIGURE 8.1 Types of antioxidants.

8.7.3.2 SOURCES OF ANTIOXIDANTS

Antioxidants are abundant in fruits, vegetables, nuts, seeds, and whole grains. Each antioxidant-rich food may contain a unique combination of compounds, contributing to a diverse range of health benefits.

8.7.4 IMPORTANCE IN COMBATING OXIDATIVE STRESS AND FREE RADICALS

8.7.4.1 OXIDATIVE STRESS

An imbalance between the body's capacity to eliminate free radicals and their creation can lead to oxidative stress. This imbalance can cause inflammation, damage to cells, and the advancement of several illnesses, including cancer, neurological diseases, and cardiovascular diseases (CVDs).

8.7.4.2 NEUTRALIZING FREE RADICALS

Antioxidants play a pivotal role in neutralizing free radicals by donating electrons to stabilize these reactive molecules. This process helps prevent oxidative damage to lipids, proteins, and DNA. By mitigating oxidative stress, antioxidants contribute to the overall health and resilience of cells and tissues.

8.7.5 ROLE IN PREVENTING CHRONIC DISEASES

8.7.5.1 CARDIOVASCULAR HEALTH

When there is an imbalance between the body's capacity to eliminate free radicals and their creation, oxidative stress results. Damage to cells, inflammation, and the advancement of several illnesses, including cancer, neurological problems, and CVDs, can result from this imbalance.

8.7.5.2 NEUROPROTECTION

The role of antioxidants in supporting brain health is evident in their ability to combat oxidative stress, which is implicated in neurodegenerative conditions such as Alzheimer's and Parkinson's diseases. Antioxidants may help protect neurons and maintain cognitive function.

8.7.5.3 CANCER PREVENTION

Antioxidants, through their anti-inflammatory and DNA-protective effects, have been studied for their potential role in cancer prevention. They may help reduce the risk of certain cancers by neutralizing free radicals that could otherwise contribute to the initiation and progression of cancerous cells.

8.7.5.4 AGING AND LONGEVITY

The cumulative effects of oxidative stress contribute to the aging process. Antioxidants may play a role in extending lifespan and promoting healthy aging by minimizing cellular damage and supporting overall cellular function. Understanding the broad spectrum of antioxidants, their sources, and their critical role in combating oxidative stress establishes a foundation for appreciating their application in functional foods and their potential impact on health and disease prevention. Subsequent sections will delve into specific antioxidants found in various foods and their associated health benefits [42, 43].

8.8 POLYUNSATURATED FATTY ACID (PUFA)

8.8.1 ESSENTIAL FATTY ACIDS

PUFAs are a category of fats characterized by the presence of multiple double bonds in their chemical structure. They include omega-3 and omega-6 fatty acids, both of which are essential, meaning the body cannot synthesize them and must obtain them from the diet. PUFAs are integral components of cell membranes and are involved in various physiological processes. The structure of saturated and unsaturated fatty acids is given in Figure 8.2.

8.8.2 OMEGA-3 FATTY ACIDS

Omega-3 fatty acids, such as alpha-linolenic acid (ALA), eicosapentaenoic acid (EPA), and docosahexaenoic acid (DHA), are well-known PUFAs with distinct health benefits. ALA is primarily found in plant sources, while EPA and DHA are commonly found in fatty fish.

8.8.3 OMEGA-6 FATTY ACIDS

Omega-6 fatty acids, including linoleic acid (LA) and arachidonic acid (AA), are also essential and are found in various vegetable oils, nuts, and seeds.

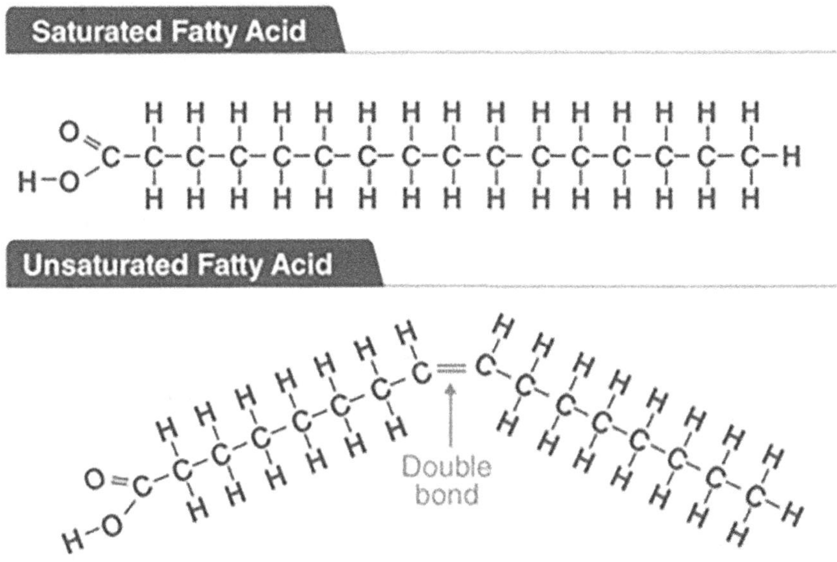

FIGURE 8.2 Types of fatty acid.

8.9 HEALTH BENEFITS AND ROLE IN CARDIOVASCULAR HEALTH

8.9.1 CARDIOPROTECTIVE EFFECTS

PUFAs, particularly omega-3 fatty acids, have been associated with a range of cardiovascular benefits. They help lower blood triglyceride levels, reduce blood pressure, and improve arterial function, collectively contributing to a reduced risk of CVDs.

8.9.2 ANTI-INFLAMMATORY EFFICACY

PUFAs play a key role in modulating the inflammatory response. Omega-3 fatty acids are known for their anti-inflammatory effects, which can help mitigate chronic inflammation implicated in various cardiovascular conditions.

8.9.3 BLOOD LIPID REGULATION

Omega-3 fatty acids contribute to the regulation of lipid metabolism by reducing the levels of harmful LDL cholesterol while increasing the levels of beneficial HDL cholesterol. This balance is essential for maintaining cardiovascular health.

8.9.4 BLOOD PRESSURE MANAGEMENT

PUFAs, especially omega-3s, have been shown to have a vasodilatory effect, helping to relax blood vessels and lower blood pressure. This effect is beneficial in preventing hypertension and its associated complications.

8.10 SOURCES OF POLYUNSATURATED FATTY ACIDS (PUFAS) AND THEIR DIETARY IMPORTANCE

8.10.1 OMEGA-3 SOURCES

Fatty fish such as salmon, mackerel, sardines, and trout are rich sources of EPA and DHA. Flaxseeds and chia seeds provide ALA, a precursor to EPA and DHA, whereas walnuts are a good source of ALA and offer additional health benefits.

8.10.2 OMEGA-6 SOURCES

Vegetable oils from sunflower, safflower, corn, and soybean are high in omega-6 fatty acids, while nuts and seeds such as almonds and sunflower seeds also contain omega-6 fatty acids.

8.10.3 DIETARY IMPORTANCE

Achieving a balanced ratio of omega-3 to omega-6 fatty acids is crucial for optimal health. The Western diet often contains an imbalance, with an overabundance of omega-6 compared to omega-3. A balanced intake supports cellular structure, brain function, and overall inflammatory balance. Understanding the fundamentals of PUFAs, their health benefits, and dietary sources sets the stage for exploring their role in functional foods and their potential impact on overall health and well-being. Subsequent sections will delve into specific PUFAs, their formulations, and their relevance in functional nutrition [44–50].

8.11 HERBS AS FUNCTIONAL FOODS

8.11.1 CLASSIFICATION OF HERBS AS FUNCTIONAL FOODS

Herbs, in the context of functional foods, refer to plants or plant parts that are used for culinary, medicinal, or therapeutic purposes due to their inherent bioactive compounds. These compounds contribute to the health-promoting properties of herbs, making them valuable components of functional foods. Herbs are classified as functional foods based on their ability to provide physiological benefits beyond basic nutrition. They contain a diverse array of phytochemicals, including polyphenols, flavonoids, terpenes, and alkaloids, which contribute to their functional properties. Culinary herbs, which are used primarily for flavoring and aroma in cooking, include basil, oregano, and thyme, whereas medicinal herbs are utilized for their therapeutic properties, addressing specific health concerns.

8.11.2 MEDICINAL PROPERTIES AND HEALTH BENEFITS OF SELECTED HERBS

Understanding the classification of herbs as functional foods and exploring the medicinal properties and health benefits of selected herbs lays the foundation for incorporating these plant-based ingredients into a functional nutrition approach. The following sections will delve into the sources, marker compounds, and specific health-promoting aspects of each herb, offering a comprehensive understanding of their role in functional foods. Table 8.1 gives an overview of the medicinal properties and health benefits of some selected herbs [51–57].

TABLE 8.1 Medicinal Properties and Health Benefits of Selected Herbs

Name	Medicinal Properties	Health Benefits
Ginseng	Adaptogenic, anti-fatigue, immune enhancing	Improved energy, stress reduction, cognitive function support
Garlic	Antimicrobial, anti-inflammatory, cardiovascular support	Lowering cholesterol, blood pressure regulation, immune system support
Turmeric	Anti-inflammatory, antioxidant, anti-cancer	Joint health, digestive support, immune modulation
Spirulina	Rich in nutrients, antioxidant	Immune support, energy boost, detoxification
Broccoli	Anticancer, antioxidant, anti-inflammatory	Detoxification, cardiovascular health, digestive support
Green and herbal tea	Antioxidant, anti-inflammatory, anti-cancer	Weight management, cardiovascular support, cognitive function
Soya bean	Cardiovascular support, hormone regulation	Protein source, cholesterol management, menopausal symptom relief
Flax seeds	Rich in omega-3 fatty acids, antioxidant	Cardiovascular health, digestive support, anti-inflammatory
Black cohosh	Hormone regulation, anti-inflammatory	Menopausal symptom relief, mood stabilization

8.12 FORMULATION AND STANDARDIZATION OF NUTRACEUTICALS

8.12.1 FORMULATION TECHNIQUES FOR FUNCTIONAL FOODS

In the formulation of functional foods, the initial step involves meticulous ingredient selection to target specific health benefits. Key functional ingredients are identified based on their inherent bioactive compounds, ensuring thoughtful consideration of their potential synergistic effects when combined. To optimize the effectiveness of these ingredients, strategies for enhancing bioavailability are employed. Techniques such as microencapsulation are harnessed to improve absorption and provide controlled release, maximizing the therapeutic impact of bioactive compounds. In addition to health benefits, the success of functional foods hinges on consumer acceptance, emphasizing the importance of texture and palatability. The sensory aspects of the product are carefully optimized, striking a delicate balance between functionality and the sensory experience, encompassing taste, texture, and appearance. This holistic approach ensures that consumers not only derive health benefits but also enjoy the overall consumption experience.

Fortification and enrichment play a pivotal role in elevating the nutritional value of functional foods. Essential nutrients, including vitamins and minerals, are incorporated strategically to fortify the product in alignment with dietary guidelines and safety standards. This process ensures that the functional foods not only deliver targeted health benefits but also contribute to overall nutritional well-being. The pursuit of innovation extends to processing methods, where novel techniques are explored to retain the maximum nutritional value of ingredients. Cold pressing and fermentation are examples of methods that preserve the integrity of bioactive compounds during production. By embracing cutting-edge technologies, the formulation of functional foods remains at the forefront of nutritional innovation, offering products that are both health-enhancing and technologically sophisticated.

8.12.2 IMPORTANCE OF STANDARDIZATION FOR QUALITY CONTROL

Achieving and maintaining consistency in bioactive content is paramount in the formulation of nutraceuticals, ensuring that the final product delivers reliable and reproducible health benefits. This involves establishing and adhering to standardized levels of key bioactive compounds, guaranteeing consistent dosages that users can depend on for their intended health-promoting effects. To uphold the highest standards of quality, stringent quality assurance measures are implemented throughout the entire production process. This includes robust monitoring of raw material quality and the application of good manufacturing practices (GMP) to guarantee the safety and efficacy of the nutraceutical product. In addition to internal quality control, nutraceutical manufacturers must prioritize regulatory compliance to meet industry standards and guidelines. This involves meticulous adherence to regulations governing the production of nutraceuticals, ensuring that the product meets the necessary safety and quality benchmarks. Providing comprehensive documentation and evidence of compliance becomes imperative in substantiating adherence to regulatory requirements.

The consistency and reliability of health-promoting properties not only satisfy regulatory demands but also contribute significantly to building consumer confidence. Trust is cultivated by consistently delivering nutraceuticals with reliable bioactive content, thereby fulfilling the promised health benefits. To further instill confidence, standardized testing methods are employed to verify the presence and concentration of bioactive compounds, assuring consumers of the efficacy and authenticity of the nutraceutical product. Through a commitment to quality, regulatory compliance, and transparency, nutraceutical manufacturers can establish a solid foundation for consumer trust and satisfaction.

8.12.3 CHALLENGES AND CONSIDERATIONS IN NUTRACEUTICAL DEVELOPMENT

Navigating the complexities of nutraceutical development requires a comprehensive approach to overcome challenges and ensure the efficacy of functional foods. Bioavailability poses a significant hurdle, demanding solutions for the poor absorption or stability of bioactive compounds. Innovative delivery systems, including nanotechnology and liposomes, offer promising avenues to enhance the bioavailability of these compounds. Taste and palatability considerations add another layer of complexity, necessitating the addressing of taste challenges associated with certain bioactive ingredients. Techniques like flavor masking or strategic selection of delivery formats are employed to enhance overall palatability.

In the realm of nutraceuticals, adherence to regulatory standards is paramount, given the complex and evolving regulatory landscapes. Ensuring compliance with health claims and labeling regulations requires a thorough understanding of the regulatory complexities in different markets. Additionally, staying abreast of evolving standards is essential to maintain product integrity.

Balancing the inclusion of high-quality ingredients with cost considerations presents a delicate challenge. Nutraceutical developers must explore formulation approaches that are cost-effective without compromising the efficacy of the final product. This strategic balance ensures that the resulting functional foods are accessible to a broader consumer base.

Scientific research and substantiation form the backbone of nutraceutical development. Crafting products based on sound scientific evidence and investing in research to substantiate health claims are pivotal. This commitment to rigorous scientific validation not only strengthens the credibility of nutraceuticals but also reinforces their potential impact on consumer health. Understanding the formulation techniques, emphasizing standardization, and addressing challenges in nutraceutical development are foundational to creating functional foods that not only meet high-quality standards but also offer reliable health benefits. The subsequent sections will delve into regulatory aspects and guidelines while exploring specific sources of nutraceuticals, such as spirulina, soybean, ginseng, garlic, broccoli, green and herbal tea, flax seeds, black cohosh, and turmeric [58–69].

8.13 REGULATORY ASPECTS AND FOOD SAFETY AND STANDARDS AUTHORITY OF INDIA (FSSAI) GUIDELINES

8.13.1 GLOBAL REGULATORY LANDSCAPE

Navigating the global regulatory landscape is essential for the development and marketing of functional foods. This involves a comprehensive exploration of regulatory frameworks established by international bodies such as the U.S. Food and Drug Administration (FDA), the European Food Safety Authority (EFSA), and the Codex Alimentarius. Understanding the nuances and variations in regulations across different countries and regions is crucial to ensure compliance with diverse standards governing functional foods.

Clearly defining functional foods within the regulatory context is foundational. This includes specifying criteria for their classification and differentiating them from dietary supplements, conventional foods, and medicinal products. By delineating these categories, regulatory compliance becomes more streamlined, allowing for a precise understanding of the regulatory requirements applicable to functional foods.

8.13.2 HEALTH CLAIMS AND LABELING

Regulations concerning the approval and use of health claims on functional food labels require careful consideration. It is imperative to evaluate and adhere to guidelines that dictate the accurate and transparent labeling of products. Understanding the intricacies of health claim approval processes and ensuring compliance with labeling regulations not only enhances product credibility but also fosters consumer trust by providing clear and truthful information.

A thorough exploration of the global regulatory landscape, coupled with precise definitions and adherence to health claims and labeling guidelines, establishes a robust foundation for the development and marketing of functional foods. This comprehensive approach ensures that products meet the necessary regulatory standards across diverse markets, fostering both compliance and consumer confidence.

8.13.3 GUIDELINES AND THEIR ROLE IN ENSURING SAFETY AND EFFICACY

8.13.3.1 ROLE OF FOOD SAFETY AND STANDARDS AUTHORITY OF INDIA (FSSAI)

Understanding the mandate and pivotal role of the Food Safety and Standards Authority of India (FSSAI) is foundational for those involved in the regulation of functional foods in India. Compliance with FSSAI regulations is paramount, ensuring not only market access but also the safety of consumers. The FSSAI plays a crucial role in setting standards, regulating food safety, and safeguarding public health, making adherence to its guidelines a cornerstone in the development and marketing of functional foods.

8.13.3.2 PRODUCT APPROVAL PROCESS

Familiarizing oneself with the intricate procedures for obtaining approval for novel ingredients or formulations is essential. This involves navigating the product approval process set forth by the FSSAI, which requires the submission of necessary documentation and scientific evidence. Providing robust support for safety and efficacy claims is a crucial aspect of this process, ensuring that products meet the rigorous standards set by the FSSAI before entering the market.

8.13.3.3 LABELING REQUIREMENTS

Adhering to FSSAI guidelines for accurate and informative product labeling is a non-negotiable aspect of regulatory compliance. This includes incorporating mandatory information on product labels, such as nutritional facts, ingredient lists, and storage instructions. Conforming to these labeling requirements not only ensures transparency but also aids consumers in making informed choices about the functional foods they consume.

8.13.3.4 CONTAMINANT LIMITS

Compliance with FSSAI regulations regarding permissible limits of contaminants in functional foods is of utmost importance. Rigorous testing for contaminants such as pesticides, heavy metals, and microbiological agents is necessary to meet these standards. Ensuring that functional foods adhere to the defined limits for contaminants safeguards both consumer health and regulatory compliance.

8.13.3.5 ADDITIVES AND INGREDIENTS APPROVAL

Obtaining FSSAI approval for the use of specific additives and ingredients is a critical step in the development of functional foods. Adhering to permissible limits and usage conditions, as defined by the FSSAI, ensures that the inclusion of additives and ingredients aligns with regulatory standards. This approval process is integral to guaranteeing the safety and quality of functional foods in the Indian market.

In conclusion, a comprehensive understanding of the FSSAI's role, coupled with meticulous adherence to its regulations, is fundamental for successfully navigating the regulatory landscape governing functional foods in India. This approach not only facilitates market access but also upholds the highest standards of safety and transparency in the food industry.

8.13.4 COMPLIANCE WITH REGULATORY STANDARDS IN THE DEVELOPMENT AND MARKETING OF NUTRACEUTICALS

8.13.4.1 QUALITY CONTROL AND ASSURANCE

Implementing robust quality control measures is imperative to ensure strict adherence to regulatory standards governing functional foods. Establishing comprehensive quality assurance protocols further guarantees consistent product quality throughout the manufacturing process. This commitment to quality control and assurance not only meets regulatory requirements but also underscores the commitment to delivering reliable and safe functional foods to consumers.

8.13.4.2 DOCUMENTATION AND RECORD-KEEPING

Maintaining meticulous records of raw materials, manufacturing processes, and quality control procedures is a foundational aspect of regulatory compliance. This comprehensive documentation not only facilitates internal quality management but also prepares the manufacturer for potential audits and inspections by regulatory authorities. The ability to provide detailed records enhances transparency and accountability in the production of functional foods.

8.13.4.3 SCIENTIFIC SUBSTANTIATION

Conducting and thoroughly documenting scientific studies that support health claims associated with functional foods is critical. It is essential to ensure that product formulations are not only innovative but also grounded in credible scientific evidence. This scientific substantiation not only strengthens the product's market position but also aligns with regulatory expectations for evidence-based claims.

8.13.4.4 ADVERSE EVENT REPORTING

Developing a robust system for monitoring and promptly reporting adverse events linked to the consumption of functional foods is a key component of responsible manufacturing. Compliance with regulatory requirements for timely reporting to relevant authorities is crucial. This proactive approach to adverse event reporting demonstrates a commitment to consumer safety and regulatory transparency.

8.13.4.5 MARKET AUTHORIZATION

Seeking necessary approvals and authorizations from regulatory bodies before introducing functional foods to the market is a fundamental step. Compliance with post-market surveillance requirements ensures ongoing adherence to regulatory standards and facilitates continuous monitoring of product safety. This proactive engagement with regulatory processes is integral to a successful and legally compliant market entry.

Understanding and adhering to regulatory frameworks, particularly those outlined by FSSAI, is essential for ensuring the safety, efficacy, and legality of functional foods. Compliance with these standards not only facilitates market access but also instills consumer confidence in the quality and reliability of nutraceutical products. The subsequent sections will delve into specific sources of nutraceuticals, including spirulina, soybean, ginseng, garlic, broccoli, green and herbal tea, flax seeds, black cohosh, and turmeric [70–73].

8.14 SPIRULINA

Spirulina, a vibrant blue-green microalgae, flourishes in warm and alkaline aquatic environments, notably in ponds and lakes. The predominant species harnessed for commercial purposes are *Arthrospira platensis* and *Arthrospira maxima*. Cultivation of Spirulina is a carefully managed process that occurs in controlled environments, ranging from open ponds to closed systems. This cultivation journey necessitates the provision of optimal conditions, ensuring an interplay of sufficient sunlight exposure, maintaining appropriate pH levels, and utilizing nutrient-rich growth media. By meticulously controlling these variables, Spirulina cultivators aim to harness its unique properties and nutritional richness for various applications in the realm of functional foods and nutraceuticals.

Spirulina boasts a distinctive biochemical profile featuring key compounds that contribute to its nutritional and functional properties. Phycocyanin, a striking blue pigment unique to Spirulina, not only imparts the characteristic blue-green color to the microalgae but also brings along potent antioxidant and anti-inflammatory properties. Extensive studies have delved into the potential of phycocyanin, revealing promising aspects such as its role in anti-cancer effects and immune system modulation. Moving to chlorophyll, Spirulina is rich in this green pigment crucial for photosynthesis. Beyond its role in plant energy conversion, chlorophyll in Spirulina serves as a robust antioxidant with detoxifying properties, potentially supporting blood health, and aiding in detoxification processes. Additionally, Spirulina shines in its carotenoid content, including beta-carotene, zeaxanthin, and lutein. Beta-carotene, a precursor to vitamin A, contributes to Spirulina's immune-boosting attributes, while zeaxanthin and lutein play crucial roles in maintaining eye health. The amalgamation of these compounds underscores Spirulina's significance as a multifaceted functional food with potential health-promoting effects.

Spirulina emerges as a nutritional powerhouse, positioned as a nutrient-dense superfood with a comprehensive profile that includes protein, essential vitamins (B-complex, including B12), vital minerals (iron and calcium), and essential fatty acids. The medicinal uses and health benefits of it are highlighted in Figure 8.3. This nutritional richness renders Spirulina invaluable for addressing deficiencies in a diverse array of essential nutrients. Beyond its nutrient content, Spirulina exhibits remarkable antioxidant and anti-inflammatory properties attributed to compounds like phycocyanin. This unique blend allows Spirulina to neutralize free radicals, mitigate oxidative stress, and potentially contribute to overall health by combating inflammation. Furthermore, Spirulina's immunomodulatory effects have been subject to scientific scrutiny, revealing potential enhancements in the activity of immune cells, with the presence of beta-glucans further contributing to immune system modulation. In the realm of cardiometabolic health, Spirulina showcases promising potential by positively influencing lipid profiles, potentially lowering cholesterol levels, and reducing blood pressure. Its chlorophyll content plays a role in detoxification processes by binding to and eliminating toxins. Additionally, some studies suggest that Spirulina supplementation may assist in weight management, fostering a sense of satiety. While further research is warranted, preliminary studies hint at potential anti-cancer effects, particularly with the investigation of phycocyanin's role in inhibiting cancer cell growth. Despite its numerous health benefits, it is prudent for individuals, especially those with pre-existing health conditions or allergies, to consult with healthcare professionals before incorporating Spirulina into their diet, recognizing the importance of personalized health considerations [74–80].

8.15 SOYA BEAN

Soybeans stand out as a nutritional powerhouse, offering a diverse array of health-promoting components. Notably, they serve as an excellent source of plant-based protein, presenting all EAAs and positioning soy protein as a high-quality alternative comparable to animal-based sources. The inclusion of soybeans in the diet contributes not only to protein intake but also to the enhancement of overall dietary fiber content. Rich in dietary fiber, soybeans support digestive health and play a crucial role in regulating

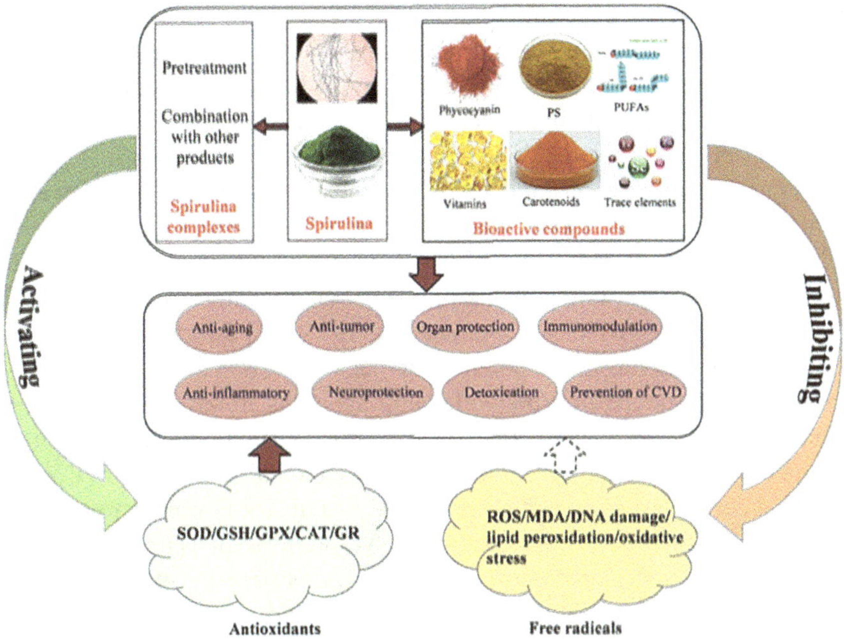

FIGURE 8.3 Medicinal uses and health benefits of spirulina.

blood sugar levels. In addition to protein and fiber, soybeans provide a healthy dose of polyunsaturated fats, encompassing both omega-3 and omega-6 fatty acids. This composition contributes significantly to cardiovascular health, emphasizing soybeans as a heart-friendly food choice. Furthermore, soybeans pack a nutritional punch with essential vitamins such as B vitamins (including folate) and an array of minerals including iron, calcium, and magnesium. The well-rounded nutrient profile of soybeans, coupled with their low saturated fat content, positions them as a multifaceted and heart-healthy addition to a balanced diet. Incorporating soybeans into one's meals not only satisfies protein requirements but also contributes to overall nutritional well-being, making them a valuable component of a health-conscious dietary regimen.

Soybeans contain bioactive compounds that contribute to their health-promoting properties. Foremost among these are isoflavones, phytoestrogens found in soybeans, with genistein and daidzein being notable representatives. Isoflavones possess estrogenic properties, potentially exerting hormone-like effects in the body. These compounds have garnered attention for their potential role in hormonal balance and their association with various health benefits. Additionally, soybeans house saponins, naturally occurring compounds that bring potential health advantages. Saponins have been studied for their ability to contribute to the prevention of certain diseases, and they particularly stand out for their investigated cholesterol-lowering effects. As part of the intricate composition of soybeans, isoflavones and saponins contribute not only to the plant's unique flavor but also to its potential as a functional food with diverse health-promoting attributes. The exploration of these bioactive compounds continues to deepen our understanding of the comprehensive health benefits offered by soybeans.

Soybeans and soy-based products emerge as a powerhouse of health benefits, showcasing their potential impact on various aspects of well-being. The presence of isoflavones and saponins in soybeans has been linked to cardiovascular advantages, with soy consumption demonstrating the potential to lower LDL cholesterol levels and reduce the risk of CVDs. Beyond cardiovascular health, the isoflavones in soy exhibit estrogen-like effects, offering relief from menopausal symptoms such as hot flashes and night sweats. Soy isoflavones also play a potential role in contributing to bone health by modulating bone turnover and mitigating the risk of osteoporosis. Moreover, soybeans show promise in cancer prevention, with studies suggesting protective effects against certain types of cancer, including breast and prostate cancers. The fiber content in soybeans contributes to blood sugar regulation, making them beneficial for individuals with diabetes, while soy protein's ability to promote satiety aids in weight management by reducing overall calorie intake. Additionally, the dietary fiber in soybeans supports digestive health by promoting regular bowel movements and preventing constipation. Furthermore, soybeans' antioxidant properties, coupled with their ability to neutralize free radicals, contribute to overall cellular health. While soy and soy-based products offer a versatile and nutritious addition to a balanced diet, individuals with soy allergies or specific medical conditions should consult healthcare professionals before incorporating significant amounts of soy into their diets. As with any food or supplement, moderation remains key, recognizing that individual responses may vary [81].

8.16 GINSENG

Ginseng, a root prized for its medicinal properties, comes in various types, each with distinct characteristics and historical uses. Asian ginseng, scientifically known as Panax ginseng, originates from East Asia, particularly China and Korea. Often referred to as Korean or Chinese ginseng, it has been a staple in traditional Chinese medicine for centuries. It comes in two main varieties: white ginseng, which is dried, and red ginseng, which undergoes a steaming and drying process, enhancing its therapeutic properties. American ginseng, or *Panax quinquefolius*, is native to North America, primarily found in the United States and Canada. While it shares similarities with Asian ginseng, American ginseng is often considered milder in its effects. It exists in wild and cultivated varieties, and like its Asian counterpart, it holds a significant place in herbal medicine. Siberian ginseng, scientifically *Eleutherococcus senticosus*, hails from Russia, China, Japan, and Korea. Despite being commonly referred to as ginseng, Siberian ginseng comes from a different botanical genus. Also known as Eleuthero, it has been traditionally used in both Russian and Chinese medicine, known for its adaptogenic properties. These different types of ginseng have been integral parts of traditional medicine systems across the globe, with each variety holding cultural significance and a history of use in promoting overall health and well-being.

Ginsenosides, the cornerstone of ginseng's pharmacological activity, are bioactive compounds that underpin the herb's therapeutic effects. These compounds, including variants like Rb1, Rg1, and Re, are found in different types of ginsengs and are responsible for eliciting various health benefits. Ginsenosides are crucial contributors to ginseng's adaptogenic properties, playing a pivotal role in assisting the body in adapting to stress. As primary active constituents, these compounds are central to understanding the diverse physiological responses and health-promoting effects associated with ginseng consumption. The intricate interplay of ginsenosides within ginseng highlights the herb's complexity and the importance of these bioactive components in unlocking its potential for supporting overall well-being.

Ginseng, recognized for its adaptogenic properties, stands out as a multifaceted natural remedy with a diverse range of health benefits rooted in both traditional medicine and contemporary scientific studies. Classified as an adaptogen, ginseng aids the body in navigating physical and mental stress, promoting resilience, heightened energy levels, and a reduction in fatigue. Scientific evidence supports its cognitive-enhancing effects, showcasing improvements in memory, concentration, and overall mental performance. The immunomodulatory effects of ginsenosides, the bioactive compounds in ginseng, contribute to the regulation of the immune system and fortify the body's defense mechanisms. As an energy booster and stamina enhancer, it finds popularity among athletes, offering a natural solution for combating fatigue and enhancing physical endurance. Ginseng's adaptogenic properties also play a role in stress reduction, mitigating both the physiological and psychological impacts of stress. Additionally, research has explored its anti-inflammatory properties and antioxidant activity, further enhancing its overall health benefits.

In the realm of specific health considerations, ginseng shows promise in diabetes management by potentially impacting blood sugar levels. Traditionally used to support sexual health, ginseng's potential benefits extend to conditions like erectile dysfunction and libido, as suggested by research. Moreover, its cardiovascular benefits, including improved blood circulation and blood pressure regulation, add another dimension to its comprehensive health-promoting profile. While ginseng's versatility and efficacy are well-established, individual responses can vary. It is advisable for individuals, especially those with existing medical conditions or taking medications, to consult healthcare professionals before integrating ginseng into their health regimens. The convergence of historical use and contemporary research underscores ginseng's standing as a valuable and versatile natural remedy [82–92].

8.17 GARLIC

Garlic, renowned for both its culinary allure and medicinal properties, derives much of its therapeutic value from key sulfur-containing compounds. Foremost among these is allicin, a bioactive compound released when fresh garlic undergoes crushing or chopping. Allicin is distinguished for its robust antimicrobial, anti-inflammatory, and antioxidant properties, making it a cornerstone of garlic's medicinal benefits. This sulfur compound is implicated in various health applications, contributing not only to the distinct flavor of garlic but also to its broad-spectrum health-promoting effects. In addition to allicin, garlic boasts other sulfur compounds such as diallyl sulfide, diallyl disulfide, and diallyl trisulfide, each imparting the characteristic aroma and flavor associated with garlic. Beyond sensory appeal, these sulfur compounds have been linked to diverse health benefits, encompassing cardiovascular support and immune system modulation. The intricate synergy of these sulfur compounds within garlic underscores the herb's rich therapeutic potential, offering a compelling blend of culinary delight and holistic well-being.

Garlic, renowned for its culinary and medicinal significance, stands as a versatile ally in promoting holistic well-being. Its therapeutic value is rooted in sulfur-containing compounds, with allicin taking center stage. Chief among its health benefits is the potential to enhance cardiovascular health by lowering blood pressure and cholesterol levels. Allicin and other sulfur compounds contribute to improved blood vessel function, reducing the risk of CVDs. Beyond its cardiovascular prowess, garlic's natural antimicrobial properties, notably driven by allicin, position it as an effective antibacterial, antiviral, and antifungal agent. The herb's anti-inflammatory effects and immune-modulating capabilities further underscore its role in supporting overall health. Studies also suggest a potential link between garlic consumption and a reduced risk of certain cancers, particularly in the digestive system, emphasizing its multifaceted contributions to well-being.

Garlic's antioxidant activity, attributed to its sulfur compounds, offers cellular protection against free radicals, contributing to overall health and safeguarding against oxidative stress. The herb's detoxification support and traditional use in respiratory health further highlight its broad spectrum of benefits. Garlic, with its rich profile of health-promoting attributes, seamlessly intertwines culinary delight with a robust contribution to holistic health, making it a valuable addition to both the kitchen and wellness regimen.

Garlic's role extends beyond the kitchen, showcasing its versatility in both culinary and therapeutic domains. Widely recognized for enhancing the flavor of diverse dishes worldwide, garlic takes center stage in soups, sauces, and marinades. Its culinary ubiquity is complemented by therapeutic applications, with supplements like garlic oil capsules and aged garlic extract offering avenues to address specific health concerns or serve as preventative measures. The nuanced interplay between raw and cooked garlic adds a layer of flexibility, with raw garlic boasting higher allicin content and various cooking methods preserving its health benefits.

Beyond ingestion, managing garlic's pungent odor becomes a consideration, prompting strategies such as consuming aged garlic supplements or parsley post-garlic consumption. Garlic's reach extends to topical applications, traditionally used for conditions like warts and fungal infections, albeit with caution to prevent skin irritation. As garlic seamlessly integrates into culinary and therapeutic practices, individuals navigating its health advantages should be mindful of their unique health contexts.

Seeking guidance from healthcare professionals, especially for those with medical conditions or medication regimens, ensures a thoughtful and tailored incorporation of garlic into their holistic well-being approach [93–99].

8.18 BROCCOLI

Sulforaphane, a robust bioactive compound abundant in cruciferous vegetables, particularly broccoli, stands out for its distinctive health properties. Its activation path is illustrated in Figure 8.4. This potent phytochemical is formed through the interaction of the enzyme myrosinase with glucoraphanin, a precursor naturally present in broccoli. Beyond contributing to broccoli's characteristic taste, sulforaphane is celebrated for its multifaceted benefits, encompassing antioxidant, anti-inflammatory, and potential anti-cancer properties. Its presence underscores the nutritional richness of broccoli and highlights the intricate biochemical processes that occur within this cruciferous vegetable, offering both flavor and functional health benefits in a single package.

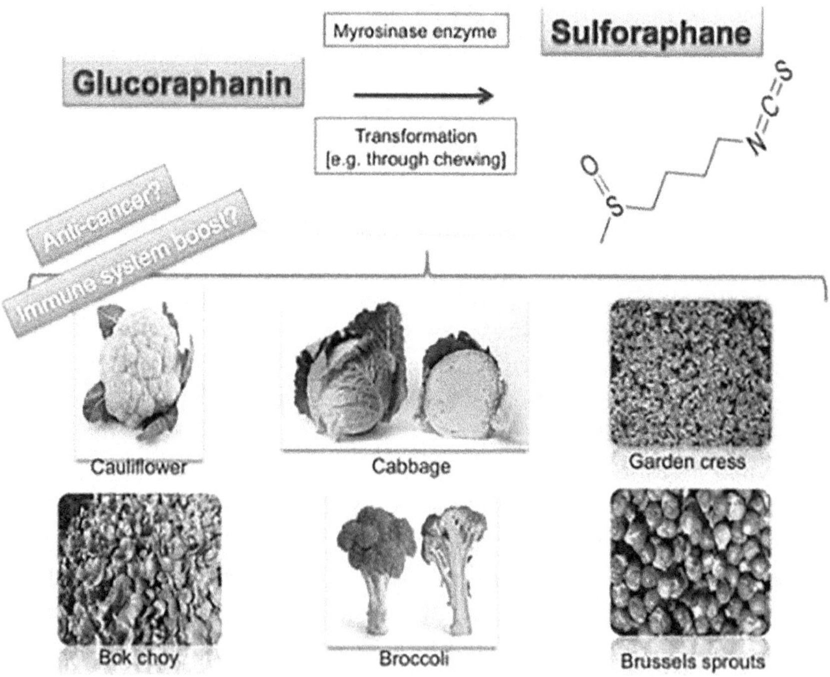

FIGURE 8.4 Structure sulforaphane.

Sulforaphane, the dynamic phytochemical abundant in broccoli, unfolds a spectrum of health benefits that extend beyond its culinary appeal. Functioning as a potent antioxidant, sulforaphane activates cellular pathways that neutralize free radicals, offering protection against oxidative stress implicated in aging and various diseases. Its role in supporting the body's natural detoxification processes adds another layer of functionality, aiding in the elimination of harmful substances. Beyond its antioxidant and detoxifying prowess, sulforaphane showcases anti-inflammatory effects, contributing to overall inflammatory balance and holding potential implications for chronic diseases associated with inflammation. The spotlight on sulforaphane intensifies when considering its potential anti-cancer properties, as it may inhibit the development and progression of certain cancers by modulating cellular processes. Sulforaphane's impact extends to cardiovascular health, with broccoli consumption, rich in this phytochemical, being associated with cardiovascular benefits. It may contribute to the reduction of risk factors for heart diseases. Additionally, preliminary studies hint at sulforaphane's neuroprotective effects, suggesting a role in supporting cognitive function and potentially reducing the risk of neurodegenerative disorders.

The multifaceted contributions of sulforaphane underscore the remarkable synergy between flavor and function in broccoli, positioning it as a nutritional powerhouse with the potential to enhance overall well-being.

Broccoli, celebrated for its nutrient density, emerges as a nutritional powerhouse, offering essential vitamins (C, K), minerals (folate, potassium), and dietary fiber that collectively contribute to overall health and well-being. Its versatility in culinary applications allows for inclusion in various dishes, from salads and stir-fries to soups and casseroles, with different cooking methods ensuring the retention of its nutrient content. Including broccoli in meal planning introduces diversity to nutrient intake, promoting a balanced diet and providing access to a broad spectrum of health-promoting compounds. The vegetable's adaptability offers both raw and cooked options, each delivering health benefits. While cooking may alter the content of certain nutrients, it enhances the bioavailability of others, emphasizing the importance of a varied approach to consumption.

Moreover, combining broccoli with other cruciferous vegetables, such as cauliflower and Brussels sprouts, amplifies the overall health impact. This strategic culinary pairing not only enhances flavor but also maximizes the synergistic effects of these vegetables, further contributing to a holistic approach to nutrition. Incorporating broccoli into one's dietary routine, guided by individual preferences and considerations, unlocks a wealth of potential health benefits, with the added advantage of sulforaphane offering protection against oxidative stress and inflammation [100–105].

8.19 GREEN AND HERBAL TEA

Catechins, a prominent group of flavonoids classified under the flavan-3-ol subgroup, stand out as crucial bioactive compounds found abundantly in tea, with green tea being a notable source. Among catechins, epigallocatechin gallate (EGCG) takes center stage as the most abundant and extensively studied member of this group. Their presence in tea contributes significantly to the beverage's antioxidant properties, providing health benefits associated with the neutralization of free radicals. Polyphenols, a broader category encompassing various plant compounds such as flavonoids and phenolic acids, play a pivotal role in the antioxidant activity observed in tea. The diverse array of polyphenols, including catechins, contributes to the overall health-promoting effects attributed to tea consumption. Understanding the significance of these bioactive compound's sheds light on the potential positive impact of tea on human health, making it a valuable addition to a balanced diet and a source of natural antioxidants.

The antioxidant activity of catechins and polyphenols found in green tea is a key aspect of the beverage's health benefits. These compounds exhibit potent antioxidant properties, effectively neutralizing free radicals and reducing oxidative stress within the body. Such antioxidative actions contribute to the overall well-being of individuals. Green tea has been linked to various cardiovascular health benefits, with regular consumption associated with improvements in lipid profiles that may reduce the risk of heart disease. Studies suggest that catechins in green tea may play a role in blood pressure regulation, promoting cardiovascular health. Additionally, the anti-inflammatory properties of polyphenols found in green tea could contribute to preventing chronic inflammatory conditions. Further benefits include positive effects on endothelial function, supporting the health of blood vessels, and potential contributions to cholesterol management. Catechins, especially EGCG, may aid in reducing LDL cholesterol levels and improving the LDL to HDL ratio. Some research also indicates favorable outcomes in terms of insulin sensitivity and blood sugar regulation, highlighting the multifaceted advantages of incorporating green tea into a balanced lifestyle.

Green tea comes in various forms, each offering unique flavors and characteristics. Sencha, a popular Japanese green tea, is known for its grassy and mildly sweet flavor. Matcha, a finely ground green tea powder used in traditional Japanese ceremonies, provides a rich and distinctive taste. Longjing, or Dragon Well, is a Chinese green tea celebrated for its smooth, chestnut-like flavor. Herbal teas, such as chamomile with its calming properties, peppermint for a refreshing taste and digestive support, and hibiscus with its tart and vibrant profile, offer diverse options.

Brewing techniques are crucial for a satisfying tea experience. For green tea, it is essential to use water below boiling temperature (around 175–185°F or 80–85°C) to prevent bitterness. Steeping time is typically 2–3 minutes, avoiding over-extraction. The tea-to-water ratio is generally one teaspoon of loose tea leaves per 8 ounces of water. Herbal tea brewing varies; boiling water is often used, with steeping times of 5–7 minutes or as specified for the herbal blend. The tea-to-water ratio for herbal infusions is typically one teaspoon of dried herbs per 8 ounces of water. To enhance the flavor, green tea can be paired with lemon or mint, while herbal teas benefit from additions like honey for sweetness or ginger for a hint of spice. Understanding the nuances of green and herbal teas, along with personalized brewing adjustments, allows individuals to tailor their tea experience to their liking while enjoying the potential health benefits associated with the bioactive compounds present in these teas [106–115].

8.20 FLAX SEEDS

Flax seeds are a notable source of ALA, a primary plant-based omega-3 fatty acid. Unlike fish oil, which contains EPA and DHA, flax seeds provide ALA, which the body can convert into EPA and DHA. This conversion process adds a plant-based dimension to omega-3 intake. The inclusion of flax seeds in the diet serves a crucial role in maintaining a balanced ratio of omega-6 to omega-3 fatty acids, contributing to overall heart health. This balance is vital for supporting various physiological functions and reducing the risk of cardiovascular issues associated with an imbalance in essential fatty acids.

Flax seeds contain a key lignan known as secoisolariciresinol diglucoside (SDG), making them one of the richest dietary sources of this compound. Lignans, including SDG, exhibit antioxidant properties, enhancing the overall health-promoting potential of flax seeds. Additionally, the phytoestrogenic properties of lignans in flax seeds introduce hormone-like compounds into the body. These phytoestrogens, through their interaction with estrogen receptors, may play a role in hormonal balance. Studies have explored potential health effects, suggesting that the presence of lignans in flax seeds might contribute to reducing the risk of hormone-related cancers, highlighting the multifaceted benefits of incorporating flax seeds into the diet.

Flax seeds, rich in ALA, contribute to heart health by reducing inflammation and supporting cardiovascular function. The presence of omega-3 fatty acids in flax seeds, including ALA, may aid in regulating cholesterol levels, specifically reducing LDL cholesterol. Additionally, the anti-inflammatory properties of omega-3s in flax seeds can benefit conditions like arthritis.

In terms of digestive health, the dietary fiber content in flax seeds, consisting of both soluble and insoluble fiber, promotes regular bowel movements and helps prevent constipation. Furthermore, the combination of dietary fiber and omega-3s in flax seeds may assist in stabilizing blood sugar levels, making them potentially advantageous for individuals managing diabetes.

Flax seeds contribute to weight management by inducing a feeling of satiety, thanks to their fiber content. The lignans present in flax seeds, particularly SDG, have been subject to studies exploring their potential role in reducing the risk of certain cancers, such as breast and prostate cancers.

Beyond their direct consumption, flax seeds can be incorporated into various functional foods. Ground flax seeds can enhance the nutritional value of bakery products like bread and muffins, and they can be added to smoothies or yogurt for increased omega-3 intake. Whole or ground flax seeds provide a nutritious addition to salads and cereals. Additionally, flaxseed oil serves as a popular omega-3 supplement, offering a concentrated source of ALA. The versatility and nutritional density of flax seeds make them a valuable component of a well-rounded and balanced diet, with consumption guided by individual preferences and moderation [116–121].

8.21 BLACK COHOSH

Black Cohosh, an herbal remedy, contains bioactive compounds known as phytoestrogens, which are plant-derived compounds that interact with estrogen receptors in the body. The relevance of phytoestrogens lies in their potential influence on hormonal balance, particularly in relation to estrogen. In women's health, Black Cohosh is often associated with addressing various issues related to hormonal changes.

Another group of key compounds found in Black Cohosh is triterpene glycosides, including actein and cimicifugoside. These compounds are believed to contribute to the herb's medicinal properties, especially concerning women's health. Black Cohosh has been traditionally used to manage symptoms associated with hormonal fluctuations, making it a popular choice for women experiencing conditions such as menopause. The combination of phytoestrogens and triterpene glycosides underscores Black Cohosh's potential in supporting women's health and well-being. As with any herbal remedy, it is essential for individuals to consult with healthcare professionals for personalized advice and guidance.

Black cohosh is commonly employed to address various menopausal symptoms, including hot flashes and night sweats. Its potential to alleviate these symptoms may be attributed to the presence of phytoestrogens, which could help modulate hormonal fluctuations associated with menopause. Beyond menopausal symptoms, black cohosh has been traditionally used to regulate menstrual cycles, offering support for women experiencing irregularities. Additionally, some women use black cohosh to address vaginal dryness, a common concern linked to hormonal changes during menopause.

Beyond its effects on physical symptoms, Black Cohosh is believed by some to have mild sedative properties, potentially contributing to its use in managing mood swings and anxiety associated with hormonal changes. Furthermore, the estrogenic influence of phytoestrogens found in Black Cohosh may have implications for bone health, which becomes particularly relevant during and after menopause when estrogen levels decline. As with any herbal remedy, individual responses may vary, and it is advisable for individuals to seek guidance from healthcare professionals for personalized advice and appropriate usage.

Individuals considering the use of Black Cohosh, particularly for menopausal symptoms or other health concerns, are strongly advised to seek consultation with healthcare professionals. This approach allows for an individualized assessment, ruling out underlying conditions and ensuring that

Black Cohosh is a safe and appropriate option for the individual's specific health circumstances. Due to its phytoestrogen content, Black Cohosh may interact with hormone therapies or medications affecting hormonal balance. This is particularly important for women with a history of hormone-related cancers, and caution should be exercised with medical advice sought. Additionally, while rare, there have been reports of liver toxicity associated with Black Cohosh use, emphasizing the importance of periodic liver function monitoring for individuals using it for an extended period.

For pregnant and breastfeeding women, limited data are available on the safety of Black Cohosh. As a precautionary measure, it is advisable for individuals in these groups to exercise caution and seek professional guidance before considering its use.

Individual responses to Black Cohosh can vary, and not all women may experience the same benefits. Monitoring for potential side effects is crucial, and individuals should discontinue use if adverse reactions occur.

For those opting for Black Cohosh supplements, ensuring the product is from a reputable source with standardized extracts is paramount. Quality assurance is crucial, as the adulteration of herbal supplements is a potential concern. Overall, a cautious and informed approach, coupled with professional guidance, is essential when incorporating Black Cohosh into one's health regimen [122–129].

8.22 TURMERIC

Turmeric, a spice commonly used in culinary practices, contains curcumin as its primary bioactive ingredient. Curcumin is a polyphenol known for its potent medicinal properties, contributing to the therapeutic benefits associated with turmeric. Notably, it imparts the bright yellow pigment that characterizes turmeric, making it easily recognizable in various dishes and traditional medicines. The inclusion of curcumin in the diet has been of interest due to its potential health-promoting effects.

Turmeric's remarkable health benefits stem from its primary bioactive ingredient, curcumin, a potent polyphenol recognized for its medicinal properties. Responsible for the vibrant yellow hue of turmeric, curcumin is renowned for its powerful anti-inflammatory effects, targeting multiple pathways within the body and potentially providing relief comparable to pharmaceutical anti-inflammatory drugs. Beyond its anti-inflammatory prowess, curcumin serves as a robust antioxidant, neutralizing free radicals and stimulating the body's intrinsic antioxidant enzymes [130, 131]. Turmeric's holistic impact extends to joint health, offering relief for conditions like arthritis, and digestive health, suggesting a role in managing inflammatory bowel diseases. Curcumin's cardiovascular benefits include improving endothelial function and reducing risk factors for heart disease. Furthermore, its neuroprotective effects, crossing the blood-brain barrier, hint at potential in preserving brain health and offering protection against conditions like Alzheimer's disease. In laboratory studies, curcumin has shown promise in cancer prevention, inhibiting the growth of cancer cells and reducing tumor spread, suggesting a supportive role in cancer treatment. Turmeric, with its versatile and impactful curcumin content, stands as a valuable natural remedy with diverse health-enhancing properties.

Turmeric, renowned for its vibrant yellow color and distinct earthy flavor, is a versatile spice that extends its influence from culinary applications to various health-related uses. Commonly used in cooking, particularly in curry powder, turmeric enriches dishes with its warm taste. The preparation of golden milk, a traditional beverage blending turmeric with milk and spices, has gained popularity for its potential health benefits, particularly anti-inflammatory properties. Beyond the kitchen, turmeric finds its way into supplements, with curcumin supplements often enhanced with piperine for improved absorption. These supplements are employed for targeted therapeutic purposes, especially in managing inflammatory conditions. Turmeric's benefits also extend to topical applications, where turmeric paste or creams are traditionally used to promote skin health and alleviate inflammation. Additionally, turmeric features in herbal teas, infusions, and oil preparations, offering diverse avenues for consumption and application. While turmeric is celebrated for its versatility and health-promoting qualities, individual responses may vary, warranting consultation with healthcare professionals, especially in specific health contexts [132–140].

8.23 CONCLUSION

The importance of antioxidants, PUFAs, and herbs as functional foods lies in their multifaceted contributions to health and well-being. Antioxidants function as a defensive shield, protecting the body from oxidative stress and reducing the risk of chronic diseases such as cardiovascular issues and neurodegenerative conditions. PUFAs, particularly omega-3 fatty acids, play a pivotal role in cardiovascular health by reducing inflammation and improving lipid profiles, with additional benefits for cognitive function. Herbs, rich in bioactive compounds, offer holistic health support, drawing from a wealth of traditional wisdom in natural remedies.

Looking ahead, future trends and research directions in nutraceutical development are poised to reshape the landscape of functional foods. Personalized nutrition, driven by tailored approaches based on individual genetics and health status, is a key focus. Advanced formulations aim to enhance the bioavailability of bioactive compounds, exploring innovative delivery systems such as nanotechnology. Functional foods designed for aging populations will address age-related health concerns, including cognitive decline and immune function. The intricate relationship between gut microbiota and immune health will drive microbiome-focused approaches, incorporating targeted prebiotics and probiotics. The integration of traditional and modern medicine is gaining momentum, combining evidence-based validation with centuries-old herbal knowledge.

Ensuring the safety and effectiveness of nutraceuticals is paramount. Regulatory efforts toward global harmonization will establish consistent standards, and transparent labeling will empower consumers to make informed choices. In conclusion, the dynamic field of functional foods is evolving toward personalized nutrition, innovative formulations, and a deeper understanding of the connections between diet and overall well-being. The integration of traditional wisdom with modern science is poised to shape a holistic approach to health and preventive medicine in the future.

KEYWORDS

- **antioxidants**
- **black cohosh**
- **broccoli**
- **flax seeds**
- **functional foods**
- **garlic**
- **ginseng**
- **green tea**
- **herbal tea**
- **herbs**
- **nutraceuticals**
- **polyunsaturated fatty acids**
- **soya bean**
- **spirulina**
- **turmeric**

REFERENCES

1. Borchers, A. T., Keen, C. L., & Gershwin, M. E. (2016). The basis of structure/function claims of nutraceuticals. *Clinical Reviews in Allergy & Immunology, 51*(3), 370–382.
2. DeFelice, S. L. (1995). The nutraceutical revolution: Its impact on food industry R&D. *Trends in Food Science & Technology, 6*(2), 59–61.
3. Aronson, J. K. (2017). Defining "nutraceuticals": Neither nutritious nor pharmaceutical. *British Journal of Clinical Pharmacology, 83*(1), 8–19.
4. Garud, S. R., Lamdande, A. G., & Gholap, S. R. (2023). Chapter 22 – Regulations on functional foods and nutraceuticals. In C. Anandharamakrishnan & P. Subramanian (Eds.), *Industrial Application of Functional Foods, Ingredients and Nutraceuticals* (pp. 785–823). Academic Press.
5. Anumala, V., Phurailatpam, A., & Sarma, P. (2021). Nutraceutical: Definition and concept. In *Fruits and Vegetables as Nutraceutical* (1st ed., pp. 1–4). CRC Press. https://doi.org/10.1201/9781003230885-5.
6. Santini, A., Cammarata, S. M., Capone, G., Ianaro, A., Tenore, G. C., Pani, L., et al. (2018). Nutraceuticals: Opening the debate for a regulatory framework. *British Journal of Clinical Pharmacology, 84*(4), 659–672.
7. Komala, M. G., Ong, S. G., Qadri, M. U., Elshafie, L. M., Pollock, C. A., & Saad, S. (2023). Investigating the regulatory process, safety, efficacy, and product transparency for nutraceuticals in the USA, Europe, and Australia. *Foods, 12*(2), 427.
8. Scientific concepts of functional foods in Europe consensus document. (1999). *British Journal of Nutrition, 81*(4), S1–S27.
9. Hardy, G. (2000). Nutraceuticals and functional foods: Introduction and meaning. *Nutrition, 16*(7), 688–689.
10. Finley, J. W. (2016). The nutraceutical revolution: Emerging vision or broken dream? Understanding scientific and regulatory concerns. *Clinical Research and Regulatory Affairs, 33*(1), 1–3.
11. Volpe, R., & Sotis, G. (2015). Nutraceuticals: Definition and epidemiological rationale for their use in clinical practice. *High Blood Pressure & Cardiovascular Prevention, 22*(3), 199–201.
12. da Costa, J. P. (2017). A current look at nutraceuticals—Key concepts and future prospects. *Trends in Food Science & Technology, 62*, 68–78.
13. Filipiak-Szok, A., Kurzawa, M., & Szłyk, E. (2015). Determination of toxic metals by ICP-MS in Asiatic and European medicinal plants and dietary supplements. *Journal of Trace Elements in Medicine and Biology, 30*, 54–58.
14. Dickinson, A., Blatman, J., El-Dash, N., & Franco, J. C. (2014). Consumer usage and reasons for using dietary supplements: Report of a series of surveys. *Journal of the American College of Nutrition, 33*(2), 176–182.
15. Santini, A., & Novellino, E. (2017). Nutraceuticals in hypercholesterolemia: An overview. *British Journal of Pharmacology, 174*(11), 1450–1463.
16. MedlinePlus. (n.d.). *MedlinePlus US National Library of Medicine.* Retrieved from: https://medlineplus.gov/minerals.html (accessed on 22 March 2025).

17. National Center for Biotechnology Information. (2023). Retrieved from: https://www.ncbi.nlm.nih.gov/books/NBK541123/ (accessed on 22 March 2025).
18. Leung, A. M., Braverman, L. E., & Pearce, E. N. (2012). History of U.S. iodine fortification and supplementation. *Nutrients, 4*(11), 1740–1746.
19. National Research Council. (1989). Water and electrolytes. In *Recommended Dietary Allowances: 10th Edition.* National Academies Press (US).
20. MedlinePlus. (n.d.). *Electrolyte Panel.* Retrieved from: https://medlineplus.gov/lab-tests/electrolyte-panel/ (accessed on 22 March 2025).
21. U.S. Food and Drug Administration. (2024). *Sodium Reduction.* Retrieved from: https://www.fda.gov/food/food-additives-petitions/sodium-reduction (accessed on 22 March 2025).
22. National Research Council. (1989). *Electrolytes.* In *Diet and Health: Implications for Reducing Chronic Disease Risk.* National Academies Press.
23. Choi, H. Y., Park, H. C., & Ha, S. K. (2015). Salt sensitivity and hypertension: A paradigm shift from kidney malfunction to vascular endothelial dysfunction. *Electrolyte & Blood Pressure, 13*(1), 7–16.
24. Mayo Clinic. (2023). *Sodium: How to Tame Your Salt Habit.* Retrieved from: https://www.mayoclinic.org/healthy-lifestyle/nutrition-and-healthy-eating/in-depth/sodium/art-20045479 (accessed on 22 March 2025).
25. National Institutes of Health, Office of Dietary Supplements. (2024). *Potassium: Fact Sheet for Health Professionals.* Retrieved from: https://ods.od.nih.gov/factsheets/Potassium-HealthProfessional/ (accessed on 22 March 2025).
26. National Institutes of Health, Office of Dietary Supplements. (2024). *Calcium: Fact Sheet for Health Professionals.*
27. National Academies of Sciences, Engineering, and Medicine. (n.d.). *Dietary Reference Intakes for Vitamin A, Vitamin K, Arsenic, Boron, Chromium, Copper, Iodine, Iron, Manganese, Molybdenum, Nickel, Silicon, Vanadium, and Zinc.* Retrieved from: https://www.ncbi.nlm.nih.gov/books/NBK222309/ (accessed on 22 March 2025).
28. Stanford University. (2017). *Ways to Boost Blood Iron Levels While Eating a Vegetarian or Vegan Diet.* Scope 10K. Retrieved from: https://scopeblog.stanford.edu/2017/10/06/ways-to-boost-blood-iron-levels-while-eating-a-vegan-or-vegetarian-diet/ (accessed on 22 March 2025).
29. Mayo Clinic. (n.d.). *Hemochromatosis.* Retrieved from: https://www.mayoclinic.org/diseases-conditions/hemochromatosis/diagnosis-treatment/drc-20351448 (accessed on 22 March 2025).
30. National Institutes of Health, Office of Dietary Supplements. (n.d.). *Zinc: Fact Sheet for Health Professionals.* Retrieved from: https://ods.od.nih.gov/factsheets/Zinc-HealthProfessional/ (accessed on 22 March 2025).
31. Bohn, L., Meyer, A. S., & Rasmussen, S. K. (2008). Phytate: Impact on environment and human nutrition. A challenge for molecular breeding. *Journal of Zhejiang University Science B, 9*, 165–191.
32. Hemilä, H. (2017). Zinc lozenges and the common cold: A meta-analysis comparing zinc acetate and zinc gluconate, and the role of zinc dosage. *JRSM Open, 8*(5), 2054270417694291.

33. Jenkins, D., Chiavaroli, L., Mirrahimi, A., Srichaikul, K., Wong, J., Jones, P., et al. (2024). *Nutraceuticals and Functional Foods for Cholesterol Reduction*, 236–245. e3.
34. Knorr, D. (2024). Food processing: Legacy, significance, and challenges. *Trends in Food Science & Technology, 143*, 104270.
35. Yang, Q., Lu, T., Yan, J., Li, J., Zhou, H., Pan, X., et al. (2021). Regulation of polyunsaturated fatty acids synthesis by enhancing carotenoid-mediated endogenous antioxidant capacity in *Schizochytrium* sp. *Algal Research, 55*, 102238.
36. Chen, H., Leng, X., Liu, S., Zeng, Z., Huang, F., Huang, R., et al. (2023). Association between dietary intake of omega-3 polyunsaturated fatty acids and all-cause and cardiovascular mortality among hypertensive adults: Results from NHANES 1999–2018. *Clinical Nutrition, 42*(12), 2434–2442.
37. Yan, C. X., Zhang, Y., Yang, W. Q., Ma, W., Sun, X. M., & Huang, H. (2024). Universal and unique strategies for the production of polyunsaturated fatty acids in industrial oleaginous microorganisms. *Biotechnology Advances, 70*, 108298.
38. Dong, Y., Wei, Y., Wang, L., Song, K., Zhang, C., Lu, K., et al. (2023). Dietary n-3/n-6 polyunsaturated fatty acid ratio modulates growth performance in spotted seabass (*Lateolabrax maculatus*) through regulating lipid metabolism, hepatic antioxidant capacity, and intestinal health. *Animal Nutrition, 14*, 20–31.
39. Agradi, S., Sulce, M., Menchetti, L., Vigo, D., Castrica, M., Barbato, O., et al. (2023). Dietary supplementation with n-3 polyunsaturated fatty acids: Effects on reproductive and productive performance and meat quality in rabbit breeding. *Animal Nutrition, 14*, 70–78.
40. Khan, I., Hussain, M., Jiang, B., Zheng, L., Pan, Y., Hu, J., et al. (2023). Omega-3 long-chain polyunsaturated fatty acids: Metabolism and health implications. *Progress in Lipid Research, 92*, 101255.
41. Shahidi, F. (2000). Antioxidants in food and food antioxidants. *Nahrung, 44*(3), 158–163.
42. Benzie, I. F. F., & Choi, S. W. (2014). Chapter 1 – Antioxidants in food: Content, measurement, significance, action, cautions, caveats, and research needs. In J. Henry (Ed.), *Advances in Food and Nutrition Research* (Vol. 71, pp. 1–53). Academic Press.
43. Akbari, B., Baghaei-Yazdi, N., Bahmaie, M., & Mahdavi Abhari, F. (2022). The role of plant-derived natural antioxidants in reduction of oxidative stress. *BioFactors, 48*(3), 611–633.
44. Ting, S. Y., Lau, N. S., Sam, K. K., Janaranjani, M., Wong, S. C., Monroig, Ó., et al. (2022). Long-chain polyunsaturated fatty acid biosynthesis in a land-crab with advanced terrestrial adaptations: Molecular cloning and functional characterization of two fatty acyl elongases. *Comparative Biochemistry and Physiology Part B: Biochemistry and Molecular Biology, 262*, 110773.
45. Ishida, Y., Furuta, S., Aiba, A., Kuzumaki, A., Miyazawa, D., & Watanabe, A. (2022). Analysis of n-6/n-3 ratio of polyunsaturated fatty acids in human serum by reactive thermal desorption-gas chromatography using a vertical microfurnace pyrolyzer. *Journal of Analytical and Applied Pyrolysis, 168*, 105758.
46. Wang, T., Fan, L., Wang, M., Zhou, J., Yang, M., & Liu, Q. (2022). Determination of polyunsaturated and omega-3 fatty acids in vegetable oils and animal fats by the

double-quantum filtered correlation spectroscopy (DQF-COSY). *Microchemical Journal, 183*, 108127.

47. Wang, Y., Li, C., Zhang, J., Xu, X., Fu, L., Xu, J., et al. (2022). Polyunsaturated fatty acids promote the rapid fusion of lipid droplets in *Caenorhabditis elegans*. *Journal of Biological Chemistry, 298*(8), 102179.
48. Mao, Y., Ji, X., Meng, Q., Xu, Z., Yuan, Y., Li, M., et al. (2022). Contribution of anthocyanin and polyunsaturated fatty acid biosynthesis to cold tolerance during bud sprouting in tree peony. *Industrial Crops and Products, 188*, 115563.
49. Mazidimoradi, A., Alemzadeh, E., Alemzadeh, E., & Salehiniya, H. (2022). The effect of polyunsaturated fatty acids on the severity and mortality of COVID patients: A systematic review. *Life Sciences, 299*, 120489.
50. Lu, C., Gao, L., Zhang, L., Liu, K., Hou, Y., He, T., et al. (2022). Selective catalytic transfer hydrogenation of polyunsaturated fatty acid methyl esters using Pd/organobentonite as catalyst under microwave heating. *Chemical Engineering and Processing–Process Intensification, 182*, 109206.
51. dos Santos Morales, P., Mantovani dos Santos, P., Evaristo de Carvalho, A., & Zanetti Corazza, M. (2022). Vortex-assisted magnetic solid-phase extraction of cadmium in food, medicinal herb, and water samples using silica-coated thiol-functionalized magnetic multiwalled carbon nanotubes as adsorbent. *Food Chemistry, 368*, 130823.
52. Zhao, J., Deng, Y., & Li, S. P. (2017). Advanced analysis of polysaccharides, novel functional components in food and medicine dual purposes Chinese herbs. *TrAC Trends in Analytical Chemistry, 96*, 138–150.
53. Hasneen, D. F., Zaki, N. L., Abbas, M. S., Soliman, A. S., Ashoush, I. S., & Fayed, A. E. (2020). Comparative evaluation of some herbs and their suitability for skimmed milk yoghurt and cast Kariesh cheese fortification as functional foods. *Annals of Agricultural Sciences, 65*(1), 6–12.
54. Liu, X., Cai, H., Niu, M., Yu, H., Wang, M., Zhu, H., et al. (2023). An integrated strategy of secondary metabolomics and glycomics to investigate multi-component variations in wine-processing of medicinal herbs and functional foods: A case study on *Fructus Corni*. *Arabian Journal of Chemistry, 16*(3), 104525.
55. Williams, C. A., & Lamprecht, E. D. (2008). Some commonly fed herbs and other functional foods in equine nutrition: A review. *The Veterinary Journal, 178*(1), 21–31.
56. Bansal, P., Maithani, M., Gupta, V., Kaur, G., & Bansal, R. (2023). *Future Prospective of Nutraceutical and Functional Food with Herbs and Spices* (pp. 361–381).
57. Venkatakrishnan, K., Chiu, H. F., & Wang, C. K. (2019). Popular functional foods and herbs for the management of type-2 diabetes mellitus: A comprehensive review with special reference to clinical trials and its proposed mechanism. *Journal of Functional Foods, 57*, 425–438.
58. Maghraby, Y. R., Labib, R. M., Sobeh, M., & Farag, M. A. (2023). Gingerols and shogaols: A multi-faceted review of their extraction, formulation, and analysis in drugs and biofluids to maximize their nutraceutical and pharmaceutical applications. *Food Chemistry: X, 20*, 100947.
59. Manocha, S., Dhiman, S., Grewal, A. S., & Guarve, K. (2022). Nanotechnology: An approach to overcome bioavailability challenges of nutraceuticals. *Journal of Drug Delivery Science and Technology, 72*, 103418.

60. Meenambal, R., & Srinivas Bharath, M. M. (2020). Nanocarriers for effective nutraceutical delivery to the brain. *Neurochemistry International, 140*, 104851.
61. Chopra, A. S., Lordan, R., Horbańczuk, O. K., Atanasov, A. G., Chopra, I., Horbańczuk, J. O., et al. (2022). The current use and evolving landscape of nutraceuticals. *Pharmacological Research, 175*, 106001.
62. Sun, W., Gregory, D. A., & Zhao, X. (2023). Designed peptide amphiphiles as scaffolds for tissue engineering. *Advances in Colloid and Interface Science, 314*, 102866.
63. Rashidi, L. (2021). Different nano-delivery systems for delivery of nutraceuticals. *Food Bioscience, 43*, 101258.
64. Gonçalves, R. F. S., Martins, J. T., Duarte, C. M. M., Vicente, A. A., & Pinheiro, A. C. (2018). Advances in nutraceutical delivery systems: From formulation design for bioavailability enhancement to efficacy and safety evaluation. *Trends in Food Science & Technology, 78*, 270–291.
65. Majumdar, S., Gupta, S., Prajapati, S. K., & Krishnamurthy, S. (2021). Neuro-nutraceutical potential of *Asparagus racemosus*: A review. *Neurochemistry International, 145*, 105013.
66. Ogino, M., Yamada, K., Sato, H., & Onoue, S. (2022). Enhanced nutraceutical functions of herbal oily extract employing formulation technology: The present and future. *PharmaNutrition, 22*, 100318.
67. Bondu, C., & Yen, F. T. (2022). Nanoliposomes, from food industry to nutraceuticals: Interests and uses. *Innovative Food Science & Emerging Technologies, 81*, 103140.
68. Rizzo, M., Colletti, A., Penson, P. E., Katsiki, N., Mikhailidis, D. P., Toth, P. P., et al. (2023). Nutraceutical approaches to non-alcoholic fatty liver disease (NAFLD): A position paper from the International Lipid Expert Panel (ILEP). *Pharmacological Research, 189*, 106679.
69. Ahmed, Z., Chen, J., Tufail, T., Latif, A., Arif, M., Ullah, R., et al. (2024). Fundamental opportunities and challenges of nutraceutical noodles enriched with agri-food by-products. *Trends in Food Science & Technology, 143*, 104299.
70. Taylor, C. L., Sempos, C. T., Davis, C. D., & Brannon, P. M. (2017). Vitamin D: Moving forward to address emerging science. *Nutrients, 9*(12), 1308.
71. Gulati, K., Thokchom, S. K., Joshi, J. C., & Ray, A. (2021). Chapter 74 – Regulatory guidelines for nutraceuticals in India: An overview. In R. C. Gupta, R. Lall, & A. Srivastava (Eds.), *Nutraceuticals* (2nd ed., pp. 1273–1280). Academic Press.
72. Shukla, S., Shankar, R., & Singh, S. P. (2014). Food safety regulatory model in India. *Food Control, 37*, 401–413.
73. Ray, A., Joshi, J., & Gulati, K. (2016). Chapter 66 – Regulatory aspects of nutraceuticals: An Indian perspective. In R. C. Gupta (Ed.), *Nutraceuticals* (pp. 941–946). Boston: Academic Press.
74. Villaró-Cos, S., Guzmán Sánchez, J. L., Acién, G., & Lafarga, T. (2024). Research trends and current requirements and challenges in the industrial production of *Spirulina* as a food source. *Trends in Food Science & Technology, 143*, 104280.
75. Ai, X., Yu, P., Li, X., Lai, X., Yang, M., Liu, F., et al. (2023). Polysaccharides from *Spirulina platensis*: Extraction methods, structural features and bioactivities diversity. *International Journal of Biological Macromolecules, 231*, 123211.

76. Vijayaram, S., Ringø, E., Zuorro, A., van Doan, H., & Sun, Y. (2023). Beneficial roles of nutrients as immunostimulants in aquaculture: A review. *Aquaculture and Fisheries, 9*(5), 707–720.
77. Ziyaei, K., Abdi, F., Mokhtari, M., Daneshmehr, M. A., & Ataie, Z. (2023). Phycocyanin as a nature-inspired antidiabetic agent: A systematic review. *Phytomedicine, 119*, 154964.
78. Nabti, B., Bammoune, N., Meliani, H., & Stambouli, B. (2023). Antioxidant and antimicrobial activities of *Spirulina* from the region of Tamanrasset, Algeria. *Journal of Herbal Medicine, 41*, 100748.
79. Rahnama, I., Arabi, S. M., Chambari, M., Bahrami, L. S., Hadi, V., Mirghazanfari, S. M., et al. (2023). The effect of *Spirulina* supplementation on lipid profile: GRADE-assessed systematic review and dose-response meta-analysis of data from randomized controlled trials. *Pharmacological Research, 193*, 106802.
80. Liao, B., Zheng, J., Xia, C., Chen, X., Xu, Q., & Duan, B. (2023). The potential, challenges, and prospects of the genus *Spirulina* polysaccharides as future multipurpose biomacromolecules. *International Journal of Biological Macromolecules, 253*, 127482.
81. Chen, J., Huang, Q., Li, J., Yao, Y., Sun, W., Zhang, Z., et al. (2023). *Panax ginseng* against myocardial ischemia/reperfusion injury: A review of preclinical evidence and potential mechanisms. *Journal of Ethnopharmacology, 300*, 115715.
82. Vijayakumar, A., & Kim, J. H. (2023). *Ginseng* and ginsenosides on cardiovascular and pulmonary diseases; Pharmacological potentials for the coronavirus (COVID-19). *Journal of Ginseng Research, 48*, 113–121.
83. Chandra Das, R., Ratan, Z. A., Rahman, M. M., Runa, N. J., Mondal, S., Konstantinov, K., et al. (2023). Antiviral activities of *ginseng* and its potential and putative benefits against monkeypox virus: A mini review. *Journal of Ginseng Research, 47*(6), 687–693.
84. Peng, Y., Pan, W., Cao, X., & Liu, C. (2023). Potential oral health benefits of *ginseng* and its extracts. *International Dental Journal, 73*(4), 473–480.
85. Huang, L., Li, H. J., & Wu, Y. C. (2023). Processing technologies, phytochemistry, bioactivities and applications of black *ginseng*—A novel manufactured *ginseng* product: A comprehensive review. *Food Chemistry, 407*, 134714.
86. Ahmad, S. S., Chun, H. J., Ahmad, K., & Choi, I. (2024). Therapeutic applications of *ginseng* for skeletal muscle-related disorder management. *Journal of Ginseng Research, 48*(1), 12–19.
87. Yi, Y. S. (2023). Pharmacological potential of *ginseng* and ginsenosides in nonalcoholic fatty liver disease and nonalcoholic steatohepatitis. *Journal of Ginseng Research, 48*(2), 122–128.
88. Li, N., Duan, Y., Chen, L., & Zhang, K. (2023). Iron metabolism: An emerging therapeutic target underlying the anti-Alzheimer's disease effect of *ginseng*. *Journal of Trace Elements in Medicine and Biology, 79*, 127252.
89. Murthy, H. N., Joseph, K. S., Paek, K. Y., & Park, S. Y. (2024). Production of biomass and bioactive compounds from cell and organ cultures of *ginseng*, *He-Shou-Wu*, *purple coneflower*, and *St. John's wort* for the use in the cosmetic industry. *South African Journal of Botany, 164*, 334–344.

90. Lee, M. Y., & Kim, M. (2024). Effects of red *ginseng* on neuroinflammation in neurodegenerative diseases. *Journal of Ginseng Research, 48*(1), 20–30.
91. Song, X., Gao, W., Shi, Y., Li, J., & Zheng, Z. (2023). *Panax ginseng* and its derivatives: Promoting angiogenesis in ischemic diseases—A mechanistic overview. *Journal of Functional Foods, 109*, 105762.
92. Wang, Z., Zhang, Z., Liu, J., Guo, M., & Li, H. (2023). *Panax ginseng* in the treatment of Alzheimer's disease and vascular dementia. *Journal of Ginseng Research, 47*(4), 506–514.
93. Sahidur, M. R., Islam, S., & Jahurul, M. H. A. (2023). Garlic (*Allium sativum*) as a natural antidote or a protective agent against diseases and toxicities: A critical review. *Food Chemistry Advances, 3*, 100353.
94. Balogun, M. A., Sobande, O. S., & Oyeyinka, S. A. (2023). Antimicrobial properties of onion and garlic extracts in beef and chicken. *Food Chemistry Advances, 3*, 100519.
95. Chidike Ezeorba, T. P., Ezugwu, A. L., Chukwuma, I. F., Anaduaka, E. G., & Udenigwe, C. C. (2024). Health-promoting properties of bioactive proteins and peptides of garlic (*Allium sativum*). *Food Chemistry, 435*, 137632.
96. Pacholczyk-Sienicka, B., Modranka, J., & Ciepielowski, G. (2024). Comparative analysis of bioactive compounds in garlic owing to the cultivar and origin. *Food Chemistry, 439*, 138141.
97. Spence, C. (2024). Garlic: Tracing its changing popularity in British cuisine. *International Journal of Gastronomy and Food Science, 35*, 100854.
98. Lu, M., Pan, J., Hu, Y., Ding, L., Li, Y., Cui, X., et al. (2024). Advances in the study of vascular-related protective effect of garlic (*Allium sativum*) extract and compounds. *The Journal of Nutritional Biochemistry, 124*, 109531.
99. Jafari, F., Khalilzadeh, S., & Nejatbakhsh, F. (2023). Therapeutic effects of garlic (*Allium sativum*) on the female reproductive system: A systematic review. *Heliyon, 9*(12), e22555.
100. Bruckner, F. P., Barbosa, T. M. C., Eiras, M., & Zanardo, L. G. (2024). Chapter 51 – Broccoli, cabbage, and cauliflower. In Awasthi, L. P. (Ed.), *Viral Diseases of Field and Horticultural Crops* (pp. 427–436). Academic Press.
101. Raeeszadeh, M., Nadia, K., & Akbari, A. (2021). The effects of broccoli and caraway extracts on serum oxidative markers, testicular structure and function, and sperm quality before and after sperm cryopreservation. *Cryobiology, 99*, 11–19.
102. Bahadoran, Z., Mirmiran, P., Yeganeh, M. Z., Hosseinpanah, F., Zojaji, H., & Azizi, F. (2014). Complementary and alternative medicinal effects of broccoli sprouts powder on *Helicobacter pylori* eradication rate in type 2 diabetic patients: A randomized clinical trial. *Journal of Functional Foods, 7*, 390–397.
103. Mohammed, A., & Mohammed, H. A. (2023). Beneficial role of broccoli and its active ingredient, sulforaphane in the treatment of diabetes. *Phytomedicine Plus, 3*(2), 100431.
104. Macharia, J. M., Mwangi, R. W., Rozmann, N., Zsolt, K., Varjas, T., Uchechukwu, P. O., et al. (2022). Medicinal plants with anti-colorectal cancer bioactive compounds: Potential game-changers in colorectal cancer management. *Biomedicine & Pharmacotherapy, 153*, 113383.

105. Abdulazeem, L., Alasmari, A. F., Alharbi, M., Alshammari, A., & Muhseen, Z. T. (2023). Utilization of aqueous broccoli florets extract for green synthesis and characterization of silver nanoparticles, with potential biological applications. *Heliyon, 9*(9), e19723.
106. Thummajitsakul, S., Nattee, K., Nathunli, P., Promprieng, C., Anekwasinchai, R., & Silprasit, K. (2023). Phytochemical composition, anti-amylase and anti-acetylcholinesterase activities of leaf extracts and herbal tea of *Dolichandrone serrulata* (DC.) Seem. *NFS Journal, 33*, 100152.
107. Bala, E., Patra, S., & Singha, S. (2023). Flavour enhancement strategy for herbal beverages and kinetic modelling of their antioxidant and sensory properties in accelerated storage conditions. *International Journal of Gastronomy and Food Science, 33*, 100788.
108. Shaik, M. I., Hamdi, I. H., & Sarbon, N. M. (2023). A comprehensive review on traditional herbal drinks: Physicochemical, phytochemicals and pharmacology properties. *Food Chemistry Advances, 3*, 100460.
109. Liu, Y., Guo, C., Zang, E., Shi, R., Liu, Q., Zhang, M., et al. (2023). Review on herbal tea as a functional food: Classification, active compounds, biological activity, and industrial status. *Journal of Future Foods, 3*(3), 206–219.
110. Silva, T. M., Fracasso, D. S., Vargas Visentin, A. P., Cassini, C., Scariot, F. J., Danetti, S., et al. (2022). Dual effect of the herbal matcha green tea (*Camellia sinensis* L. Kuntze) supplement in EA.hy926 endothelial cells and *Artemia salina*. *Journal of Ethnopharmacology, 298*, 115564.
111. Abdullah, R., Zaheer, S., Kaleem, A., Iqtedar, M., Aftab, M., & Saleem, F. (2023). Formulation of herbal tea using *Cymbopogon citratus, Foeniculum vulgare*, and *Murraya koenigii* and its anti-obesity potential. *Journal of King Saud University–Science, 35*(6), 102734.
112. Ruchika, & Sehgal, A. (2022). An update on disease-preventing potential of green tea in comparison with some tisanes. *South African Journal of Botany, 144*, 92–96.
113. Ghosh, A., Majumder, S., Samadder, R., Sarkar, S., Nandi, S., Subba, P., et al. (2023). Study of *in vitro* antioxidant and antibacterial potential of different tea clones. *Pharmacological Research–Modern Chinese Medicine, 9*, 100312.
114. Jin, L., Li, X. B., Tian, D. Q., Fang, X. P., Yu, Y. M., Zhu, H. Q., et al. (2016). Antioxidant properties and color parameters of herbal teas in China. *Industrial Crops and Products, 87*, 198–209.
115. Villaescusa, L., Zaragozá, C., Zaragozá, F., & Tamargo, J. (2023). Herbal medicines for the treatment of cardiovascular diseases: Benefits and risks—A narrative review. *International Journal of Cardiology, 385*, 44–52.
116. Motyka, S., Skała, E., Ekiert, H., & Szopa, A. (2023). Health-promoting approaches of the use of chia seeds. *Journal of Functional Foods, 103*, 105480.
117. Bakowska-Barczak, A., Larminat, M. Ad., & Kolodziejczyk, P. P. (2020). The application of flax and hempseed in food, nutraceutical, and personal care products. In Kozłowski, R. M., & Mackiewicz-Talarczyk, M. (Eds.), *Handbook of Natural Fibers (Second Edition)* (pp. 557–590). Woodhead Publishing.
118. Rashid, F., Ahmed, Z., Hussain, S., Huang, J. Y., & Ahmad, A. (2019). *Linum usitatissimum* L. seeds: Flax gum extraction, physicochemical and functional characterization. *Carbohydrate Polymers, 215*, 29–38.

119. Bozan, B., & Temelli, F. (2008). Chemical composition and oxidative stability of flax, safflower, and poppy seed and seed oils. *Bioresource Technology, 99*(14), 6354–6359.
120. Pappu, R., Varghese, J., Koteshwara, K. B., Kamath, V., Lobo, R., & Nimmy, K. (2019). Evaluation of biodegradable gel containing flax seed extract (*Linum usitatissimum*) as a targeted drug delivery for management of chronic periodontitis. *Journal of Herbal Medicine, 15*, 100254.
121. Cakmak, H., Ilyasoglu-Buyukkestelli, H., Sogut, E., Ozyurt, V. H., Gumus-Bonacina, C. E., & Simsek, S. (2023). A review on recent advances of plant mucilages and their applications in food industry: Extraction, functional properties and health benefits. *Food Hydrocolloids for Health, 3*, 100131.
122. Borrelli, F., & Ernst, E. (2008). Black cohosh (*Cimicifuga racemosa*): A systematic review of adverse events. *American Journal of Obstetrics & Gynecology, 199*(5), 455–466.
123. Romm, A., Hardy, M. L., & Mills, S. (2010). Black cohosh. In A. Romm, M. L. Hardy, & S. Mills (Eds.), *Botanical Medicine for Women's Health* (pp. 523–527). Churchill Livingstone.
124. Wuttke, W., Rauš, K., & Gorkow, C. (2006). Efficacy and tolerability of the Black cohosh (*Actaea racemosa*) ethanolic extract BNO 1055 on climacteric complaints: A double-blind, placebo- and conjugated estrogens-controlled study. *Maturitas, 55*, S83–S91.
125. Shulman, L. P., Banuvar, S., Fong, H. H. S., & Farnsworth, N. R. (2011). Discussion of a well-designed clinical trial which did not demonstrate effectiveness: UIC center for botanical dietary supplements research study of black cohosh and red clover. *Fitoterapia, 82*(1), 88–91.
126. Hui, Z., Xiaoyan, M., Mukun, Y., Ke, W., Liyuan, Y., & Sainan, Z., et al. (2012). Effects of black cohosh and estrogen on the hypothalamic nuclei of ovariectomized rats at different temperatures. *Journal of Ethnopharmacology, 142*(3), 769–775.
127. Roberts, H. (2010). Safety of herbal medicinal products in women with breast cancer. *Maturitas, 66*(4), 363–369.
128. Bokelmann, J. M. (2022). Black cohosh (*Actaea racemosa/Cimicifuga racemosa*): Root. In J. M. Bokelmann (Ed.), *Medicinal Herbs in Primary Care* (pp. 225–233). Elsevier.
129. Murray, M. T., & Nowicki, J. (2020). *Cimicifuga racemosa* (Black cohosh). In J. E. Pizzorno & M. T. Murray (Eds.), *Textbook of Natural Medicine* (5th ed., pp. 510–514. e1). Churchill Livingstone.
130. Singh, S., Supaweera, N., Nwabor, O. F., Chaichompoo, W., Suksamrarn, A., Chittasupho, C., et al. (2024). Poly (vinyl alcohol)-gelatin-sericin copolymerized film fortified with vesicle-entrapped demethoxycurcumin/bisdemethoxycurcumin for improved stability, antibacterial, anti-inflammatory, and skin tissue regeneration. *International Journal of Biological Macromolecules, 258*, 129071.
131. Patel, R., Singh, S., Singh, S., Sheth, N., & Gendle, R. (2009). Development and characterization of curcumin loaded transfersome for transdermal delivery. *Journal of Pharmaceutical Sciences and Research, 1*(4), 71.
132. Kumar, S., Chauhan, N., Tyagi, B., Yadav, P., Samanta, A. K., & Tyagi, A. K. (2023). Exploring bioactive compounds and antioxidant properties of twenty-six Indian

medicinal plant extracts: A correlative analysis for potential therapeutic insights. *Food and Humanity, 1*, 1670–1679.

133. Zhu, M. Z., Yang, M. F., Song, Y., Xu, H. M., Xu, J., Yue, N. N., et al. (2023). Exploring the efficacy of herbal medicinal products as oral therapy for inflammatory bowel disease. *Biomedicine & Pharmacotherapy, 165*, 115266.
134. Okwunodulu, I. N., Obioma, V. N., Okwunodulu, F. U., Ndife, J., & Wabali, V. (2023). Functional combo juice drink from ginger, garlic, turmeric, and pineapple juice blends: Bioactive compounds, antioxidant activity, physicochemical elucidation, and their sensorial expectations. *Food Chemistry Advances, 3*, 100391.
135. Wang, Z., Wang, X., Li, X., Lu, K., Wang, L., Ma, X., et al. (2024). Antioxidant effects of the aqueous extract of turmeric against hydrogen peroxide-induced oxidative stress in spotted seabass (*Lateolabrax maculatus*). *Aquaculture and Fisheries, 9*(1), 71–77.
136. Iweala, E. J., Uche, M. E., Dike, E. D., Etumnu, L. R., Dokunmu, T. M., Oluwapelumi, A. E., et al. (2023). *Curcuma longa* (Turmeric): Ethnomedicinal uses, phytochemistry, pharmacological activities, and toxicity profiles—A review. *Pharmacological Research–Modern Chinese Medicine, 6*, 100222.
137. Islam, M., Prottay, A. A. S., Sultana, I., Al Faruq, A., Bappi, M. H., Akbor, M. S., et al. (2023). Phytochemical screening and evaluation of antioxidant, anti-inflammatory, antimicrobial, and membrane-stabilizing activities of different fractional extracts of *Grewia nervosa* (Lour.) Panigrahi. *Food Bioscience, 54*, 102933.
138. Joshi, P., Yadaw, G. S., Joshi, S., Semwal, R. B., & Semwal, D. K. (2020). Antioxidant and anti-inflammatory activities of selected medicinal herbs and their polyherbal formulation. *South African Journal of Botany, 130*, 440–447.
139. Zubaidah, E., Susanti, I., Sujuti, H., Martati, E., Rahayu, A. P., Srianta, I., et al. (2023). The distinctive hepatoprotective activity of turmeric kombucha (*Curcuma longa*) induced by diethylnitrosamine in Balb/C mice. *Food Bioscience, 55*, 103043.
140. Vafaeipour, Z., Razavi, B. M., & Hosseinzadeh, H. (2022). Effects of turmeric (*Curcuma longa*) and its constituent (curcumin) on the metabolic syndrome: An updated review. *Journal of Integrative Medicine, 20*(3), 193–203.

CHAPTER 9

Biological Screening, Toxicity, and Regulations of Herbal Drugs

ANUJ K. SRIVASTAVA[1], AJAY KUMAR[1], and DEEPAK KUMAR[2]

[1]*Department of Pharmacology, Sardar Patel College of Pharmacy, Gorakhpur, Uttar Pradesh, India*

[2]*Faculty of Pharmaceutical Sciences, Mahayogi Gorakhnath University Gorakhpur, Uttar Pradesh, India*

*Corresponding author

ABSTRACT

For millennia, the use of herbal treatments generated by plants has been a crucial aspect of human healing. Because of their possible medical advantages, herbal treatments have seen a rise in popularity in recent years. Nonetheless, there are frequently concerns about the effectiveness and safety of herbal medications. This abstract provides an overview of the key aspects of biological screening, toxicity assessment, and regulatory guidelines for plants and their natural origins.

Biological screening is a critical step in the evaluation of the pharmacological activities of herbal drugs. The field involves several *in vitro* and *in vivo* methodologies in order to identify biologically active compounds, evaluate their processes of action, and ascertain their possible medicinal advantages. These screenings are essential for understanding the physiological effects of herbal drugs.

Toxicity assessment is another fundamental aspect of herbal drug research. It entails determining and measuring any possible negative consequences connected to the usage of herbal remedies. This assessment helps in establishing safe dosage levels and minimizing the risks associated with herbal drug consumption.

The Essentials of Herbal Drugs. Varsha Tiwari, Abhishek Tiwari, and Ajay Sharma (Eds.)

DOI: 10.1201/9781998511778-9

Regulations are essential for guaranteeing the effectiveness, security, and efficacy of herbal remedies. Different countries have distinct regulatory frameworks to oversee the marketing and distribution of herbal products. Harmonization of these regulations is an ongoing challenge, as it can enhance the global trade of herbal drugs while safeguarding consumer health.

In this chapter, we cover the aspects of biological screening and toxicity of herbal drugs, coupled with robust regulatory frameworks to harness the therapeutic potential of these natural remedies while ensuring their safety. An evidence-based approach, focusing on scientific validation and adherence to international standards, is essential to promote the responsible use of herbal drugs in modern healthcare.

9.1 INTRODUCTION

It has long been known that using plants, plant parts, and isolated phytochemicals can help prevent and treat a variety of medical diseases. This old custom still has a significant influence on modern medicine today. More than 25% of all prescription drugs utilized worldwide are made from plants; there are a total of 121 active ingredients in use at this moment in time. Surprisingly, just 11% of the drugs on the WHO list of vital medicines are derived from plants [1].

Traditionally, medications, which are often an essential part of standard treatment, are used by about 80% of the population, especially in Asia and Africa. India, in particular, has a rich heritage of utilizing medicinal herbs and indigenous medical systems, with over 80% of the rural population supporting these methods [2]. The Indian herbal industry uses about 960 plant species, 178 of which are substantial producers that yield in excess of 100 metric tons annually [3].

The herbal market of India is expanding rapidly, and by 2012, it is expected to increase to a value of Rs 145,000 million. In addition, exports are anticipated to reach Rs 90,000 million, exhibiting noteworthy Compound Annual Growth Rates (CAGRs) of 20% and 25%, respectively, according to ASSOCHAM's 2008 study. This underscores the growing recognition and economic significance of herbal remedies in contemporary healthcare systems.

The first category of therapeutic medicines includes over-the-counter medications (OTC). The second group consists of active ingredients that are extracted from plant materials after a certain amount of processing, which represents a more advanced form of herbal medications. These fractionated substances usually have higher pharmacological activity and greater purity. The third category includes medications made from herbs, for which extensive information on toxicity tests conducted on animals, both abruptly and over an extended time, is available [4].

A system of classification for herbal drugs was proposed by the WHO Geographic Regions Center for the Southeast Asian Region during a 2003 workshop on regulating the use of herbal products in the local area. Herbal medications were methodically divided into four groups: imported products with a basis in herbal medicine, genetically modified medicinal products, natural therapies within recognized frameworks, and traditional herbal products [5]. Traditional natural products (NPs) have a long history of use in the communities where they are used, which distinguishes them with their well-known composition, therapeutic methods, and dosage.

Because herbal remedies have an extensive record of usage in established systems like Ayurveda, Unani, and Siddha, there is no need to conduct local efficacy studies. The form, shape, dosage, route of administration, herbal constituents, preparation techniques, and medicinal indications of native plants are all altered in modified herbal medicines. These modifications must adhere to national regulatory safety and efficacy standards, with the necessity for pre-clinical and clinical data contingent on the nature of the modifications. Herbal medicines that are imported, both as unfinished and finished products, must be registered and approved for sale in their native countries. The importing country's national authority mandates the submission of safety and efficacy data. Compliance with good manufacturing practices (GMP) is particularly crucial for the last two categories of herbal drugs.

India, renowned for its export of standardized herbal extracts and raw materials, notably ships herbal medicines rooted in systems like Ayurveda globally. Despite the increasing global adoption of herbal drugs, concerns have been raised regarding reported side effects and adulteration, casting a shadow on their widespread use and commercial viability. Additionally, the lack of uniform regulatory procedures for these drugs across different countries further compounds these challenges. The purpose of this research is to identify the advancement of technical guidelines in the production of herbal medications and to create a system of oversight for their sale [6].

9.2 HISTORY OF HERBAL MEDICINE

The historical evolution of herbal medicine has been extensively chronicled in various texts authored by scholars throughout the ages. Here are noteworthy books and authors who have significantly contributed to our understanding of herbal medicine: "De Materia Medica" by Dioscorides (circa 40–90 CE): A Greek physician and pharmacologist, Dioscorides authored this influential work during the Roman Empire. This comprehensive compilation details medicinal plants and their applications, serving as a foundational text in herbal medicine. "Huangdi Neijing" (Yellow Emperor's Inner Canon): Traditionally attributed to the Yellow Emperor (Huangdi), this ancient Chinese text is a cornerstone of traditional Chinese medicine. Comprising the Suwen (Basic Questions) and the Lingshu (Spiritual Pivot), it provides insights into acupuncture, herbal remedies, and Chinese medical principles. "Avicenna's Canon of Medicine" by Avicenna (Ibn Sina) (980–1037): Avicenna, a Persian polymath, synthesized contemporary knowledge in this influential medical encyclopedia. The work delves into herbal medicine, diagnosis, and treatment, impacting both Eastern and Western medicine [7].

Many different writers from the medieval and Renaissance periods wrote "Herbarium." The term "herbarium" refers to a collection of several European herbal writings from the times of the medieval and Renaissance. These books provide a detailed description of the characteristics and use of medicinal herbs. Nicholas Culpeper's "The Complete Herbal" (1616–1654): English doctor and herbalist Culpeper promoted the use of herbs for treatment in his approachable herbal guide. For the general population, it offered useful information regarding the therapeutic qualities of numerous herbs. Harvey Wickes Felter (1865–1932) and John Uri Lloyd (1849–1936) wrote "The Eclectic Materia Medica, Pharmacology and Therapeutics": This extensive treatise, which emphasizes herbal cures among other things, is a component of the American medical tradition known as eclectic medicine. James A. Duke's book "The Green Pharmacy" (1929–2017): renowned American botanist James A. Duke [8].

9.3 SOURCES OF DRUGS

9.3.1 PLANT SOURCES

Due to a decline in new drug approvals and escalating costs, numerous obstacles confront the field of novel medication research. More successful outcomes for newly developed chemical entities (NCEs) were first expected with the introduction of sequential chemistry. However, despite this scientific advancement, the success rate for new drug discovery remains unimproved. In response to this, a novel integrated drug discovery approach has been developed, merging Ayurvedic knowledge with plant-based drug discovery. The identification of NCEs stands as a crucial initial step in discovering new drugs, which can be achieved through chemical synthesis or biological activity-guided fractionation, separating them from NPs. To develop new plant-based drugs, the selection of candidate plants should be informed by Ayurvedic knowledge, traditional reported use, tribal non-documented use, and thorough literature searches. Analyzing ancient documented formulations can provide insights into the predominance of specific Ayurvedic characteristics, aiding in the selection of candidate plants for bioactivity-based fractionation. It is necessary to transition the method for extraction from sequential to parallel extraction in order to combine drug research with Ayurvedic wisdom. A standardized extract or isolated bioactive curative aspect from the identified plant may be created as a novel medicine via bioassay-guided fractionation. This integrated approach not only saves time and money but also increases the success rate of drug discovery. Herbal drugs predominantly derive from various plant parts, including leaves, roots, seeds, and bark, with the choice of plant parts contingent on the desired therapeutic properties [7, 9].

9.3.2 ANIMAL SOURCES

Although minerals are seldom encountered in herbal remedies, several minerals have long been utilized in traditional medicine due to their antacid or absorbent qualities. Major (P and K), secondary (Ca, Mg, S), and micro, trace, or rare (B, Cl, Cr, F, I, Fe, Mn, Mo, Ni, Se, Na, V, Zn) minerals are among the groups of essential nutrients from minerals that are vital to human health maintenance [10]. Two cytotoxins from Naja kaouthia (NK-CTX) and Naja sumatrana (NS-CTX) have been found by Chong et al. [11] to be effective in stopping the proliferation of cell lines associated with lung cancer. Nevertheless, their cytotoxic character, which has evolved and adapted to food, could restrict their safe and effective usage as drugs [11]. De Avelar Júnior et al.'s [12] research indicates that the peptide LyeTx I-b has potential as a combination chemotherapy approach for breast cancer. To validate its effectiveness as a curative medication candidate, either alone or in conjunction with cisplatin, more *in vivo* research is required [12]. Yang and colleagues conducted a comprehensive metabolomic analysis, identifying 26 biomarkers regulated by folic acid with potential therapeutic targets for preventing ischemic stroke. In a rat ischemic stroke model, folic acid demonstrated significant protective effects against pathological development [12]. Certain traditional medicines, including Traditional Chinese Medicine (TCM), incorporate animal-derived ingredients. Tiger bones, tiger urine, bear gallbladder, and rhino horn have been historically used in TCM for various medicinal purposes [13].

9.3.3 MINERAL SOURCES

Although minerals are seldom encountered in herbal remedies, several minerals have long been utilized in traditional medicine due to their antacid or absorbent qualities. Major (P and K), secondary (Ca, Mg, S), and micro, trace, or rare (B, Cl, Cr, F, I, Fe, Mn, Mo, Ni, Se, Na, V, Zn) minerals are among the groups of essential nutrients from minerals that are vital to human health maintenance [14, 15].

9.3.4 MARINE SOURCES

Marine organisms, both plants and animals, serve as sources of bioactive compounds for potential medicinal or herbal uses. These marine sources often contain unique compounds that show promise in pharmaceutical research. Numerous natural compounds and unique chemical compounds that have potential therapeutic applications are found in the sea owing to its great biodiversity. Certain compounds produced from marine sources have the ability to target specific ion channels, which show promise for use as analgesics, anesthetics, and in the therapy of diseases like epileptic seizures, coronary artery disease, and mental health issues [16, 17].

9.4 TRADITIONAL USES OF HERBAL DRUGS

Natural medications have a long history of usage for a variety of objectives in many different cultures throughout the world. Although these treatments have historically been used for possible medicinal benefits, it is important to recognize that there can be variations in their safety as well as effectiveness. Not every herbal remedy has been proven to work by reliable science.

Many different plants have been utilized traditionally to cure specific ailments. Some examples of herbs that may help with issues related to the kidneys are the plants *Allium sativum* (garlic/Bawang), *Blumea balsamifera* (Nagal camphor/sambong), and *Clinopodium douglasii* (mint/yerba Buena), which, when mixed with oregano, is known to have anti-asthmatic properties. Herbal remedies range from the antidiabetic properties of *Momordica charantia* (bitter melon/AMPALAYA) to the use of Peperomia to treat rheumatism and gout [18, 19].

9.5 TOXICITY STUDIES

Traditional herbal medicine (THM) has evolved through centuries of trial and error, with accumulated knowledge forming the basis for today's traditional medicine. While a long history of traditional use may suggest safety and efficacy, it is crucial to acknowledge its limitations, particularly in identifying subtle reactions with prolonged latency periods. Numerous studies have highlighted the association between herbal medicine and adverse effects [20, 21].

Toxicity testing for medicinal plants can follow OECD guidelines, utilizing female rodents under ideal conditions. Acute and subacute toxicity studies, along with the determination of lethal dose and IC_{50}, are crucial aspects. Organ toxicity, often a result of chronic exposure to toxic agents, poses challenges to the widespread use of herbal medicine. Advanced analytical techniques, *in vitro* and *in vivo* test systems, and a systems biological approach aid in toxicological studies and safety evaluations [22].

Assessing the long-term effects of herbal drugs over months to years is essential for understanding potential chronic diseases or toxicities. Evaluation methods include determining effects on DNA, assessing potential carcinogenicity through long-term animal studies, and investigating impacts on fertility, pregnancy, and offspring development [23, 24].

Understanding the dose-response relationship is critical, distinguishing between intrinsic effects related to active chemical constituents and extrinsic effects attributed to contamination, adulteration, or misidentification of herbal products. Despite the increasing popularity of herbal medicines, many are marketed without reliable scientific evidence and mandatory safety evaluations, raising concerns about their safety and toxicity [25–27].

Reports of adverse drug reactions (ADRs) related to herbal medicine have increased, prompting countries to publish guidance documents for herbal products. Ethical concerns in chronic and subacute toxicity testing highlight the need for alternative approaches. The International Conference on Harmonization (ICH) advocates for reduced animal use in genotoxicity studies, utilizing *in vitro* models [28, 29].

9.5.1 ACUTE TOXICITY STUDIES

1. **OECD Guideline:** During toxicity studies, OECD standards for the investigation of acute oral toxicity have been adhered to. These consist of guidelines 420, 423, and 425. Initially, Standard 423 was implemented in March 1996 as a substitute for the conventional acute toxic overload test. This guideline describes a step-by-step protocol for the severe toxic class approach that uses three single-sex animals for each phase. The technique may categorize chemicals similarly to other acute toxicology (to determine Standards 420 and 425), is repeatable, and requires the least number of animals. In order to classify and evaluate a substance's hazards, an acute toxicity category technique is predicated on biological measurements using fixed dosages that are appropriately isolated [30].
2. **Principle:** The acute toxic method evaluates acute oral toxicity by identifying the dose level causing mortality. This involves administering a single dose of test substances to rodents via oral gavage, observing them for up to 15 days, recording all animal body weights, and conducting necropsy. Fixed doses of the test substances are used, and the method aims to identify toxicity without causing death [31].
3. **Objective:** The objective of conducting acute toxicity studies is to determine the therapeutic index (TI) of a particular drug and ensure *in vivo* safety. Acute toxicity studies are typically conducted in experimental animals to determine the LD_{50} value.

4. **Validation of Toxicological Data:** General Parameters: In accordance with mainstream research, safety claims regarding the health of humans should be backed by data, especially for natural remedies with a lengthy history of traditional use. It is anticipated that planning for experimental toxicity research will be guided by the history of the plant material's traditional use. Since these effects might not show up during traditional practice, some specific toxic consequences, such as genotoxicity, carcinogenicity, and toxicity to development and reproduction, should be assessed for THMs. Further pre-clinical testing may be needed if there is a lack of information on traditional medicines made from herbs or if there are issues related to these goods [11, 12].
5. **Selecting Appropriate Test Models:** To accumulate information that is scientifically valid, it is crucial to select appropriate animal models or other test systems. Animal models, as well as *ex vivo* and *in vitro* preparations, can be employed as test platforms. Selection is based on factors including species, tissues, organs, cells, and endpoints of interest. While it is important to take into account the limits of propagation of cell techniques, complementary research may make use of *in vitro* techniques. Experimental animal *in vivo* evaluations are sometimes more useful than *in vitro* research when assessing toxic effects. However, 3R (elimination, reduction, and refinement of assessment animals) initiatives recommend using approved alternative test systems in place of some animal tests [2].
6. **Quantity of Sample:** The European Authorities, the FDA, and the OECD have all established uniform official recommendations that address sample size concerns. It is essential that the experimental design includes both favorable and adverse groups of controls. To ensure that there is sufficient power to detect potential effects, statistical considerations should be taken into account while determining the sample size.
7. **Administrative Approach of Herbal Drugs (*In Vivo*):** The results of ethno-medical research on the traditional application of the plant as a treatment have an impact on the technique through which it is administered, selected for a toxic examination. Since the majority of THMs are taken orally, it is necessary to look into

their effects on tissues and organs, as well as their gastrointestinal toxicity. Although there are alternatives, including intraperitoneal injection, their applicability to actual hazards needs to be taken into account. When assessing the efficacy of any item, choosing its handling method is crucial.

8. **The Doses of Plant Extract:** To describe the dose-response relationship, *in vivo* trials should be designed, while *in vitro* investigations aim to identify a concentration-activity link. In order to determine the envisioned curative impact on individuals or the primary physiological action in experimental animals, it is crucial to distinguish between the doses that result in adverse effects.
9. **Methods of Testing:** Long-term, repeated administration of a THM might result in beneficial effects; however, it enhances the prospect of toxicity.
10. **Contaminants in THMs:** During cultivation or processing, THMs may come into contact with heavy metals, microbes, agricultural residues, and industrial wastes, among additional risks to the environment. It is imperative to keep an eye out for contaminants prior to subjecting THMs to toxicity testing. Mycotoxins, pesticide residues, and heavy metal pollution are regarded as major hazards for plant materials and can affect how toxicological test results are evaluated.
11. **Determining the Toxicity of THMs:** THMs with potentially harmful compounds may give rise to safety concerns notwithstanding their extensive history of usage. Certain components, such as pyrrolizidine alkaloids, ephedrine alkaloids, and aristolochic acid, have been linked to particular health problems. As a result, in order to identify potential dangers, toxicological investigations—including acute to chronic toxicity tests—may be necessary. Herbal medicinal products' (HMPs) toxicity evaluation should adhere to global recommendations published by relevant authorities, such as the WHO, EU officials, ICH standards, or OECD.
12. **Unit Dose Toxicity (Acute Effect of Toxicity):** The unit dose toxicity examines the acute toxic effects of THMs in accordance with pertinent international criteria. Determining a dose that is

obviously hazardous but not lethal is the goal, as it provides information for further repeated dose toxicity studies. The test involves giving experimental animals escalating dosages, monitoring for significant, life-threatening toxicity, and figuring out the LD_{50} level. Recent revisions have favored various acute toxicity tests that require fewer experimental animals, such as the fixed dosage technique, acute toxic group strategy, and up-and-down procedure.

13. **Repeated Lethal Dose:** The major objective of repetitive dosage toxicity testing is to determine the *in vivo* effects resulting from repetitive everyday administration of THMs for a minimum of 28 days. These investigations need to identify potential toxicity targets to promote the ascertainment of dose-response correlations. One should never disregard the risks related to repeated dose exposure, not even with conventional drugs that possess an extensive record of safe usage.

9.5.2 SUB-ACUTE TOXICITY

Sub-acute toxicity studies aid in the development of dosage schedules for longer-term treatments and offer details on potential hazards associated with repeated oral exposure. The specimen being tested is administered orally to the animals being studied every day for a total of 28 days at gradually increasing doses. This test provides details on the dose-response correlation and produces the overall no-observed adverse effect level (NOAEL).

9.5.3 CHRONIC TOXICITY

In chronic toxicity investigations, the research animal groups receive the test drug daily at increasing doses, as was previously indicated in the multiple dose tests for toxicity. In testing for chronic toxicity, rats are the preferred species; however, specific legislation may also call for non-rodent species. ICH has recently made an effort to carry out harmonization assessments within the European Region, Japan, and the US. However, there is a lack of uniformity in management periods between international organizations. Consequently, the ICH recommendation [32] specifies this time frame as nine months for non-rodents and a total of six months for rodents; however, the recommendations of the OECD describe this period as up to 12 months, with different durations. Although the oral route is the most common route of administration, depending on how the drug is normally administered, more superficial or aerosol methods may also be used for traditional drugs. One or more interim kills, for example, at three and six months, may also be an aspect of the study design. Animals are constantly monitored for symptoms of illness or mortality during the administration phase. Necropsies are carried out on animals that pass away during the study or are sacrificed at its conclusion, as previously explained in the sub-acute toxicity test (Figure 9.1).

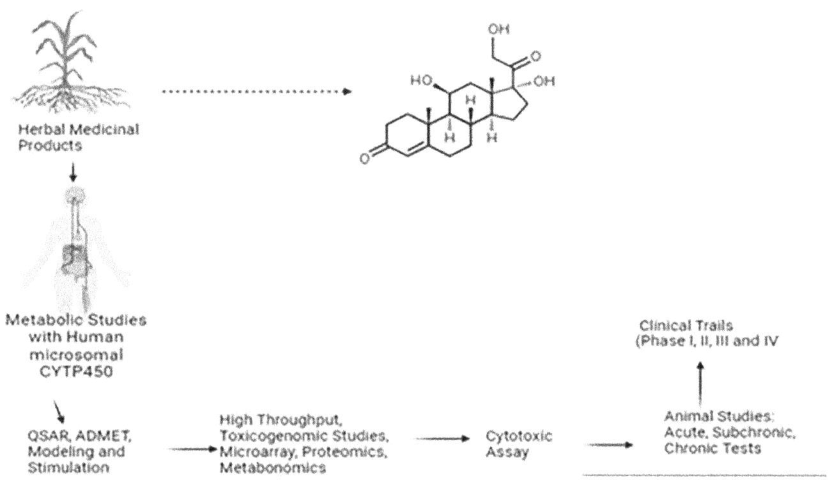

FIGURE 9.1 Animal study of herbal drugs.

9.6 MICROBIAL, PESTICIDES, RADIOACTIVE, AND HEAVY METALS CONTAMINATION

External factors, including microbial contamination, mycotoxins, pesticides, radioactive contamination, and heavy metals, can enhance the toxicity of herbal medicine. Mycotoxins, such as aflatoxin B1, pose significant health risks, leading to established regulations for their permissible limits. Chromatographic techniques and immunological assays are employed for mycotoxin detection, ensuring the safety of HMPCs [33–35].

Pesticide residues in medicinal herbs, especially in Asian herbal medicines, are a concern. Maximum residual levels (MRLs) have been established for pesticides, and chromatographic methods are commonly used for their identification and quantification. Immunological assays, such as IC-ELISA, offer rapid screening for pesticide residues. Heavy metal contamination, particularly in Asian traditional medicines, can lead to negative health effects. Quantification of heavy metals through techniques like ICP-MS, ICP-OES, and AAS is essential to ensure consumer safety [36–41] (Table 9.1).

TABLE 9.1 Standard Limits of Heavy Metals Contamination

Test For Heavy/ Toxic Metals	AYUSH, India	USA, FDA	WHO	HAS, Singapore
Lead	10.00 ppm	10.00 ppm	10.00 ppm	20.00 ppm
Mercury	1.00 ppm	1.00 ppm	1.00 ppm	0.50 ppm
Arsenic	10.00 ppm	10.00 ppm	10.00 ppm	5.00 ppm

9.7 REGULATIONS OF HERBAL DRUGS

A significant percentage—approximately 80% to even 90%—of the community depends on natural healers for their therapeutic needs. However, it is notable that in these populations, herbal drugs often lack state regulation. In contrast, developed countries, where natural healers are produced and used following GMP and good clinical practices, contribute significantly to the trade. It is noteworthy that certain nations, such as China, India, and Korea, regulate natural healers, where traditional medicine is treated with the same respect as modern pharmaceuticals. The approval process involves clinical trials, marketing approval, and certification of manufacturers and marketers by local drug regulatory authorities. Stress is laid on GMP and good supply practices. Regulatory authorities' quality control, data analysis, and post-marketing compliance must be established. Good laboratory practices (GLP), good agriculture and collection procedures (GACP), and other standards must be followed by manufacturers to ensure that products exceed the required standards. The monitoring of quality includes a number of analytical techniques, particularly high-performance liquid chromatography (HPLC) and gas chromatography-mass spectrometry (GC-MS), and so forth.

The registration of herbal products requires detailed information, including a list of ingredients, product formula, manufacturer details, dosage information, adverse effects, and storage conditions. Pharmacovigilance centers for herbal products are essential for assessing safety and efficacy by monitoring ADRs. However, there is a need for national systems for monitoring the safety of natural remedies.

To ensure that herbal medication safety is maintained, adverse event reporting and post-market surveillance must be put into place. Post-marketing surveillance for medication safety involves a range of techniques, such as proactive surveillance and prescribed event tracking. Suspected adverse reactions are often identified through spontaneous reports provided by healthcare providers and occasionally by customers. Patient conduct, practitioner inefficiencies, and an absence of associative recognition all play a part in this issue of understatement, which is problematic when it comes to herbal medicines. To address particular issues with herbal medications, pharmacovigilance techniques must be modified [42, 43] (Figure 9.2).

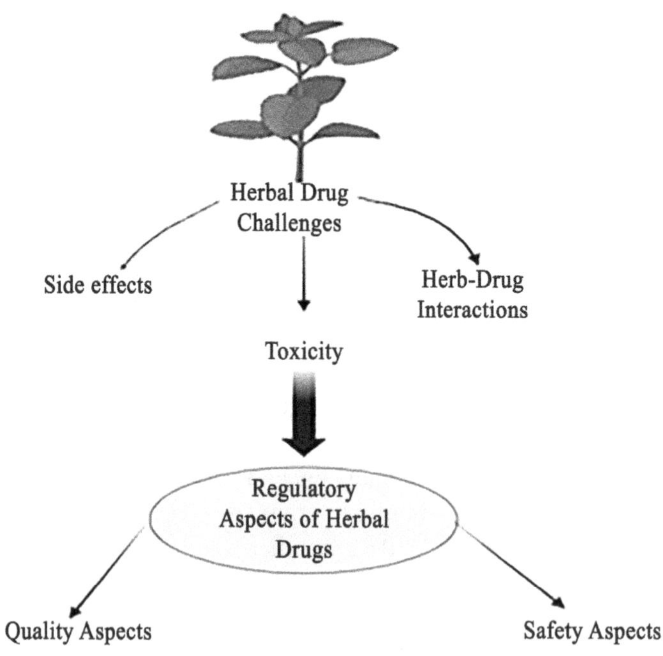

FIGURE 9.2 Regulatory aspects of herbal drugs.

9.7.1 GUIDELINES FOR THE DEVELOPMENT OF HERBAL MEDICATIONS

The importance underlying conventional healing, including its implementation in general medical care, was initially acknowledged internationally with the Alma Ata, Ethiopia Statement. It states, among other items, that primary medical treatment is dependent upon medical specialists at the district and reference stages, including medical professionals, nurses, midwives, and other support workers, as well as community service providers, in addition to conventional healers if necessary [44]. The reason for the safety concerns surrounding herbal therapeutic goods is the absence of reliable quality assurance in a rapidly expanding sector. The main differences between various regulatory regimes are their expertise with alternative and complementary medicine (TM/CAM) and mainstream medicine, as well as their lack of specific standards for quality assurance, safety monitoring, and efficacy and safety evaluation.

Under some regulatory frameworks, herbs can be categorized as foods, functional foods, nutritional supplements, or herbal medicines. According to the World Health Organization, herbal medicines consist of plant parts, plant-based substances, medicinal substances, and finished herbal remedies that contain combinations of plant parts, plant material alone, or other plant parts as active ingredients. Similarly, in the European Union (EU), whole, broken, or sliced organisms, components of plants, microorganisms, and mushrooms in their natural state, unprocessed form—typically in dry or fresh form—are categorized as herbal remedies by the EMEA. Unprocessed exudates are also included in herbal remedies. Herbal pharmaceutical preparations are characterized as substances made from herbs that undergo procedures comprising extraction, distillation, separation, purification, concentration, or fermentation. This includes concentrated juice and tinctures, as well as extracts from plants, essential oils, and herbal medicines in powder form.

In the US, almost all herbal products are regarded as foods because they are nutritional supplements. A natural merchandise that originates from a variety of organisms such as algae, plants, or microscopic fungal organisms is produced through one or several methods that include crushing, decoction, water-based extraction, ethanol-based extraction, or other procedures meant to be administered as a medicinal product. This can be referred to as a Natural Drugs Product (Article 201(g)(1)(B),

Federal Food, Drug, and Cosmetic Act). National health authorities have implemented restrictions to ensure the safe use of herbal medicines due to global concerns about their safety.

WHO launched a worldwide survey in 2001 covering national TM/ CAM and herbal medicine regulations in 191 member states. The most crucial elements for the field of herbal medicine regulation are found to be research data, suitable regulatory mechanisms, provider education, and knowledge [3]. According to the report, until 2003, 37% of member states had rules and regulations pertaining to natural remedies; 42% of member states had laws and regulations that were unique to them. Additionally, it was noted that about 35% of member states treat natural remedies as prescription medications and that almost 68% of member countries offer them as OTC medications.

Herbal medication can be legally sold, with the most prevalent forms of claims being medical, health, and nutrient content claims. Just 24% of the countries that responded indicated they had a national pharmacopoeia for herbal drugs that was in use, and 18% claimed one was being prepared.

Around 51% of the countries indicated that the production of herbal products is subject to the same GMP regulations as that of conventional pharmaceuticals. Just 15% of the 142 member nations that explained had herbal medicines on their list of essential medications. China ranked first in the vital drug list with 1242 herbal medicines [45]. Some of the elements that help identify how a country's regulation of herbal drugs has evolved include the overall regulatory structure, the medicine licensing system, the pharmacist's manual expansion, national manuals, participation in the prescribed medicine list, and prescription type (prescription or OTC).

We have compared the regulations controlling herbal drugs in several Western Pacific and Southeast Asian nations using these parameters. With the exception of Bhutan, Sri Lanka, and the Maldives, all 18 countries under investigation have systems in place for regulating and registering herbal drugs. Nine countries—China, the Philippines, Vietnam, Malaysia, Myanmar, the Indian Ocean Territory, Sri Lanka, Thailand, and Korea—have national monographs on herbal medicines. In Bhutan, Nepal, and the Philippines, monographs are now being developed. Except for Singapore, Malaysia, and the Maldives, 15 nations have produced pharmacopoeias for herbal remedies.

The vital drug list of seven countries comprises herbal remedies: China, Bhutan, India, Thailand, Korea, the Philippines, and Vietnam. The Philippines is first on the list with 2000 natural pharmaceuticals, followed by China with 1242 medications made from herbs. India keeps separate medicinal product lists for Ayurvedic and Unani herbal treatments. Almost every nation except Bhutan offers herbal medications as OTC products.

Herbal pharmaceuticals are exclusively sold as prescription medications in Bhutan, as there is no specific legislation governing them. The EU, US, and India have different regulations regarding the registration and marketing of natural medicaments.

9.7.1.1 RULES ASSOCIATED WITH MEDICINAL HERB REGISTRATION AND MARKETING AUTHORIZATION

The European Medicines Agency (EMEA) Committee on HMPCs has streamlined the registration process for traditional HMPC in EU member states. Insofar as it provides adequate proof that the product has been used medicinally for not less than 30 years in total, comprising at least 15 of those decades in the Community, according to Directive 2001/83/EC's Article 16c (1) (c), the streamlined process enables the certification of herbal medical products without the need for specificity and documentation of safety and efficacy testing and studies. Regarding the quality, nonclinical features, clinical safety, and efficacy of natural drugs, EMEA has established a number of guidelines. The Dietary Supplement Health and Education Act of 1994 regulated herbal medications in the US. In the US, an herbal drug may be supplied under its official OTC drug monograph, authorized NDA, or ANDA (21 CFR sections 331–358) [46].

9.7.2 INDIAN REGULATIONS

With the exception of allopathy, herbal medicines are a fundamental component of all known traditional Indian medicine systems. The Central Council of Indian Medicine Act, Research Councils, Department of AYUSH, and the D&C Act of 1940 (Amendment) govern herbal medicine in India. The ICMR, the CSIR, and the AYUSH department collaborate to develop novel pharmaceuticals in India and to accomplish the objective of safe and effective AYUSH products for identified ailments. The D&C Act of 1940 and the Rules of 1945 apply to herbal drugs.

All medications used internally or externally for the diagnosis, treatment, mitigation, or cure of any disease or disorder in humans or animals are generally considered Ayurvedic, Unani, or Siddha drugs. These drugs are made entirely in accordance with the formulae described in the recognized books of Siddha, the system of Ayurvedic and Unani medicine, which are listed in the First Schedule. The D&C Act increases the authority over export, quality, labeling, packing, manufacture, licensing, and composition of formulation. GMP standards are outlined in Schedule "T" of the Act and are applicable to the production of herbal medications [47] and CDSCO natural remedies [Schedules 92].

The Ministry of AYUSH was established on November 9, 2014, with the goal of ensuring the excellent growth and distribution of AYUSH health care systems. The Department of AYUSH was renamed as part of ISM & H in November 2003. The department was founded in March 1995, and its main objective was to develop education and research in the fields of traditional Indian systems of medicine.

9.7.2.1 AIM OF AYUSH

1. The primary goal of AYUSH is to raise the educational bar for the nation's homoeopathic colleges and universities and the traditional Indian system.
2. To strengthen the already established research institutes and ensure that a one-time study program on diseases that can be identified has an effective therapy available for these systems.
3. To create a plan for the propagation, cultivation, and regrowth of medicinal plants used in the systems discussed in sections 9.7.2.
4. To provide pharmacopeial criteria for medicines employed for the traditional Indian system.

Regulating medicine quality, establishing pharmacopeial standards, monitoring the operations of the IMPL under the auspices of the QCI, and monitoring the operations of IMPCL are the goals of AYUSH. Along with regulating the implementation of GMPs, AYUSH also sets up shared facilities using the cluster approach and implements the Drug Quality Control scheme, which includes revealing herbal drug formulations, knowledge, and manuscripts, documenting, and promoting local health customs. A certification program for AYUSH medicine goods is established by the QCI and the AYUSH government. People have always been concerned about the efficacy, safety, and quality standards of AYUSH products. A new voluntary certification program for AYUSH formulation has been launched by the QCI in response to these concerns. Typically, the data related to formulations contains the following kinds of information:

9.7.2.2 AYUSH ACCREDITATIONS

There are two degrees of AYUSH certification:

1. The AYUSH Standard Mark is dependent upon compliance with national regulations.
2. AYUSH Premium Mark, which is established by the selections made below:
    - **i. Option A:** The certification standards' contamination limits and WHO guidelines-recommended GMP requirements are met.
    - **ii. Option B:** Compliance with the laws of the country of import, provided that they are stricter than Option A's [47].

9.7.2.3 DEVELOPMENT OF HERBAL DRUGS

When developing new medications, the following details are typically included:

1. Chemical alteration and identification of biological activity components.
2. Assessment of efficacy as well as safety.
3. The approval of the FDA associated with the therapeutic ingredient whenever it concerns new medications.
4. Clinical investigations of medications.

After the drug becomes uniform, preliminary safety and biological impact studies are conducted. For every formula, the standardization method is included in the accompanying supplements.

9.7.3 CLINICAL STUDIES ON HERBAL MEDICINES

Regulations for good clinical practice state that herbal medicines are first explored on animals before being examined and tested on people. Herbal remedies and therapeutic plants must go through scientific evaluation before being employed in the medical system and finally in allopathic hospitals. The DCGI office's standards for allopathic medications must be followed. This is in no way related to the guidelines developed by experts in both traditional, Unani, or Siddha medicine for conducting clinical trials on these medications, which they can then apply in their own clinics [47].

9.7.3.1 PHASES OF A CLINICAL TRIAL

1. **Phase I Studies:** Since there is a good likelihood that herbal therapies may be safely administered to a relatively small number of clinical animals under observation in phase II trials, phase I studies are not necessary for herbal treatments. Phase I research usually takes many months.
2. **Phase II:** These investigate the dosage range for patients (100–300) with specific conditions. This step determines appropriate dose categories or protocols and outlines dose-response relationships, providing a comprehensive framework for the design of major treatment studies. At this point, it is imperative to confirm tolerance. A comprehensive analysis regarding clinical safety considerations should be the focal point of both the literature review and the protocol's parameters. Trials in phase II might involve up to a few 1000 persons and extend across numerous weeks to a year.
3. **Phase III:** This trial phase, which is carried out after phase 2 dose-ranging data have been established, includes comprehensive risk and benefit assessments. This phase involves approximately 1000 to 3000 volunteers with the specific illness who are at clinics or hospitals. In order to evaluate the impacts of the herbal remedies and detect any possible adverse effects, patients are closely examined. At this point in the trial, the drug's effectiveness and efficacy have been verified. This phase could take more than three years.

In order to compare different treatment modalities, patients are divided into two groups in several randomized phase 2 and phase 3 trials. A placebo is given to one group, and an experimental treatment under test is given to the other group.

The following are the Standards for standardized clinical practice for medicinal products containing herbs and items for conducting clinical studies in India:

1. Plants and herbal remedies that are currently in use should be disclosed in the literature of reputed traditional systems of medicine and processed in accordance with the guidelines provided in the literature for good manufacturing practices (GMPs) to ensure that the procedure is standard.
2. Including the phase 1 clinical trial studies is not necessary. Nonetheless, it is essential that the chemicals under examination are found in the Indian System of Medicine and described in their texts; additionally, it is required to determine whether or not the drugs' toxicity to animals has decreased.
3. The phase 2 clinical trial's toxicity study is not as crucial until a report indicating toxicity or the best time to take herbal medications—likely three months or less—is available. Under all these conditions, it is imperative that the two types of animals conduct a 4- to 6-week toxicity assessment.
4 Clinical trials using herbal medications should only be conducted if they have been standardized to guarantee that the indicators found for treatments under evaluation are consistent every time.
5. Clinical studies involving plant drugs must also adhere to the following regulations: informed consent, issues, benefits for participation, facts to be specified to participants, and those obtaining from research and study, which include young people or individuals with reduced independence; these studies must be approved by the relevant academic and ethical councils of concerned institutes. It is necessary, however, that clinical trials including plant drugs be conducted with the involvement of an indigenous Siddha, Ayurvedic, or Unani physician as a co-investigator.
6. Any allopathic physician conducting plant clinical trials without having any formal instruction or experience in all of these medical

systems would be unethical. As a result, the clinical examination should be conducted collaboratively with the presence of an expert from these systems.

9.7.4 AMONG THE LATIN AMERICAN COUNTRIES

The leading countries in the herbal market are Mexico, Argentina, and Brazil. Brazil has regulated herbal drugs since 1967. Herbal remedies are available OTC and through prescription. Directive 6 outlines the legal requirements for the registration of phyto-pharmaceutical drugs in Brazil. It was released in 1995 by the Brazilian Drug Division (DIMED), which is responsible for enforcing drug regulations.

In 2004, the RDC/48/2004 rule was released in its fourth iteration. The directive states that registration of phytopharmaceutical products is contingent upon full verification of safety, efficacy, and consistently defined quality. In accordance with the Federal Health Agency's Directive 116, human efficacy and safety test findings are also necessary for registration. The national pharmacopoeia and monographs are legally binding for the manufacturers [48].

The requirements for safety assessments are the same in Mexico and Argentina: traditional use without proven harmful effects; citation to published scientific research on comparable products; toxicological studies in cases where traditional use cannot be proven; and submission of a comprehensive toxicological and pharmacological dossier. Regular inspections guarantee adherence to these regulations [45].

The Eastern Mediterranean Region's most often utilized form of traditional medicine is herbal medicine. Iran's vast population relies on locally manufactured herbal medications for primary healthcare.

The majority of herbal products used in other countries, such as the UAE, come from Europe, Asia, or the United States. In this context, herbal therapies are generally categorized as "conventional herbal medicines" if they have been used widely, have a solid track record of safety and effectiveness, or have been a fixture in the community for a minimum of 51 years. "New herbal remedies" are those made with innovative blends of natural components that have never been used together before, or they are used very infrequently (a few times in a limited number of patients). Few nations in the area have laws in place to guarantee standards of quality.

A recent survey conducted in this area also revealed that adequate management and licensing of herbal medicines are required [49].

Significant information about efficacy, safety, and quality assurance is frequently lacking or missing. Herbal medicines are either not included in safety monitoring systems or are not covered by them in the majority of countries. Drug regulatory authorities received broad direction in 1999 and 2001 from the Eastern Mediterranean Drug Regulatory Authorities Conferences about the creation and execution of draft regulatory frameworks for herbal medicines. The WHO created guidelines in 2006 about the minimal standards for herbal medicine products registered in the Eastern Mediterranean region [3].

A summary of the general requirements for both safety and effectiveness is given in this guideline for both new and conventional HMPCs, as well as features of quality control, pharmacovigilance, and regulation over herbal medicine marketing. Globally, monographs for medicinal plants are being developed, but there is not currently agreement on how these should be implemented. There is no interlinking of the monographs for herbal raw materials published by various publications, such as the USP, BHC, BHP, CP, PDR for herbal medicines, and API. The monograph for a certain plant may differ across publications. Different national regulations for the same composition present challenges for herbal medicine makers.

9.7.5 WORLDWIDE HARMONIZATION

Harmonizing initiatives concerning the pharmacopoeial specifications, standardization, and grouping of herbal pharmaceuticals have been initiated in order to achieve agreement on the safety, efficacy, and effectiveness of natural drugs throughout nations. The pharmaceutical manuals of the three Asian nations describe similar herbal medicines; however, their standards differ slightly. The primary botanical family or species might have changed, but the identical raw plant material can still be described. Furthermore, despite the fact that the same raw material from plants is stated, the term suggested by the Chinese traits, the Latin generic pharmacopoeia identity, or the portion employed for the herbal cure may differ [50].

In an effort to promote the international commercialization of safe and efficacious herbal drugs, the basic drug monographs in the pharmacopoeias of six Asian countries—Japan, China, Korea, Singapore, Vietnam, and Hong Kong—were intended to be harmonized by the Pacific Western Global Framework for the Harmonization of Herbal Medicine (FHH). In 2000, the American countries started to harmonize their procedural criteria for herbal product registration.

The objective of the working group of the Pan American Network of Drug Regulatory Harmonization (PANDRH) on medicinal plants is to advance a shared knowledge of the different categories of herbal products, terminology, protocols, and minimal standards for herbal product registration [51].

The WHO Concepts on Traditional Medical Treatment in the Pacific Northwest Region" have produced a global standard vocabulary. This will aid in creating a shared scientific foundation for various traditional medicine systems. There are roughly 4000 traditional medicine phrases in this compilation. This is supposed to help with the development of clinical practice standards for traditional medicine that are based on evidence. It has been suggested to classify herbal remedies using an anatomical therapeutic chemical (ATC) approach that is completely compatible with prescription medications. With a few modifications, this method has since been approved and included in the Herbal ATC Index and Standards for Medicinal ATC Classification [3].

There are approximately 8000 herbal medication enterprises in India, most of which are small or medium-sized enterprises. Of them, 5000 have production facilities that comply with GMP regulations. Around 30% of manufactured goods, including extracts from herbs, make up the remaining 30% of Indian herbal industry exports, which mainly consist of raw materials [52].

In India, there are 55 significant business organizations that export herbal drugs. We have conducted an initial investigation using a 25-product questionnaire to determine the difficulties these businesses encounter when producing and shipping herbal medications. One of the main obstacles to commercialization is recognized as compliance with various national regulatory norms. A common technical document (CTD) needs to be created or embraced for the purpose of being eligible for approval for marketing in different countries, according to 33% of the industries surveyed, who also stated that it takes a long time to accomplish compliance with regulatory requirements to different country standards.

9.8 CONCLUSIONS

The expanding herbal medicine market has triggered concerns about the safety of herbal remedies, largely due to the insufficient availability of adequate pharmacological and toxicological data. The increasing evidence pointing to adverse effects associated with herbal medicine emphasizes the urgent need for toxicological evaluation. Recent strides in technologies and molecular biology offer the capability to analyze complex reactions to a multitude of herbal products at the molecular level. This advanced "-omic-" technology holds promise for predicting and conducting preclinical toxicity testing of herbal medicine in the future.

Our comprehension of the connection between specific substances and their effects has grown as a result of technological advancements in the detection and quantification of herbal medicine constituents. An increasing number of research investigations in developed nations are challenging the idea that long-standing conventional utilization is a sufficient indicator of the efficacy of herbal medicines due to growing concerns about the unanticipated or negative consequences of these treatments.

During the commercialization process, manufacturers face the issue of verifying the validity and effectiveness of herbal medicinal formulations, especially in Southeast Asia. The use of marker-based criteria to recognize and validate the ingredients of herbal drugs is growing in favor. However, because herbal medications are plant extracts, it is important to use a multi-marker approach and take storage conditions into account.

Plant-specific characteristics and quality standards vary significantly between countries, as may be seen by comparing pharmacopoeial standards generally. Although regional and national standards and recommendations have been produced, their acceptance is still uneven. The creation of a CTD is a major step in the right direction, even though there is disagreement over the application of a single, uniform strategy for either drugs or systems.

India stands out as one of the top countries in Southeast Asia when it comes to generating pharmacopoeial standards and updating current regulatory frameworks. The incorporation of many pharmacopoeial monographs, supported by evidence submissions for authorization from regulators, would enable herbal firms to reach more regulated markets globally.

KEYWORDS

- **bioactive**
- **biological screening**
- **good manufacturing practices**
- **herbal**
- **regulatory guidelines**
- **toxicity**

REFERENCES

1. Rates, S. M. K. (2001). Plants as sources of drugs. *Toxicon, 39*(5), 603–613.
2. Mukherjee, A., Mukhi, S., & Pakman, A. (2007). FZZ algebra. *Journal of High Energy Physics, 2007*(1), 025.
3. Sahoo, N., Manchikanti, P., & Dey, S. (2010). Herbal drugs: Standards and regulation. *Fitoterapia, 81*(6), 462–471.
4. Iwu, M. W., Duncan, A. R., & Okunji, C. O. (1999). New antimicrobials of plant origin. In *Perspectives on New Crops and New Uses* (pp. 457–462). ASHS Press.
5. World Health Organization. (2004). *Guidelines for the Regulation of Herbal Medicines in the South-East Asia Region.* WHO Regional Office for South-East Asia.
6. Ravishankar, B., & Shukla, V. J. (2007). Indian systems of medicine: A brief profile. *African Journal of Traditional, Complementary and Alternative Medicines, 4*(3), 319–337.
7. Katiyar, C., Gupta, A., Kanjilal, S., & Katiyar, S. (2012). Drug discovery from plant sources: An integrated approach. *Ayu, 33*(1), 10.
8. Sharma, A., Sabharwal, P., & Dada, R. (2021). Herbal medicine—An introduction to its history. In R. Henkel & A. Agarwal (Eds.), *Herbal Medicine in Andrology* (pp. 1–8). Academic Press.
9. Nasim, N., Sandeep, I. S., & Mohanty, S. (2022). Plant-derived natural products for drug discovery: Current approaches and prospects. *The Nucleus, 65*(3), 399–411.
10. Kwok, H. F. (2022). Drug discovery from natural sources: Animal venoms, plants, bacteria, and fungi. *Frontiers in Molecular Biosciences, 9*, 998676.
11. Chong, H. P., Tan, K. Y., & Tan, C. H. (2020). Cytotoxicity of snake venoms and cytotoxins from two Southeast Asian cobras (*Naja sumatrana, Naja kaouthia*): Exploration of anticancer potential, selectivity, and cell death mechanism. *Frontiers in Molecular Biosciences, 7*, 583587.
12. Avelar Júnior, J. T. d., Sousa, D. F., Melo, M. M., Alves, N. C. L., Silva, J. S., & Castro, M. E. B., et al. (2022). LyeTxI-b, a synthetic peptide derived from a spider

venom, is highly active in triple-negative breast cancer cells and acts synergistically with cisplatin. *Frontiers in Molecular Biosciences, 9*, 876833.

13. Still, J. (2003). Use of animal products in traditional Chinese medicine: Environmental impact and health hazards. *Complementary Therapies in Medicine, 11*(2), 118–122.
14. Gupta, U., & Gupta, S. (2014). Sources and deficiency diseases of mineral nutrients in human health and nutrition: A review. *Pedosphere, 24*(1), 13–38.
15. Rajurkar, N., & Damame, M. (1998). Mineral content of medicinal plants used in the treatment of diseases resulting from urinary tract disorders. *Applied Radiation and Isotopes, 49*(7), 773–776.
16. Galaris, D., Barbouti, A., & Pantopoulos, K. (2019). Iron homeostasis and oxidative stress: An intimate relationship. *Biochimica et Biophysica Acta (BBA)–Molecular Cell Research, 1866*(12), 118535.
17. Haefner, B. (2003). Drugs from the deep: Marine natural products as drug candidates. *Drug Discovery Today, 8*(12), 536–544.
18. Passioti, M., Maggina, P., Megremis, S., & Papadopoulos, N. G. (2014). The common cold: Potential for future prevention or cure. *Current Allergy and Asthma Reports, 14*, 1–11.
19. Khan, M., Shah, A. J., & Gilani, A. H. (2015). Insight into the bronchodilator activity of *Vitex negundo*. *Pharmaceutical Biology, 53*(3), 340–344.
20. De Smet, P. A. (1995). Health risks of herbal remedies. *Drug Safety, 13*, 81–93.
21. De Smet, P. A. (1997). Adverse effects of herbal remedies. *Adverse Drug Reaction Bulletin, 183*(1), 695–698.
22. Subramanian, K., Sankaramourthy, D., & Gunasekaran, M. (2018). Toxicity studies related to medicinal plants. In *Natural Products and Drug Discovery* (pp. 491–505). Elsevier.
23. Jha, V., & Rathi, M. (2008). Natural medicines causing acute kidney injury. In *Seminars in Nephrology*. Elsevier.
24. Mahmoodian, S., Ahmadian, G., Tarrahimofrad, H., Katalani, C., & Hoseini, Z. S. (2023). *Development and Commercialization of Biopesticides: Costs and Benefits* (p. 403).
25. Drew, A. K., & Myers, S. P. (1997). Safety issues in herbal medicine: Implications for the health professions. *Medical Journal of Australia, 166*(10), 538–541.
26. Edwards, I. R., & Aronson, J. K. (2000). Adverse drug reactions: Definitions, diagnosis, and management. *The Lancet, 356*(9237), 1255–1259.
27. Bandaranayake, W. M. (2006). Quality control, screening, toxicity, and regulation of herbal drugs. In *Modern Phytomedicine: Turning Medicinal Plants into Drugs* (pp. 25–57).
28. Shaw, D. (2010). Toxicological risks of Chinese herbs. *Planta Medica, 76*(17), 2012–2018.
29. Wang, X., Hou, J., Su, X., Xie, X., & Yu, J. (2008). Analysis of the constituents in the rat plasma after oral administration of *Yin Chen Hao Tang* by UPLC/Q-TOF-MS/MS. *Journal of Pharmaceutical and Biomedical Analysis, 46*(3), 477–490.
30. Jonsson, M., Jestoi, M., Nathanail, A. V., Kokkonen, M., & Anttila, M. (2013). Application of OECD Guideline 423 in assessing the acute oral toxicity of moniliformin. *Food and Chemical Toxicology, 53*, 27–32.

31. Jothy, S. L., Zakaria, Z., Chen, Y., Lau, Y. L., Latha, L. Y., & Sasidharan, S. (2011). Acute oral toxicity of methanolic seed extract of *Cassia fistula* in mice. *Molecules, 16*(6), 5268–5282.
32. Santos, L., Marín, S., Sanchis, V., & Ramos, A. J. (2009). Screening of mycotoxin multicontamination in medicinal and aromatic herbs sampled in Spain. *Journal of the Science of Food and Agriculture, 89*(10), 1802–1807.
33. Huff, J. (2002). IARC monographs, industry influence, and upgrading, downgrading and under grading chemicals. *International Journal of Occupational and Environmental Health, 8*(3), 249–270.
34. Ałtyn, I., & Twarużek, M. (2020). Mycotoxin contamination concerns of herbs and medicinal plants. *Toxins, 12*(3), 182.
35. Ashiq, S., Hussain, M., & Ahmad, B. (2014). Natural occurrence of mycotoxins in medicinal plants: A review. *Fungal Genetics and Biology, 66*, 1–10.
36. Shaban, N. S., Abdou, K. A., & Hassan, N. E. H. Y. (2016). Impact of toxic heavy metals and pesticide residues in herbal products. *Beni-Suef University Journal of Basic and Applied Sciences, 5*(1), 102–106.
37. Tripathy, V., Basak, B. B., Varghese, T. S., & Saha, A. (2015). Residues and contaminants in medicinal herbs—A review. *Phytochemistry Letters, 14*, 67–78.
38. Wang, Y., Wu, Y., Li, Y., Wang, J., & Zhang, Q. (2022). Levels and health risk of pesticide residues in Chinese herbal medicines. *Frontiers in Pharmacology, 12*, 818268.
39. Chen, L., Zhou, X., Shi, Y., Wu, Y., & Liu, D. (2012). Multi-residue method for fast determination of pesticide residues in plants used in traditional Chinese medicine by ultra-high-performance liquid chromatography coupled to tandem mass spectrometry. *Journal of Chromatography A, 1225*, 132–140.
40. Elvin-Lewis, M. (2005). Safety issues associated with herbal ingredients. *Advances in Food and Nutrition Research, 50*, 219–313.
41. Rao, M. M., KumarMeena, A., & Galib. (2011). Detection of toxic heavy metals and pesticide residue in herbal plants which are commonly used in herbal formulations. *Environmental Monitoring and Assessment, 181*, 267–271.
42. Ameh, S. J., Obodozie, O. O., Inyang, U. S., Abubakar, M. S., & Garba, M. (2010). Current phytotherapy – An inter-regional perspective on policy, research, and development of herbal medicine. *Journal of Medicinal Plants Research, 4*(15), 1508–1516.
43. Vlietinck, A., Pieters, L., & Apers, S. (2009). Legal requirements for the quality of herbal substances and herbal preparations for the manufacturing of herbal medicinal products in the European Union. *Planta Medica, 75*(7), 683–688.
44. World Health Organization. (1978). *Declaration of Alma-Ata*. World Health Organization, Regional Office for Europe.
45. World Health Organization. (2005). *National Policy on Traditional Medicine and Regulation of Herbal Medicines: Report of a WHO Global Survey*. World Health Organization.
46. U.S. Department of Health and Human Services. (2004). *Guidance for Industry: Botanical Drug Products*. Retrieved from: http://www.fda.gov/cder/guidance/4592fnl.htm.

47. Singh, S., & Shukla, V. K. (2021). Current regulations for herbal medicines in India. *International Journal of Drug Regulatory Affairs, 9*(2), 30–34.
48. Petrovick, P. R., Marques, L. C., & De Paula, I. (1999). New rules for phytopharmaceutical drug registration in Brazil. *Journal of Ethnopharmacology, 66*(1), 51–55.
49. Azaizeh, H., Saad, B., Cooper, E., & Said, O. (2006). The state of the art of traditional Arab herbal medicine in the Eastern region of the Mediterranean: A review. *Evidence-Based Complementary and Alternative Medicine, 3*, 229–235.
50. Choi, D. W., Jung, B. H., Lee, S. H., Kang, S. H., & Chung, B. C. (2002). Regulation and quality control of herbal drugs in Korea. *Toxicology, 181*, 581–586.
51. Chan, K., Leung, K. S., & Zhao, S. S. (2009). Harmonization of monographic standards is needed to ensure the quality of Chinese medicinal materials. *Chinese Medicine, 4*, 18.
52. Government of India Planning Commission. (2006). *Working Group on "Access to Health Systems Including AYUSH."* New Delhi.

CHAPTER 10

Pharmacovigilance of Natural Products

JAYANT KUMAR,[1] ASHIMA THAKUR,[2] and ANOOP KUMAR[3]

[1]*Department of Pharmaceutical Sciences, Hemwati Nandan Bahuguna Garhwal University (A Central University), Srinagar, Jammu and Kashmir, India*

[2]*Faculty of Pharmaceutical Sciences, ICFAI University, Baddi, Himachal Pradesh, India*

[3]*Department of Pharmacology, Delhi Pharmaceutical Sciences and Research University (DPSRU), New Delhi, India*

*Corresponding author

ABSTRACT

Natural products (NPs) play a significant role in the management of various diseases, particularly lifestyle disorders such as type 2 diabetes, obesity, and hypertension. Many people assume that these medicines are safe; however, various studies have reported the adverse drug reactions (ADRs) of these drugs. The regulatory authorities are concerned about the community's use of NPs without a prescription. They also advocate for adequate phytochemical surveillance. However, the main concern is that the existing pharmacovigilance paradigm and its related tools were designed for synthetic medications, and using these approaches to monitor the safety of NPs brings additional issues in addition to those mentioned for conventional medicines. Some of the major obstacles in evaluating the safety of these medicines are low rates of adverse reaction (AR) reporting, chemical complexity, many constituents, and a lack of clinical evidence. Therefore, a proper pharmacovigilance system for NPs

The Essentials of Herbal Drugs. Varsha Tiwari, Abhishek Tiwari, and Ajay Sharma (Eds.)

DOI: 10.1201/9781998511778-10

is required to ensure patient safety. This chapter provides an overview of NPs and their associated ADRs, followed by the pharmacovigilance system of NPs. Finally, the chapter summarizes the current challenges and future perspectives.

10.1 INTRODUCTION

From ancient times, Natural products (NPs) have made a remarkable contribution in the field of drug discovery for various diseases, mainly cancer and other infectious diseases. There is a growing demand for the use of NPs in the management of different health issues worldwide. They are generally believed to be safer drugs than conventional medical therapies. Nevertheless, there is increasing evidence of the side effects and adverse effects associated with these NPs [1].

Some of the main issues regarding the safety of herbal products are listed below:

1. First is the complex nature of these herbal formulations. Intermolecular interactions of different biologically active ingredients present within the herbal formulation.
2. Second, intramolecular interactions or extrinsic interactions in the herbal formulation are another source of concern. For example, in herbal products, many metals are found in higher concentrations than their prescribed limit.
3. Wrong identification of medicinal plants and their use.
4. Drug interactions between synthetic medicines and natural medicines consumed by the patients [2] (Figure 10.1).

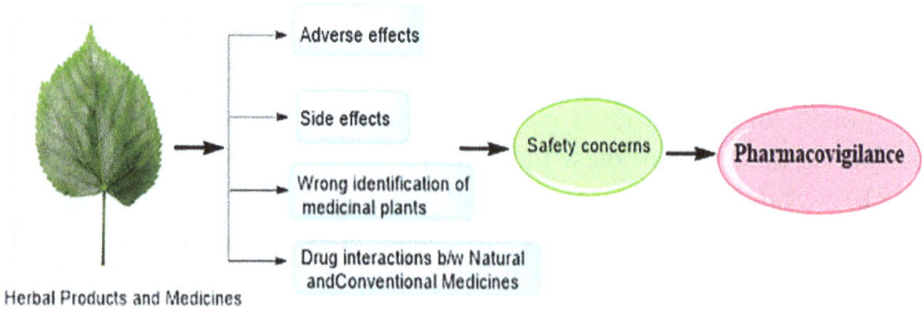

FIGURE 10.1 Main concerns regarding the safety of natural products.

These safety concerns make the evaluation more difficult than that of conventional medicines.

Pharmacovigilance is a branch of science related to the monitoring, evaluation, and prevention of adverse effects of various drugs. The World Health Organization (WHO) introduces guidelines for regulatory authorities and national pharmacovigilance centers regarding the safety of NPs. Yet, no system has been developed that ensures the safety of herbal drugs, and an initiative has been taken up by the pharmacovigilance centers to incorporate the coverage of herbal medicines [3]. Here are examples of some NPs and their adverse drug reactions (ADRs) listed in Table 10.1.

The regulations were created with the idea that successful monitoring of herbal medicines could be made possible by improving and expanding drug safety monitoring within the framework of the current pharmacovigilance systems. Given the rising usage of NPs and herbal formulations worldwide, it is becoming increasingly crucial to include herbal medicines in pharmacovigilance systems. For instance, in the United States of America, around 158 million people spent about US$ 17 billion in 2000. Additionally, a new study found that over 70% of Germans reported using "natural medicines," with the majority of them choosing to treat minor illnesses or disorders with herbal medicinal goods as their first option [4].

10.1.1 THE KEY OBJECTIVES OF PHARMACOVIGILANCE'S PRACTICE OF NATURAL PRODUCTS

1. Enhance the safety of patients and health regarding medication use.
2. Enhance public health and safety.
3. Assist with the evaluation of the risks, benefits, effectiveness, and harms associated with NPs.
4. Encourage public awareness, education, and clinical training in pharmacovigilance and its efficient dissemination [5] (Figure 10.2).

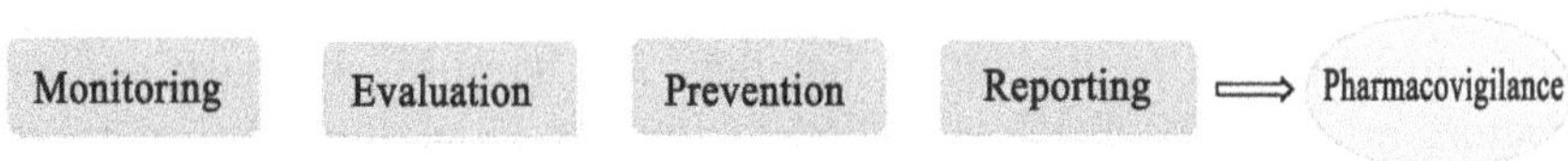

FIGURE 10.2 Parameters of pharmacovigilance.

10.2 NATURAL PRODUCT (NP)

NPs have historically played an important role in drug development, such as diabetes, cancer, cardiac disease, brain disorders, and lifestyle disorders [6]. When compared with traditional synthetic compounds, NPs have unique properties that provide both benefits and difficulties in the drug discovery process. The scaffold variety and structural complexity of NPs are immense. When compared to synthetic compound libraries [7], they generally follow the Lipinski rule of five, usually have higher molecular mass, a greater number of SP^3 carbon atoms and oxygen atoms, but fewer nitrogen and halogen atoms, a greater number of H-bond acceptors and donors, lower partition coefficients (cLogP values, indicating higher hydrophilicity), and greater molecular rigidity. In drug discovery involving protein-protein interactions, herbal products are very useful [7]. NPs represent a significant source of oral medicines that are "over the Lipinski's rule of five." The rise in molecular mass of approved oral medications over the last 20 years demonstrates the growing importance of drugs that do not follow this rule [8]. Evolution has structurally "optimized" NPs to perform certain biological functions, such as endogenous defensive mechanisms and interactions with other species, which explains their significant importance for infectious illnesses and cancer. In addition, their application in conventional medicine may reveal information about efficacy and safety. In general, the NP pool is richer with "bioactive" molecules that cover a larger area compared with synthetic small-molecule libraries [9]. The pharmaceutical industry has reduced its use of NP-based drug discovery programs due to several limitations associated with NPs, despite these benefits and numerous examples of effective drug discovery. A library of extracts from natural sources is commonly used in NP screens, and this may not work well with conventional target-based assays. It can be difficult to identify the bioactive molecules of interest, and to prevent the rediscovery of existing compounds, dereplication techniques must be used. It can also be difficult to obtain enough biological material to separate and describe a bioactive NP [10].

The general population views NPs as safe and helpful, including "health foods" and herbal medicines. The fact that these drugs are mostly uncontrolled adds to the myth that they are harmless because neither doctors nor patients feel compelled to inquire about their use of these substances from time to time. However, these items can change how some

TABLE 10.1 ADR Associated with Natural Products

SL. No.	Natural Product	Pharmacological Effect	Plant Source	Adverse Effects/Side Effects	References
1.	Acetyldigoxin	Cardiotonic effect	*Digitalis lanata* (Grecian foxglove)	Nausea, Vomiting, Vision disturbances Allergic reactions	[13]
2.	Atropine	Anticholinergic	*Atropa belladonna* (deadly nightshade)	Blurred near vision, flush and fever	[14–16]
3.	Anabesine	Skeletal muscle relaxant	*Anabasis sphylla*	Cleft palate formation	[17]
4.	Caffeine	CNS Stimulant	*Camellia sinensis*	Addiction, insomnia, migraine, and other side effects	[18]
5.	Curcumin	Choleretic	*Curcuma longa* (turmeric)	Nausea, diarrhea, headache, rash, and yellow stool on long-term exposure	[19]
6.	Colchicine	Antitumor, antigout	*Colchicum autumnale* (autumn crocus)	Sensorimotor neuropathy, alopecia, abdominal pain, aplastic anemia	[20]
7.	Digitoxin	Cardiotonic	*Digitalis purpurea* (purple foxglove)	Heart failure, Nodal block, Anaphylaxis associated with digibind	[21]
8.	L-Dopa	Antiparkinsonism	Mucuna species	Fluctuations, dyskinesias, toxicity, or loss of efficacy	[22]
9.	Emetine	Amoebicide, emetic	*Cephaelis ipecacuanha*	Cardiotoxicity	[23]
10.	Ephedrine	Sympathomimetic, antihistamine	*Ephedra sinica*	Palpitation, excitation, insomnia, and dysuria	[24]
11.	Etoposide	Antitumor agent	*Podophyllum peltatum*	Myelosuppression, alopecia, nausea and vomiting, mucositis, and hypotension after rapid intravenous administration.	[25]
12.	Glaucine	Antitussive	*Glaucoum flavum* (sea poppy)	Acute glaucine syndrome (AGS) include fatigue, sleepiness	[26]

TABLE 10.1 *(Continued)*

SL. No.	Natural Product	Pharmacological Effect	Plant Source	Adverse Effects/Side Effects	References
13.	Glycyrrhizin	Sweetener, treatment for Addison's disease	*Glycyrrhiza glabra* (licorice)	Glycyrrhizin poisonings include hypertension, fluid retention, and hypokalemia with metabolic alkalosis and increased kaliuresis	[27]
14.	Hyoscyamine	Anticholinergic	*Hyoscyamus Niger* (black henbane, stinking nightshade, henpin)	Sinus tachycardia	[28]
15.	a-Lobeline	Smoking deterrent, respiratory stimulant	*Lobelia aritim* (Indian tobacco)	Dizziness, nausea, vomiting and throat infection	[29]
16.	Morphine	Analgesic	*Papaver somniferum* (poppy)	Constipation, dysphoria, myoclonus, nausea, and sedation	[30]
17.	Nicotine	Insecticide	*Nicotiana tabacum* (tobacco)	Irritation and burning sensation in the mouth and throat, increased salivation, nausea, abdominal pain, vomiting and diarrhea	[31]
18.	Noscapine	Antitussive	*Papaver somniferum* (poppy)	Nausea and abdominal discomfort	[32]
19.	Pachycarpine	Oxytocic	*Sophora pschycarpa*	Permanent damage, birth defects	[33]
20.	Papavarine	Smooth muscle relaxant	*Papaver somniferum* (opium poppy, common poppy)	Discomfort and dizziness with venous leakage	[34]
21.	Physostigmine	Cholinesterase inhibitor	*Physostigma venenosum* (Calabar bean)	Hypersalivation (206; 9.0%) and nausea and vomiting (96; 4.2%) were the most common adverse effects.	[35]
22.	Podophyllotoxin	Antitumor, anticancer agent	*Podophyllum peltatum* (mayapple)	A slight-to-moderate tenderness, pain, burning, or all of the above in the treated areas was noted by more than 60% of the women who were treated with the podophyllotoxin cream	[36]

TABLE 10.1 *(Continued)*

SL. No.	Natural Product	Pharmacological Effect	Plant Source	Adverse Effects/Side Effects	References
23.	Quinine	Antimalarial, antipyretic	*Cinchona ledgeriana* (quinine tree)	Gastrointestinal disturbances, vasodilatation, sweating, and headache occur with moderately elevated plasma quinine concentration. As these rise, increasingly severe visual disturbances and then cardiac and neurologic features occur	[37]
24.	Rererpine	Circulatory disorders	*Rauwolfia serpentina*	Sedation, Lethargy, Gastric ulceration, Skin rashes	[38]
25.	Salicin	Analgesic	*Salix alba* (white willow)	Anaphylactic reactions in people with a history of allergy to salicylates may occur	[39]
26.	Scillarin A	Cardiotonic	*Urginea aritime* (squill)	Cardiac dysfunction, Arrhythmia	[40]
27.	Scopolamine	Sedative	Datura species (e.g., Jimsonweed)	Blurred vision, Salivation, bradycardia	[41]
28.	Silymarin	Antihepatotoxic	*Silybum marianum* (milk thistle)	Mild allergic reactions, GIT disturbances, nausea, headache	[42]
29.	Taxol	Antitumor agent	*Taxus brevifolia* (Pacific yew)	Hypersensitivity-like reactions	[43]
30.	Theophylline	Diuretic, bronchodilator	*Theobroma cacao* and others (cocoa, tea)	Nausea, vomiting and tachycardia	[44]
31.	Thymol	Topical antifungal	*Thymus vulgaris* (thyme)	Pulmonary and renal damage	[45]
32.	Tubocurarine	Skeletal muscle relaxant	*Chondodendron tomentosum* (curare vine)	Flushing, hypotension, and tachycardia	[46]

medications work, occasionally with unfavorable clinical outcomes [11]. Herbal products combined with conventional medicines show interactions that alter biological mechanisms such as metabolism and excretion. The cytochrome P450s (CYPs) enzyme family is a major player in the metabolism of pharmaceuticals. CYP3A4 is one of the most significant of its numerous variants, and we will use it to demonstrate how interactions between natural items and pharmaceuticals might occur. An enzyme can be inhibited by a natural substance, which modifies its activity. The first discovery by our research was that grapefruit can significantly lower enteric CYP3A4 activity, increasing the bioavailability of medications metabolized by enteric CYP3A4 to potentially hazardous levels [12]. Therefore, a proper clinical and toxicological investigation is needed before practices in the clinics or over the counter (Figure 10.3).

10.3 WHY PHARMACOVIGILANCE NEEDED OF NATURAL PRODUCTS

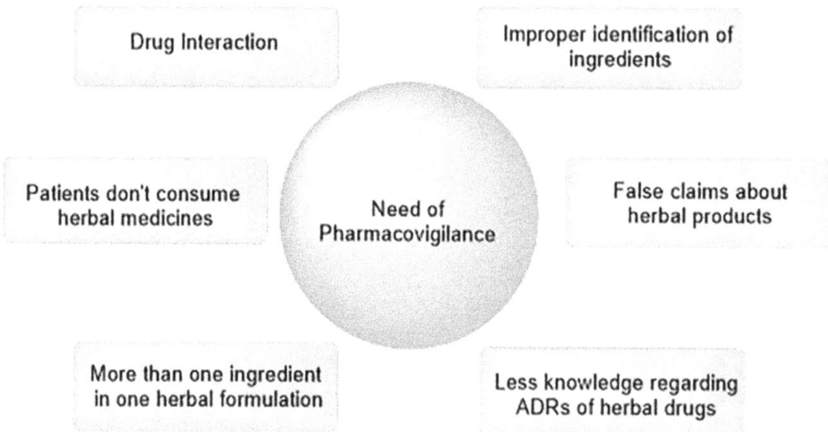

FIGURE 10.3 Factors that influence the need of pharmacovigilance.

The safety of herbal medications is a crucial public health concern. It is important to recognize the hazards involved in using NPs. Herbal medicines are often used in combination with other medications. It is important to know the potential risks associated with this practice and to keep an eye out for any negative effects. Most easily, this can be accomplished within the current pharmacovigilance systems. In order to manage herbal medications and, specifically, investigate the reasons behind adverse events, the national pharmacovigilance centers (or similar establishments) must acquire specialized technical knowledge. This will comprise skilled workers in the necessary technical fields and facilities to examine the products in question, about which there is frequently limited knowledge and restricted access. The WHO Collaborating Centre for International Drug Monitoring has suggested the application of proper scientific binomial names for medicinal herbs in the coding of adverse reaction (AR) reports to ensure consistency in the naming of herbs in AR reports. By doing this, reports from different international pharmacovigilance databases would be comparable to one another. The precise product(s) involved, together with label and manufacturer information, specific constituents, and the dosage used, should all be identified by the authors of published AR case reports. An examination of the suspected product used for adulteration and contamination, as well as, if feasible, species identification, would be beneficial for published case reports.

10.4 AVAILABLE METHODS AND PROCESS OF PHARMACOVIGILANCE FOR NATURAL PRODUCTS

10.4.1 PASSIVE SURVEILLANCE SPONTANEOUS REPORTING

"Spontaneous reporting" is a methodology used to collect global pharmacovigilance data and depends on healthcare professionals for the recognition and reporting of potential undesirable drug reactions to the manufacturer or National Pharmacovigilance Centre. The majority of the time, spontaneous reports are provided voluntarily. Spontaneous reports are a significant aspect of finding safety signals following the marketing of a pharmaceutical product. They alert to unusual adverse events that were not found in previous clinical trials or other premarketing investigations. This provides critical information on at-risk populations, risk factors, and clinical characteristics of documented major adverse responses. Underreporting is one of the main problems with the system, but estimates differ greatly between countries and between minor and serious ADRs. Medical professionals who are overworked may not always prioritize reporting, and even in cases where symptoms are severe, they might not be identified as a side effect of a particular medication. Yet spontaneous reports constitute the backbone of the WHO Database, which has over

3.7 million reports and is growing at a rate of approximately 250,000 per year, and are a crucial component of the worldwide pharmacovigilance effort. A case report is a notification from a practitioner about a patient who has a problem that may be caused by drugs. When multiple doctors independently report the same unknown and unexpected bad effects from a medicine, it can be a warning indicator.

10.4.2 OTHER REPORTING METHODS

Some countries require physicians to report spontaneously. Most nations compel manufacturers to submit reports received from healthcare providers to the government authority. Others have an aggressive, concentrated program that focuses on new pharmaceuticals, especially contentious drugs, as well as the prescribing behaviors of groups of doctors, with pharmacists reporting to provide potentially useful information.

10.4.3 STIMULATED REPORTING

Stimulated reporting is a method of encouraging and facilitating the reporting of adverse events by health professionals in certain contexts (e.g., in-hospital settings) for new products or for limited time periods by following a pre-planned procedure. One more of these methods is online reporting of adverse events. Stimulated adverse event reporting in the early post-marketing period may result in corporations notifying health-care professionals of novel pharmaceuticals and disseminating safety information to the public early in usage (e.g., Early postmarketing period vigilance, EPPV in Japan).

10.4.4 ACTIVE SURVEILLANCE

Active surveillance, as an alternative to passive surveillance, uses a continuous, planned method to determine the exact number of unfavorable events. Active surveillance refers to monitoring patients receiving a certain medication as part of a risk management scheme. In addition to providing their consent for future contact, patients are requested to fill out a quick survey form [47, 48].

10.5 REGULATORY ASPECTS OF HERBOVIGILANCE

Furthermore, the regulatory framework for NPs might vary globally, with certain regions having less strict clearance requirements. This variation in regulatory criteria can have an impact on the consistency with which adverse occurrences are monitored and reported. The lack of a thorough and consistent post-marketing surveillance mechanism adds to the difficulties in NP pharmacovigilance [49]. Herbal medicines, unlike conventional pharmaceuticals, may not be subjected to the same amount of examination following market approval, resulting in the late detection of safety concerns and a lack of detailed safety data [50].

10.5.1 QUALITY ASSURANCE AND QUALITY CONTROL MEASURES

Every country where NPs are regulated should implement quality assurance and control parameters such as specifications and standards for herbal materials, GMP for herbal medicines, labeling, and licensing schemes for manufacturing, imports, and marketing. These control parameters are essential for guaranteeing the effectiveness and safety of herbal medicines, as inadequate regulation of control parameters may lead to a high incidence of AR and result in low quality of herbal medicines [2].

10.5.2 SAFETY EVALUATION

Clinical trials and spontaneous reports on marketed medicinal products are the most popular sources of information on adverse effects and reactions to medications. A significant percentage of natural remedies are over-the-counter (OTC) medications, and several of them are integrated into this category as prescription medications without first undergoing post-marketing safety monitoring. Thus, it is crucial to boost pharmacovigilance efforts in the context of non-prescription drugs. Customers' participation in the usage of herbal remedies and medications in healthcare, as well as their concern over potential negative consequences of herbal drugs, ought to be respected in a good way. Reports from customers regarding negative reactions should be acknowledged as a reliable source of data, which can aid in the identification of AR of NP remedies [51].

10.5.3 IDENTIFICATION OF NATURAL MEDICINES

WHO recommended the use of the WHO Drug Dictionary (WHO-DD) to preserve organized, classified information on the names of herbal products and their constituents in a manner similar to those of other medicines. The Uppsala Monitoring Centre (UMC) suggests the herbal anatomic–therapeutic–chemical (HATC) classification for the therapeutic classification of herbal products. This classification is structurally identical to the anatomic–therapeutic–chemical (ATC) classification used for chemical substances in alternative therapies. In order to improve the clarity and correctness of reports, the UMC recommends that the national pharmacovigilance centers make use of the WHO-DD, the HATC categorization, and the checklist as helpful resources. To enhance the quality of reports, pharmacovigilance centers should work in conjunction with university pharmacognosy departments as well as botanists, zoologists, and other related departments when it comes to botanical and chemical identification because NPs usually contain various constituents [52].

10.6 CHALLENGES WITH CURRENT METHODS

The pharmacovigilance of natural and herbal formulations presents a number of significant challenges due to the intrinsic complexity, diversity, and unique properties of these compounds. To begin with, the wide varieties of natural items, such as herbs, botanicals, and traditional drugs, pose a substantial problem. It is difficult to develop standardized procedures for monitoring and analyzing the safety of the aforementioned drugs due to a wide range of chemical constituents. The lack of defined manufacturing techniques for herbal goods is a significant barrier [53]. Variations in cultivation, harvesting, and processing can lead to discrepancies in product quality, purity, and potency. This lack of uniformity hinders efforts to establish universal safety assessment processes and makes identifying causative agents responsible for adverse effects more difficult. The ambiguity around the active components in herbal preparations adds further complications. Herbal medications, unlike conventional drugs with well-defined chemical structures, may contain complex combinations of substances. This makes determining the particular elements responsible for therapeutic effects or unfavorable reactions difficult, hampering proper safety assessments [54]. The challenges in herbal product pharmacovigilance are exacerbated by analytical issues in quality control. Because herbal products contain complex mixtures of substances, the identification of contaminants and adulterants can be difficult. The analytical methodologies and quality control standards for herbal products may not be as well-established as those for conventional pharmaceuticals, complicating efforts to ensure product safety and uniformity. The use of herbal items in combination with conventional drugs adds another degree of complication to the pharmacovigilance of herbal drugs. Many people utilize herbal medicines alongside prescription drugs, which raises concerns regarding potential interactions and synergy between natural and synthetic chemicals. Unfortunately, complete data on such interactions is still unavailable, leaving medical practitioners with little information to guide safe and successful treatment approaches. This lack of knowledge of potential herb-drug interactions adds another element of risk, especially for people with chronic diseases who may need both herbal and pharmacological interventions [55].

Under-reporting of adverse events is a common problem in herbal product pharmacovigilance. Many customers believe that natural and herbal products are fundamentally safe, leading them to think that adverse effects are rare or insignificant. Because AR may go unreported and due to gaps in pharmacovigilance, important safety steps may be delayed as a result of under-reporting. The scarcity of meaningful clinical trial data is a significant barrier in herbal product-based pharmacovigilance. Traditional knowledge and subjective proof may not provide enough information on infrequent or long-term adverse effects, making a full assessment of the safety profile difficult [56]. The qualitative and quantitative aspects of the chemical profile can be influenced by several circumstances, such as:

- Origin geographical factors: soil, climate, and photoperiod.
- The genotype.
- Plant components, such as leaves, stems, roots, and root bark.
- Harvesting conditions and time (year, season, and time of day).
- Processing, extraction, and storage.
- Herb combinations and/or the preparation of the resulting medicines [57].

10.7 IMPORTANT METHODS USED TO BOOST PHARMACOVIGILANCE PROGRAMME

NPs as medicine need to be integrated into national health care systems in developing nations. Traditional herbal therapy is accepted and integrated into all facets of health care delivery in an integrative approach. This means that the nation's national drug policy should cover THM; all suppliers and manufacturers of herbal medicine should be registered and subject to regulation; traditional herbal therapies should be offered at both public and private hospitals and clinics; and treatment with THM should be covered by health insurance. The following tactics can be developed for the successful implementation of a pharmacovigilance program for herbal and traditional medicines:

1. The legal proprietor of NPs encompassing formulations must provide users with information about the safe and effective use of herbal medicines. By analyzing these data, regulatory agencies will be better equipped to identify the benefits and risks of medications, as well as what steps, if any, need to be taken to ensure their safe use.
2. NP manufacturer license bearers need to provide concise brief details in addition to a critical review of the product's risk-benefit balance in light of new or updated comprehension. This examination will determine whether additional investigations are necessary, and it will also determine whether revisions to the registration and product information are required.
3. A consistent categorization and/or coding system for herbal treatments should be developed, including standardized terminology and meanings. Relevant research must be conducted in order to thoroughly explore the pharmacogenetics and pharmacoepidemiology of herbal medications. The provision of emoluments and research funds is expected to boost conventional herbal medicine education.
4. To support the capacity of national pharmacovigilance centers to monitor herbal medications, it is necessary to promote workforce technical proficiency, ensure access to facilities for product analysis suspected of producing ARs, and facilitate access to trustworthy information.

5. A nationwide safety monitoring program for herbal medicines should be run with the intention and capability of responding to signals emitted by reports of adverse effects of herbal medicines and enacting appropriate regulatory measures.
6. A wider range of traditional and complementary/alternative medicine providers, as well as manufacturers of herbal medicines, should be included in case reporting sources. Additionally, systems of information exchange involving drug information centers, poison centers, consumer organizations, and manufacturers should be developed. Manufacturers should also be included in the process, enhancing awareness and communication on all fronts (local, national, regional, global, and community).
7. For the purpose of cultivating widespread reporting behavior among herbal users, an interactive reporting pattern should be created.
8. Additionally, sample reporting forms with all the template questions and queries needed for the best reporting of herbal ADRs should be made available online. The public will find it easier and more comfortable to report ADRs related to NPs.
9. Health care professionals and providers of NPs should ask patients directly, respectfully, and persistently what other medicines they are taking, including prescription medicines, herbal medicines, and other health products for self-care.
10. The goal of safe herbals will be closer to reality if all medical professionals—a physician, surgeons, dentists, chemists, nurses, and others—are involved in herbal pharmacovigilance.
11. Monitoring the consequences of any steps taken against the reporting of adverse events is critical for the effective implementation of the pharmacovigilance system. To monitor safety elements, the manufacturer, regulatory bodies, CDSCO, and WHO can all collaborate.
12. The PSUR application for NPs must be made mandatory, encompassing all dosage forms and formulations, as well as all indications associated with an active ingredient. Within the PSUR, separate data presentations for different dosage forms, indications, or demographics (e.g., children vs. adults) may be appropriate, but a summary of the combined data should also be provided.

13. Periodic Safety Update Reports (PSURs) must be submitted after a traditional NP is registered, even if it is not sold. PSURs must be prepared at regular intervals over the life of the product.
14. Depending on the circumstances, safety information for a fixed combination of chemicals that are likewise registered individually may be reported either in a distinct PSUR or as a different presentation in the PSUR for one of the independent components. It is critical to cross-reference all applicable PSURs [48].

10.8 CONCLUSION AND FUTURE PERSPECTIVE

Emerging herbovigilance is playing a crucial role in ensuring that NPs are safe, effective, and of high quality for general public use. Since the existing pharmacovigilance model and sophisticated instruments utilized to evaluate the safety of NPs are not very useful, as they were all developed for synthetic molecules, NPs, which are very complex molecules, may create more difficulties even when using these methods. A number of problems arise related to the process by which natural drugs are identified, perceived, obtained, and administered. The current regulatory system for herbal medicines in resource-constrained nations also poses challenges. With herbal remedies, unreported ADRs are likely to be serious because consumers usually do not seek medical guidance before using them or disclose side effects. It can be difficult to communicate with them through the standard routes used by medical professionals (such as pharmacies) because a large number of individuals do not buy their products from licensed or registered pharmacies. At present, a number of additional techniques used in traditional pharmaceutical pharmacovigilance, such as computerized health record databases and prescription-event monitoring, are inadequate for evaluating the safety of herbal and other OTC drugs. To effectively promote the use of NPs as a means of enhancing healthcare, it is imperative to identify the safest and most effective remedies and make efforts toward promoting their rational usage. In many nations, it is an issue for natural remedies to be adulterated with prescription medications. Even with the widespread and meticulous ADR monitoring programs in place today, relatively few ADRs involving herbs are being reported. NPs have different legal statuses and approval processes in different nations, and there are higher risks when they are used irrationally. The WHO or other organizations should establish a drug reaction monitoring center for herbal medications. The herbal regulatory system should incorporate herbal pharmacovigilance, and authorities should document different elements of individual herbs and/or compound herbal formulations, such as ADRs, immediate or delayed harmful effects, allergies, and so forth. The reporter must be asked for the precise information needed because forms intended for spontaneous reporting are not designed to gather data on herbal remedies. It would be ideal to have a reporting form that has been updated to more effectively gather data on suspected herbal ADRs. The ultimate objective of providing safer and more effective natural medicine treatments could be reached with correct risk-benefit ratios of NPs and their formulations. It is also recommended that regulatory organizations and legal manufacturers offer safety information about the product and educate practitioners, paramedics, and even patients.

KEYWORDS

- **adverse drug reactions**
- **herbal medicine**
- **natural products**
- **pharmacovigilance**
- **risk-benefit analysis**
- **safety monitoring**

REFERENCES

1. Heydari, M., et al. (2022). Editorial: Clinical safety of natural products, an evidence-based approach. *Frontiers in Pharmacology, 13*, 960556.
2. Ekor, M. (2014). The growing use of herbal medicines: Issues relating to adverse reactions and challenges in monitoring safety. *Frontiers in Pharmacology, 4*, 177.
3. Hamid, A. A. A., Rahim, R., & Teo, S. P. (2022). Pharmacovigilance and its importance for primary health care professionals. *Korean Journal of Family Medicine, 43*(5), 290–295.
4. Shetti, S., et al. (2011). Pharmacovigilance of herbal medicines: Current state and future directions. *Pharmacognosy Magazine, 7*(25), 69–73.

5. Nour, S., & Plourde, G. (2019). Pharmacovigilance. In S. Nour & G. Plourde (Eds.), *Pharmacoepidemiology and Pharmacovigilance* (pp. 7–23). Academic Press.
6. Atanasov, A. G., et al. (2021). Natural products in drug discovery: Advances and opportunities. *Nature Reviews Drug Discovery, 20*(3), 200–216.
7. Tzvetkov, N. T., et al. (2023). Natural product drug discovery and drug design: Two approaches shaping new pharmaceutical development. *Nephrology Dialysis Transplantation, 39*(3), 375–378.
8. Newman, D. J., & Cragg, G. M. (2020). Natural products as sources of new drugs over the nearly four decades from 01/1981 to 09/2019. *Journal of Natural Products, 83*(3), 770–803.
9. Naeem, A., et al. (2022). Natural products as anticancer agents: Current status and future perspectives. *Molecules, 27*(23), 8367. https://doi.org/10.3390/molecules27238367.
10. Amirkia, V., & Heinrich, M. (2015). Natural products and drug discovery: A survey of stakeholders in industry and academia. *Frontiers in Pharmacology, 6*, 237.
11. Fu, P. P., et al. (2009). Quality assurance and safety of herbal dietary supplements. *Journal of Environmental Science and Health, Part C: Environmental Carcinogenesis & Ecotoxicology Reviews, 27*(2), 91–119.
12. Wanwimolruk, S., Phopin, K., & Prachayasittikul, V. (2014). Cytochrome P450 enzyme-mediated herbal drug interactions (Part 2). *EXCLI Journal, 13*, 869–896.
13. Patocka, J., et al. (2020). Digoxin: Pharmacology and toxicology—A review. *Environmental Toxicology and Pharmacology, 79*, 103400.
14. Gallasch, G., et al. (1982). Side effects of atropine: Pharmacological, allergic, pseudo-allergic, or toxic reactions? *Klinische Monatsblätter für Augenheilkunde, 181*(2), 96–99.
15. Sun, H., et al. (2023). Incidence of adverse events induced by atropine in myopic children: A meta-analysis. *Journal of Clinical Pharmacology, 63*(12), 1377–1386.
16. Wakayama, A., et al. (2018). Incidence of side effects of topical atropine sulfate and cyclopentolate hydrochloride for cycloplegia in Japanese children: A multicenter study. *Japanese Journal of Ophthalmology, 62*(5), 531–536.
17. Peng, Z., et al. (2011). An experimental study on chemically induced animal model of goat cleft palate in uterus. *Zhongguo Xiu Fu Chong Jian Wai Ke Za Zhi, 25*(2), 235–238.
18. Saimaiti, A., et al. (2023). Dietary sources, health benefits, and risks of caffeine. *Journal of Clinical Pharmacology, 63*(29), 9648–9666.
19. Hewlings, S. J., & Kalman, D. S. (2017). Curcumin: A review of its effects on human health. *Foods, 6*(10), 92.
20. Thompson, P. L., & Nidorf, S. M. (2018). Colchicine: An affordable anti-inflammatory agent for atherosclerosis. *Current Opinion in Lipidology, 29*(6), 467–473.
21. Rehman, R., & Hai, O. (2023). *Digitalis Toxicity*. In StatPearls. StatPearls Publishing. https://www.ncbi.nlm.nih.gov/books/NBK537162/ (accessed on 22 March 2025).
22. Marsden, C. D. (1994). Problems with long-term levodopa therapy for Parkinson's disease. *Clinical Neuropharmacology, 17*(Suppl 2), S32–S44.
23. Marino, A., Costa, R., & De Natale, G. (1990). Cardiotoxicity of emetine. *Clinica Terapeutica, 133*(3), 131–143.

24. Odaguchi, H., et al. (2019). The adverse effects of Ephedra herb and the safety of ephedrine alkaloids-free Ephedra herb extract (EFE). *Yakugaku Zasshi, 139*(11), 1417–1425.
25. Fleming, R. A., Miller, A. A., & Stewart, C. F. (1989). Etoposide: An update. *Clinical Pharmacy, 8*(4), 274–293.
26. Rovinskiĭ, V. I. (2006). Acute glaucine syndrome in the physician's practice: The clinical picture and potential danger. *Klinicheskaia Meditsina (Mosk), 84*(11), 68–70.
27. Caré, W., et al. (2023). Adverse effects of licorice consumed as food: An update. *Revue de Médecine Interne, 44*(9), 487–494.
28. Marshall, J. B., et al. (1999). Benefit of intravenous antispasmodic (hyoscyamine sulfate) as premedication for colonoscopy. *Gastrointestinal Endoscopy, 49*(6), 720–726.
29. Stead, L. F., & Hughes, J. R. (2012). Lobeline for smoking cessation. *Cochrane Database of Systematic Reviews, 2012*(2), Cd000124.
30. Glare, P., Walsh, D., & Sheehan, D. (2006). The adverse effects of morphine: A prospective survey of common symptoms during repeated dosing for chronic cancer pain. *American Journal of Hospice and Palliative Medicine, 23*(3), 229–235.
31. Mishra, A., et al. (2015). Harmful effects of nicotine. *Indian Journal of Medical and Pediatric Oncology, 36*(1), 24–31.
32. Rida, P. C., et al. (2015). The Noscapine chronicle: A pharmaco-historic biography of the opiate alkaloid family and its clinical applications. *Medical Research Reviews, 35*(5), 1072–1096.
33. Erina, E. V. (1957). Effect of pachycarpine in arrhythmias. *Terapevticheskii Arkhiv, 29*(2), 65–70.
34. Wespes, E., & Schulman, C. C. (1988). Systemic complication of intracavernous papaverine injection in patients with venous leakage. *Urology, 31*(2), 114, 115.
35. Arens, A. M., & Kearney, T. (2019). Adverse effects of physostigmine. *Journal of Medical Toxicology, 15*(3), 184–191.
36. von Krogh, G., & Hellberg, D. (1992). Self-treatment using a 0.5% podophyllotoxin cream of external genital condylomata acuminata in women: A placebo-controlled, double-blind study. *Sexually Transmitted Diseases, 19*(3), 170–174.
37. Bateman, D. N., & Dyson, E. H. (1986). Quinine toxicity. *Adverse Drug Reactions and Acute Poisoning Reviews, 5*(4), 215–233.
38. Lobay, D. (2015). Rauwolfia in the treatment of hypertension. *Integrative Medicine (Encinitas), 14*(3), 40–46.
39. Matyjaszczyk, E., & Schumann, R. (2018). Risk assessment of white willow (*Salix alba*) in food. *EFSA Journal, 16*(Suppl 1), e16081.
40. Zou, D., et al. (2022). Bufadienolides originated from toad source and their anti-inflammatory activity. *Frontiers in Pharmacology, 13*, 1044027.
41. Parrott, A. C. (1989). Transdermal scopolamine: A review of its effects upon motion sickness, psychological performance, and physiological functioning. *Aviation, Space, and Environmental Medicine, 60*(1), 1–9.
42. Karimi, G., et al. (2011). "Silymarin," a promising pharmacological agent for treatment of diseases. *Iranian Journal of Basic Medical Sciences, 14*(4), 308–317.
43. Price, K. S., & Castells, M. C. (2002). Taxol reactions. *Allergy and Asthma Proceedings, 23*(3), 205–208.

44. Skinner, M. H. (1990). Adverse reactions and interactions with theophylline. *Drug Safety, 5*(4), 275–285.
45. Fuentes, C., & Fuentes, A. (2021). Relevant essential oil components: A minireview on increasing applications and potential toxicity. *Natural Product Research, 31*(8), 559–565.
46. Ostergaard, D., Engbaek, J., & Viby-Mogensen, J. (1989). Adverse reactions and interactions of the neuromuscular blocking drugs. *Medical Toxicology and Adverse Drug Experience, 4*(5), 351–368.
47. Liu, X., & Chen, H. (2015). A research framework for pharmacovigilance in health social media: Identification and evaluation of patient adverse drug event reports. *Journal of Biomedical Informatics, 58*, 268–279.
48. Fokunang, E. T., et al. (2020). Pharmacovigilance of natural herbal medicines research for efficacy, safety, and quality assurance of phytomedicine products. *Journal of Complementary and Alternative Medical Research, 12*(1), 21–37.
49. Sen, S., Chakraborty, R., & De, B. (2011). Challenges and opportunities in the advancement of herbal medicine: India's position and role in a global context. *Journal of Herbal Medicine, 1*(3), 67–75.
50. Barnes, J. (2003). Quality, efficacy, and safety of complementary medicines: Fashions, facts, and the future. Part II: Efficacy and safety. *British Journal of Clinical Pharmacology, 55*(4), 331–340.
51. Coleman, J. J., & Pontefract, S. K. (2016). Adverse drug reactions. *Clinical Medicine (London), 16*(5), 481–485.
52. Lagerlund, O., et al. (2020). WHODrug: A global, validated, and updated dictionary for medicinal information. *Therapeutic Innovation & Regulatory Science, 54*(5), 1116–1122.
53. Hong, J. (2011). Role of natural product diversity in chemical biology. *Current Opinion in Chemical Biology, 15*(3), 350–354.
54. Onyegbule Okubuiro, E., & Okoli, C. E. (2018). Is quality of life improved by neurolytic coeliac plexus block in pancreatic cancer pain management? *International Research in Medical and Health Sciences, 1*(2), 1–5.
55. Pai, V., et al. (2024). Issues and challenges in pharmacovigilance of herbal formulations. *Current Drug Safety, 19*(1), 19–23.
56. Sanghvi, K., et al. (2023). Pharmacovigilance in herbal drugs: A challenge. *Current Drug Safety, 18*(2), 138–142.
57. Pandey, A., & Savita, R. (2017). Harvesting and post-harvest processing of medicinal plants: Problems and prospects. *The Pharma Innovation Journal, 6*(12), 229–235.

CHAPTER 11

Conclusion and Future Trends in Phyto-Pharmaceutical Research

VILAS SHIVAJI SAWALE,[1] SHOHEB S. SHAIKH,[2] HARSHAL A. VISHE,[3] KRISHNA G. KHAMKAR,[4] TEJASWINI T. ASAWE,[1] SAVITA S. DEOKAR,[4] TOMY M. JOSEPH,[5,*] and DEBARSHI KAR MAHAPATRA[6,*]

[1]*Pathrikar Institute of Pharmacy, Aurangabad, Maharashtra, India*

[1]*NN Sattha College of Pharmacy, Ahilyanager, Maharashtra, India*

[2]*Department of Pharmaceutical Quality Assurance, Siddhi's Institute of Pharmacy, Thane, Maharashtra, India*

[3]*Department of Pharmaceutics, Siddhi's Institute of Pharmacy, Thane, Maharashtra, India*

[4]*Department of Pharmaceutics, School of Pharmacy, Pimpri Chinchwad University, Vadgaon, Sate Maval, Pune, Maharashtra, India*

[5]*Department of Polymer Technology, Faculty of Chemistry, Gdańsk University of Technology, Gdańsk, Poland*

[6]*Chitkara College of Pharmacy, Chitkara University, Rajpura, Punjab, India*

*Corresponding author

ABSTRACT

Natural products (NPs) have historically served as a valuable reservoir of pharmaceutical agents targeting cancer, a disease that is anticipated to emerge as the primary contributor to mortality in the current era.

The Essentials of Herbal Drugs. Varsha Tiwari, Abhishek Tiwari, and Ajay Sharma (Eds.)

DOI: 10.1201/9781998511778-11

There exists a minimum of 250,000 plant species, out of which over 1000 plants have been verified to possess medicinal characteristics. Among the current array of 10,121 prescription medications, 1090 are sourced from plant species. Several plants have undergone clinical evaluation and are now undergoing phytochemical investigation to comprehend their effects. Alkaloids, terpenoids, flavonoids, and lignans are the primary categories of anticancer chemicals. The focus of this book chapter was on the pharmacotherapeutic properties of various compounds, including carotenoids (specifically α- and β-carotene and xanthophyll), limonoids (specifically *d*-limonene and *β*-terpineol), saponins (specifically shatavarin), flavonoids (specifically resveratrol, rutin, hesperidin, naringin, and quercetin), phenolic acids (specifically ellagic acid), vitamins (including A, B_1, B_2, B_5, B_6, B_7, B_9, B_{12}, C, D, E, and K), and miscellaneous bioactive compounds (andrographolide, glycolipid, gugulipid, withanolides, and vasicine). The content provides a complete overview of the sources, technology, history, regulatory issues, drug development methodologies, and regulatory viewpoints, aiming to enhance readers' comprehension.

11.1 INTRODUCTION

Plants are abundant in a diverse array of natural substances that exhibit a multitude of medicinal attributes and are consistently investigated for the purpose of creating innovative pharmaceuticals. Natural ingredients have long been relied upon by traditional treatments for the management of many disorders. Currently, the majority of pharmaceutical treatments are derived from natural ingredients. Bioactive compounds constitute the majority of natural products (NPs). The aforementioned bioactive compounds have biological activity against several pathogenic organisms. Thus far, a multitude of secondary metabolites with varied structures and pharmacological effects have been detected in plants. The adherence to knowledge within the traditional medicine system has facilitated the continuous investigation of medicinal plants for the purpose of producing pharmaceutical products. A significant proportion, exceeding 85–90%, of the global population relies on the traditional medical system as a means of addressing many ailments [1].

The commencement of the age of drug exploration was initiated by the extraction of morphine, the first naturally occurring and unadulterated substance produced from *Papaver somniferum*, in the year 1803. In India, around 20% of the total plant population is used for medicinal applications. The medicinal plants provide a vast reservoir of ethnobotanical compounds that are now being used in several medication delivery initiatives (Table 11.1).

TABLE 11.1 Phyto-Pharmaceuticals with Their Clinical Uses

Constituent	Plant	Clinical Use
(–)-Δ^9-trans-Tetrahydrocannabinol	*Cannabis sativa*	Central analgesic
Artemisinin	*Artimisia annua*	Anti-malarial
Atropine	*Atropa belladonna*	Parasympathomimetic
Camptothecin	*Camptotheca acuminata*	Anticancer
Combretastatin	*Combretum caffrum*	Anticancer
Curcumin	*Curcuma longa*	Anticancer
Digitoxin	*Digitalis purpurea*	Congestive Heart Failure
Digoxin	*Digitalis lanata*	Congestive Heart Failure
Etoposide	*Hexandrum*	Anticancer
Galanthamine	*Galanthus species*	Anti-Alzheimer
Morphine	*Papaver somniferum*	Central analgesic
Paclitaxel	*Taxus brevifolia*	Anticancer
Quinine	*Cinchona ledgeriana*	Anti-malarial
Vinca	*Catharanthus species*	Anticancer

11.2 RECAP OF KEY CONCEPTS

11.2.1 VIBRANT HISTORY

In the contemporary era, the enhanced effectiveness of pharmacological properties shown by medicinal plants has led to the recognition of herbal medicine as a potentially advantageous avenue for healthcare treatment. Throughout history, medicinal plants have been used and are well-respected globally as a valuable reservoir of therapeutic substances for the prevention of illnesses and afflictions. The medical use of plants has been documented in ancient Chinese and Egyptian papyrus inscriptions dating back to 3000 BC. Herbs have been used in healing rituals among indigenous societies such as African and Native American communities. In contrast, Siddha, Ayurveda, Unani, and traditional Chinese medicine

(TCM) are other well-established traditional medical systems that have effectively used herbal remedies. Approximately two centuries ago, the predominant focus of our therapeutic practices revolved around the use of plant-based remedies. However, the Western population saw a significant decrease in the use of herbs for therapeutic purposes with the advent of synthetic medications, which offered more predictable results and convenient accessibility [2].

Conversely, several underdeveloped countries have persisted in reaping the advantages of the abundant wisdom of herbal therapy. A significant majority of people continue to use Siddha and Ayurveda remedies in India, Kampo medicine in Japan, as well as TCM and Unani medicine throughout the Middle East and South Asia. In contemporary times, there is a growing inclination towards the use of plant-based medications, health products, dietary supplements, and cosmetics in both developing and developed nations. The rationale for this phenomenon stems from the increasing acknowledgment that NPs possess non-toxic properties, exhibit fewer side effects, and are readily accessible at low-cost points [3].

Medicinal plants are regarded as abundant reservoirs of phytochemical constituents that are crucial for the advancement of novel pharmaceuticals. For millennia, people have relied on plants as a form of medicine without scientific expertise or appropriate supervision. Scientific evidence has substantiated the notion that many components of plants, such as roots, stems, leaves, flowers, fruits, and seeds, possess therapeutic characteristics. Nevertheless, it has been observed that many plants are deemed unsafe for food due to their toxicity and the negative impact they have on the body. Hence, in order to facilitate the development of pharmaceuticals derived from phytocompounds (Figure 11.1), it is essential to standardize the bioactive extract based on the active compound and conduct comprehensive safety investigations. In recent times, there has been a renewed inclination towards the exploration of medicinal plants as a possible reservoir of pharmaceutical candidates [4].

Traditional medicine encompasses a range of health practices and methodologies that are grounded in knowledge and beliefs, involving the use of plants as medicinal agents, spiritual treatments, and physical therapy. These techniques are used either independently or in conjunction to address, diagnose, and prevent diseases, as well as to promote overall well-being. Complementary and alternative medicine refers to the modifications of conventional medicine in industrialized nations.

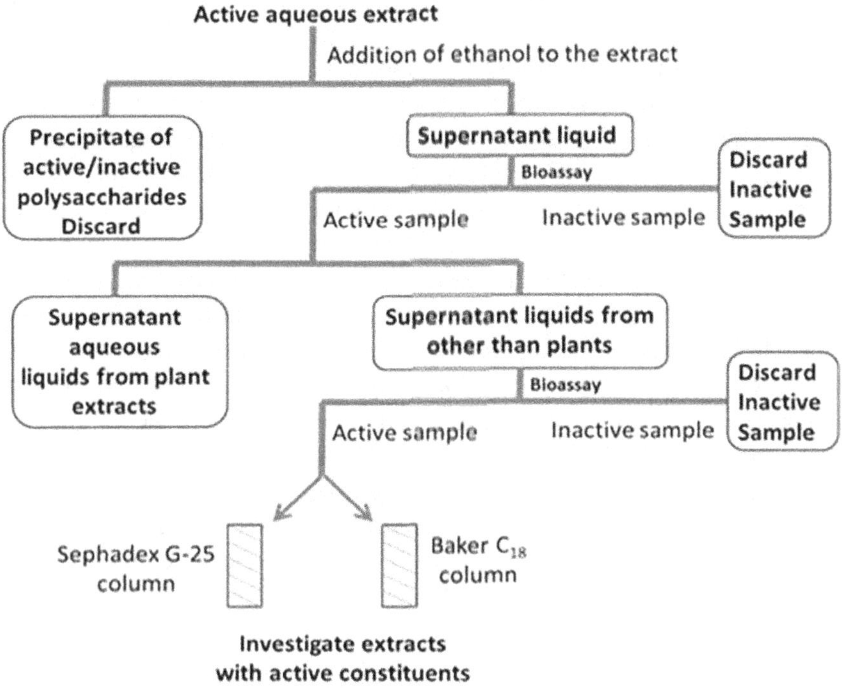

FIGURE 11.1 Fractionation process of an extract.

Herbal medicine, also known as phytomedicine, refers to the use of plants for medical and therapeutic purposes, with the aim of treating ailments and enhancing human well-being. The definition of herbal medicines, as provided by the World Health Organization (WHO), includes medical products that are labeled and contain an active component, as well as aerial or subterranean sections of the plant or other plant materials, either alone or in combination. Herbal medicines can be categorized at the pharmacodynamics level into three groups: (i) herbal drugs that have demonstrated efficacy and possess known active compounds and dosages; (ii) herbal drugs that are expected to have efficacies and require standardization of active compounds; and (iii) herbal drugs that have uncertain efficacies but have a documented history of traditional use [5].

Plants used as a source of sustenance or as primary constituents in traditional medicinal practices have a higher propensity to produce pharmacologically active chemicals. Additionally, plants serve as abundant dietary supplies of macromolecules, vitamins, and minerals that play a vital role in sustaining optimal bodily health. The practice of herbal therapy has been prevalent for generations, with individuals seeking natural cures to alleviate common diseases like colds, allergies, stomach upsets, and toothaches. The demand for herbal medicines is steadily increasing. Nevertheless, around the mid-20th century, herbal medications were abandoned from traditional medical use. This phenomenon may be attributed not only to their lack of efficacy but also to their comparatively lower economic viability in comparison to more recent synthetic pharmaceuticals. Subsequently, when scientific techniques progressed, herbal remedies could be subjected to investigation and recorded for their efficacy like pharmaceuticals. Moreover, throughout the 1960s, apprehensions over the harmful and unnecessary consequences of traditional medicine led to a need for safer and more cost-effective medications that would support "natural health." Consequently, there has been a notable transition in the global trajectory from synthetic pharmaceuticals to natural remedies. In addition, herbal medicine gained global recognition when the WHO encouraged poor nations to use traditional plant medicine to address unmet requirements in contemporary healthcare systems [6].

According to the WHO, around 4 billion individuals, which accounts for 80% of the global population, use herbal medicines for various aspects of primary healthcare. The existence of metabolites, which are organic substances categorized into primary and secondary metabolites, is responsible for the pharmacological actions of plants. The growth and development of the human body are facilitated by primary metabolites, including glucose, starch, polysaccharides, proteins, lipids, and nucleic acids. Plants, in order to defend themselves against microbial infections or insect invasions, create secondary metabolites such as alkaloids, flavonoids, saponins, terpenoids, steroids, glycosides, tannins, volatile oils, and more. The medicinal effectiveness of plants may be attributed to the presence of secondary metabolites, sometimes referred to as "phytocompounds." Phenolically active substances are used as pharmaceutical agents due to their medicinal characteristics. These substances have effectively decreased the likelihood of several human ailments, such as cardiovascular illnesses, hepatorenal diseases, diabetes, malignancies, and neurological disorders. In addition, plants possess many pharmacological properties, including antioxidant, antiviral, antibacterial, and antiparasitic effects, which may be used by humans. In particular, alkaloids have been documented to exhibit antispasmodic, antimalarial, analgesic, and diuretic properties. Terpenoids, on the other hand, are recognized for their antiviral, anthelmintic, antibacterial, anticancer, antimalarial, and anti-inflammatory characteristics. Phenols and flavonoids have been found to possess antioxidant, antiallergic, and antibacterial properties. Lastly, saponins have demonstrated anti-inflammatory and antiviral activities [7].

11.2.2 SOURCE OF MODERN MEDICINE

Medicinal plants are crucial for the development of novel pharmaceuticals. According to the WHO, around 25% of contemporary medications have been obtained from plants that were used in traditional medicine. Numerous synthetic analogues have been developed based on model molecules that have been identified from plants. The WHO has officially acknowledged herbal medicine as an essential element of basic healthcare. Plant-derived medications have made a revolutionary contribution to contemporary therapies. Vinblastine, derived from *Catharanthus roseus*, has shown efficacy in the treatment of many malignancies, including Hodgkin's disease, choriocarcinoma, non-Hodgkin's lymphomas, pediatric leukemia, testicular cancer, and neck cancer. Phophyllotoxin, derived from the plant species *Podophyllum emodi*, has shown significant effectiveness in the treatment of testicular cancer, lung cancer, and lymphomas. In the treatment of metastatic ovarian cancer and lung cancer, Taxol, derived from *Taxus brevifolia*, is used. Furthermore, the chemical serpentine, which was extracted from the root of *Rauwolfia serpentina* in 1953, represents a significant breakthrough in the field of hypertension therapy and blood pressure reduction. Approximately 100 novel plant-derived medications were launched into the US pharmaceutical industry between 1950 and 1970, such as deserpidine, reserpine, vinblastine, and vincristine. Between the years 1971 and 1990, a number of novel pharmaceutical compounds were extracted from various plant sources, including etoposide, guggulsterone, teniposide, nabilone, plaunotol, Z-guggulsterone, lectinan, artemisinin, and ginkgolides. Between 1991 and 1995, more plant-derived medications such as paclitaxel, topotecan, gomishin, and irinotecan were introduced into the pharmaceutical industry. Furthermore, several scholars in the last few decades have identified various other chemical compounds obtained from botanical origins, such as quinine, digoxin, aspirin, ephedrine, atropine, and colchicine [8].

11.2.3 INCREASING USE AND POPULARITY

Presently, herbal medicine remains highly favored in the majority of developing nations, and its use is rapidly spreading in industrialized nations as well. According to estimates, a significant proportion of medical practitioners in France and Germany, over 70%, engage in the regular prescription of herbal medicine. Globally, it is projected that over 80% of the populace utilizes herbal remedies, with potential rates reaching as high as 95% in poorer nations. Traditional herbal medicine (THM) accounts for around 30% to 50% of the overall medication usage in China. Herbal medications provide 60% of the primary therapeutic options in Ghana, Mali, Nigeria, and Zambia. Herbal formulations are used by 75% of HIV/AIDS-affected individuals in San Francisco, London, and South Africa. In both Canada and Germany, around 70% and 90% of the respective populations have reported using herbal remedies at least once in their lifetime. Herbal medicine usage among adults in the United States is estimated to encompass approximately 158 million individuals, showcasing a steady upward trajectory in its prevalence. The worldwide market for herbal medicines presently exceeds US $60 billion per year and is seeing steady growth. Furthermore, it is noteworthy to observe that the adult demographic has a higher propensity for using both conventional and herbal remedies in an equitable manner. The escalating prevalence of chronic illnesses in this demographic group often obstructs the sustained utilization of advanced conventional pharmacological treatments, primarily due to the enduring adverse effects they entail. In contrast, herbal medications provide a therapeutic approach that is devoid of any adverse effects when used over an extended period. Due to its special characteristics, herbal medicine has garnered significant attention and is experiencing a more rapid global acceptance [9].

11.2.4 THE FUTURE TREND

For many decades, THM practitioners have been transmitting spoken instructions on the preparation of medication using plants. Typically, they do not maintain records, although the WHO has recently made efforts to document the use of medicinal herbs by traditional practitioners worldwide. Consequently, several developing nations have intensified their endeavors to record ethnomedical information about plants. The scientific validation of their pharmacological properties has been facilitated. Once the scientific evaluation and adequate dissemination of these local ethnomedical preparations are conducted, individuals will experience enhanced awareness and satisfaction with regard to the effectiveness of pharmacological therapy and the subsequent improvement in their health state. Plants continue to possess the potential to serve as a valuable reservoir of medicinal agents while also functioning as a fundamental resource for the extraction of semisynthetic chemical compounds used in several sectors, including cosmetics, fragrances, and food. Furthermore, there has been a growing acceptance and use of plant-derived health care products within the beauty business. Hence, medicinal plants play a significant role in the broader economic development process by serving as both a healthcare resource and a source of commercial revenue. The need for herbal supplements and therapies is expected to increase in the future, creating a thriving market for herbal products. This implies that scholars, medical professionals, and pharmaceutical enterprises will be examining nations such as China, India, and other emerging economies as potential sources of supply. Due to their extensive range of medicinal plant species and status as leading exporters of herbal raw materials, these nations possess the most diversity. The future will see the continued exploitation of plants, both in their whole form and as pharmaceuticals, due to their growing appeal as a safer and more cost-effective alternative to traditional medicinal treatments [10].

11.3 EMERGING TRENDS IN PHYTO-PHARMACEUTICALS

11.3.1 NATURAL PRODUCTS DRUG DISCOVERY

The medicinal potential of plants may be harnessed via several conceptual approaches. The most often inferred use is the utilization of homemade treatments, namely herbal teas. Plant extracts, whether in their crude form or standardized fractions, find use in a diverse range of medicinal products, including powders, tinctures, tablets, and other similar formulations. Plants have yielded several bioactive chemicals that are used as pharmaceuticals [11] (Figure 11.2).

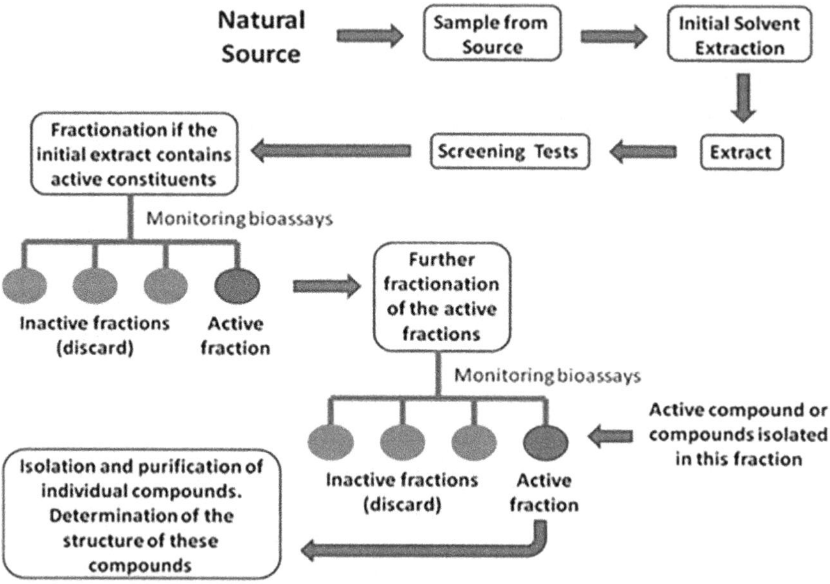

FIGURE 11.2 The overall process of drug discovery.

11.3.1.1 SMALL MOLECULES

Various conceptual methods may be used to exploit the therapeutic potential of plants. The most commonly implied use is the use of homemade remedies, especially herbal infusions. A wide variety of therapeutic preparations, such as powders, tinctures, pills, and similar formulations, use plant extracts, whether in their unrefined state or standardized fractions. Plants have been found to produce several bioactive compounds that are used in the field of medicine [12].

11.3.1.2 PLANT-MADE BIOLOGICS

Advancements in biotechnology have facilitated the harnessing of botanical resources for producing therapeutic proteins. These proteins are instrumental in developing pharmaceuticals and biotechnological therapies to combat life-threatening conditions such as cancer, diabetes, HIV, cystic fibrosis, heart disease, and Alzheimer's disease. Plant-derived biologics (PDBs) or plant-derived pharmaceuticals (PDPs) offer a more efficient, safer, and economically viable alternative for producing therapeutic proteins compared to conventional methods reliant on animal cell cultures and microbial fermentation, which entail costly infrastructure. Additionally, plants have a low susceptibility to infection by animal or human pathogens, making them a highly capable and rapidly expanding platform for pharmaceutical production. PDBs have significantly improved patients' access to medications, with the potential to facilitate the production of numerous life-saving drugs.

Elelyso, the first authorized PDB, also known as taliglucerase alfa, is an enzyme derived from carrot cells genetically modified for treating Gaucher's disease. Ongoing clinical studies are exploring the use of plant-derived proteins for influenza vaccines, and plant-derived lectins are being developed for novel anti-cancer biologics. Given the global pandemic caused by the COVID-19 virus, there is an urgent need to employ cost-effective technology in PDB production to mitigate its impact. Currently, there is anticipation for a promising biopharmaceutical candidate, with announcements of vaccines based on virus-like particles (VLPs) being made [13].

11.3.1.3 PHYTOPHARMACEUTICAL DRUGS

A phytopharmaceutical drug (PPD) is a new category of herbal medications formulated in accordance with guidelines established by the Department of Ayurveda, Unani, Siddha, and Homoeopathy (AYUSH) and the Central Drugs Standards Control Organization (CDSCO) in India. These medicines are derived from botanical species with a rich historical background in traditional remedies, though comprehensive documentation regarding their preparation is often lacking. PPDs are standardized and purified portions of medicinal plant extracts containing at least four bioactive phytoconstituents. They are utilized for treating and preventing various disorders. Recognizing the lack of oversight and regulation in the production of herbal drugs, procedures have been implemented to analyze and standardize these medications for safe usage.

PPDs consist of enriched extracts containing phytomolecules, flavonoids, carotenoids, polyphenols, lycopene, anthocyanidins, omega-3 fatty acids, phytoestrogens, and glucosinolates, which possess distinct pharmacological properties against numerous human health issues such as allergies, inflammation, diabetes, and more [14].

11.3.1.4 NEED FOR PRODUCTION OF PLANT-BASED DRUGS

The pharmaceutical business has always been drawn to natural goods, particularly PDPs and alternative treatments, due to many compelling factors. While synthetic medications provide rapid alleviation, they are often accompanied by many unwanted effects. The production process of synthetic medicine incurs significant costs, rendering it potentially unavailable to a substantial portion of the global population. In contrast, conventional drugs are often benign, highly efficacious with few adverse reactions, and readily metabolized and assimilated by the body. The widespread acceptance, affordability, and accessibility of these products may be attributed to the cultural and societal beliefs held by the population. Evidence-based treatments have been made available via an escalation in scientific investigations and clinical trials conducted by academics and pharmaceutical businesses. Additionally, the process of purifying and standardizing a singular component offers greater convenience, consequently enhancing its applicability within contemporary medication delivery systems [15].

11.3.1.5 CHALLENGES IN PRODUCTION OF PHYTOPHARMACEUTICAL DRUGS

Despite several benefits, the manufacturing of PPDs faces numerous obstacles. India's insufficient regulation of NPs can lead to subpar quality and ineffectiveness of plant-derived goods, resulting in reduced trade and reluctance to prescribe PPDs. Additional challenges include:

- low yield of plant material;
- solubility issues of plant extracts in water and other solvents;
- presence of cytotoxic components in the extract;
- limited bioavailability of the sample;
- inappropriate use of available phytomedicines leading to toxic incidents;
- errors in botanical identification of plants and their use;
- unauthorized usage of popular remedies;
- domestic accidents due to the consumption of decorative plants containing cardiotonic components;
- hemorrhagic and hypertensive accidents due to coumarin derivatives present in certain plants.

- presence of estrogenic components in plants;
- use of plants causing allergic reactions due to pollens or volatile components [16].

11.3.2 NATURAL PRODUCTS DRUG DEVELOPMENT

Several strategies have been devised for drug development, each tailored to the specific goal and intended application, whether it involves herbal medicine or incorporation into different formulations.

11.3.2.1 ETHNOPHARMACOLOGY

The selection of the plant is a crucial and pivotal phase in every pharmacological investigation. Typically, there is a preference for plants that have a historical record of use in traditional medicinal practices across many ethnic communities. This particular method is sometimes referred to as ethnobotany or ethnopharmacology. This strategy is based on a range of extraction processes and herbal formulations used by different ethnic groups. Herbal formulations provide succinct details pertaining to the medical characteristics inherent in the herbal recipe. The consumption method and dosage of the medicine are also recognized. Nevertheless, it is important to conduct thorough screening of the herbal medication due to the diverse health beliefs and healthcare systems across various ethnic groups. Therefore, it is important to accurately assess the symptoms prior to using any herbal composition for medicinal purposes. The extensive historical record of therapeutic use enhances the likelihood of achieving bioactivity in a novel pharmacological candidate. Therefore, it streamlines the process of drug selection, making it the most efficient search engine for the identification of natural medications [17].

During the drug development process, plant extracts are subjected to isolation in order to obtain biologically active ingredients that exhibit pharmacological characteristics. In several instances, the whole plant extract exhibits more activity compared to a single component. Plant extracts are composed of several chemically different components that may exist in varying amounts and play a crucial role in quality determination. The isolation and identification of bioactive chemicals require the use of bioactivity-guided fractionation techniques for these extracts. The use of bioactive standardized extracts is imperative in cases when the pharmacological impact arises from the synergistic interaction of many substances, rather than being influenced by a solitary constituent. The "standardized extract" of Ginkgo is composed of ginkgolides A, B, C, and M, which possess the ability to impede platelet aggregation generated by platelet aggregation factor (PAF). In contrast, it was shown that the bioactive standardized saponin fractions derived from Panax ginseng exhibited more activity compared to the isolated components. Additionally, a number of bioactive standardized compounds have been identified [18].

11.3.2.2 REVERSE PHARMACOLOGY

The conventional approach to drug development has facilitated novel avenues for pharmacological exploration; nonetheless, it sometimes exhibits inefficiencies and incurs high costs. There has been a recent emergence of a transdisciplinary strategy that offers cost-effectiveness, decreased time, and lower toxicity levels in comparison to the traditional way. The novel methodology is referred to as reverse pharmacology (RP). RP relies on the empirical verification of reported results to discover efficacious medications. The document encompasses the records of the clinical trials conducted on herbal mixtures used in traditional medicine. Subsequently, investigations are conducted pertaining to medication dosage, drug tolerance, as well as *in vitro* and *in vivo* evaluation of the formulation's efficacy in targeting the desired drug. The last stage encompasses clinical and experimental investigations conducted at various levels of biological systems. Therefore, it is important to accurately identify and validate the RP research in connection to the safety and effectiveness of the herbal medication. Consequently, RP has substituted the conventional journey from the laboratory to the clinic with the road from the clinic to the labs. RP serves as the intermediary between contemporary technology and conventional medications, enhancing their cooperation. The RP technique is founded upon the focused screening of prospective compounds with functional activity, hence enabling their further use in the field of drug development. The process of drug development in RP is centered on people, ensuring their safety and effectiveness [19].

11.3.2.3 HIGH THROUGHPUT SCREENING

For decades, pharmaceutical screening has focused on natural compounds to uncover potential medications. However, high-throughput screening (HTS) has emerged as a prevalent and contemporary method extensively used in drug delivery endeavors. HTS integrates premium components and assays to investigate the biological activity of numerous samples. A wide range of bioactive natural compounds and their derivatives have demonstrated anti-cancer, anti-diabetic, and anti-inflammatory properties. Additionally, over 100 natural compounds are currently undergoing clinical evaluation. There is a growing inclination towards exploring the potential of analyzing these naturally occurring chemicals derived from traditional medicinal sources. The screening of natural chemicals has been aligned with HTS due to progress in analytical instruments and fractionation procedures for the identification, isolation, and purification of these products [20].

11.3.2.4 FRAGMENT-BASED DRUG DISCOVERY

This is a novel paradigm used as a substitute for HTS within the pharmaceutical sector. The proposed methodology is grounded in the principles of structure-based drug design, using X-ray crystallography or NMR spectroscopy as analytical techniques to ascertain the potency of pharmacological compounds. FBDD has the ability to decrease attrition and identify leads for biological targets that were previously difficult to address. It can detect minuscule molecules (fragments) with a low molecular weight ($\leq$150 Da) that attach to larger molecules or potential therapeutic candidates. In order to expand the use of FBDD to further labs, researchers are now working on the development of advanced computational tools and biophysical methodologies, as well as the creation of new fragment libraries [21].

11.3.2.5 POLYPHARMACOLOGY

Over the last several years, drug research has undergone many substantial changes. Recently, several medications have been pulled from the market shortly after their debut. Therefore, the development of innovative drug discovery methodologies has emerged as a significant problem. Numerous bioactive compounds derived from medicinal plants, such as alkaloids, phyllanthins, piperidines, bacosides, and curcumin, have shown efficacy in the treatment of various human ailments. In addition, it is essential to use a multi-targeted strategy when addressing complicated illnesses such as cancer, heart disorders, multiple sclerosis, and diabetes. Therefore, a new method called polypharmacology has arisen, which relies on a multi-target strategy. This methodology entails the development of pharmaceuticals capable of modulating many targets, in contrast to the conventional notion of a single gene, medicine, and illness. The identification of important targets in these illnesses has been facilitated by advancements in omics technology and bioinformatics [22].

There are various benefits associated with multitarget medication methods as compared to current combinational medicines. A single molecule that acts on several targets provides superior effectiveness and minimizes harm compared to medication combinations. Furthermore, the use of combination medications may give rise to unfavorable synergistic effects, hence presenting significant hurdles in the context of testing. Nevertheless, the regulatory obstacles that cause delays in clinical trials are minimal when dealing with individual drugs. Moreover, it is well recognized that natural compounds exhibit greater polypharmacological profiles in comparison to synthesized drugs. Various research investigations have used the polypharmacology methodology to gain insights into the underlying processes of TCM. The research conducted demonstrated the polypharmacological characteristics of five naturally occurring compounds, namely curcumin, epigallocatechin gallate, quercetin, resveratrol, and berberine. Additionally, several methodologies were used to investigate the interactions between these compounds and their targets. In a similar vein, a virtual screening technique based on machine learning was used to ascertain the polypharmacological profile of galantamine, a natural substance. The acceleration and enhancement of polypharmacology-based investigations may be facilitated by the construction of databases and the creation of novel bioinformatics tools. Polypharm-DB has been recently created to find potential medication candidates for COVID-19. Therefore, polypharmacology presents a promising avenue for the future repurposing of drugs [23].

11.3.2.6 NETWORK PHARMACOLOGY

The popularity of the "one-disease, one-target therapy" model is diminishing due to advancements in systems biology, which have highlighted the challenges associated with treating complex disorders. Therefore, the emerging ideas of polypharmacology and network pharmacology, which include targeting numerous targets, are gaining momentum. Network pharmacology is a theoretical framework that draws upon principles from systems biology, network analysis, redundancy, connectedness, and pleiotropy. This research provides strategies for enhancing the clinical effectiveness of pharmaceuticals via the monitoring of side effects and toxicity levels, as well as the examination of the drug's kinetic and biological characteristics. The network biology hypothesis posits that bioactive chemicals with the ability to interact with many targets exhibit greater efficiency compared to those that only interact with single targets. Therefore, network pharmacology emerges as a promising paradigm in the field of drug development due to its cost-effective framework and comprehensive elucidation of network theory and systems biology concepts. The network pharmacology method serves as the foundation for several case studies pertaining to traditional medicines. The use of network pharmacology is also utilized in the examination of many biological systems, illnesses, medications, and pathways, including complex proteins, genes, and diseases, drawing upon the principles of network biology [24].

11.3.3 NATURAL PRODUCTS DRUG DEVELOPMENT

The increasing popularity of herbal medications may be attributed to their reduced toxicity and enhanced therapeutic effects. However, as a result of the volatile acidic pH and challenges related to solubility, the concentration of the medication in the blood plasma may diminish, resulting in decreased therapeutic efficacy. Although plant metabolites such as flavonoids and glycosides possess medicinal properties, their absorption across lipid-rich cellular membranes is constrained by their polar nature and large molecular size, resulting in decreased bioavailability. A unique medicine delivery mechanism for plants has been implemented, resulting in a reduction in drug loss and degradation inside the target tissues. The negative effects have been reduced, leading to increased therapeutic effectiveness and enhanced medication absorption [25].

Nanotechnology has been recognized as a very effective approach for addressing the challenges associated with the stability, solubility, and bioavailability of herbal medications. Surface-engineered nanoparticles are used in the method to enhance the therapeutic efficacy of phytochemicals by selectively targeting certain anatomical locations within the body. Nanoparticles generated from plant viruses, namely the tobacco mosaic virus, are successfully used as carriers for drugs in the activation of immune cells associated with tumors, both in immunotherapy and chemotherapy. The use of nanoparticles in drug delivery systems has facilitated the transportation of phytochemicals across biological membranes, enabling precise administration to specific targets while minimizing degradation. Various phytochemicals that have been formulated at the nano level include hypericin, curcumin, silymarin, and others [26].

11.3.3.1 BIOADHESIVE MICROSPHERES (BMS)

BMs are distinctive types of drug delivery systems that provide close interaction between the medication and the biological membrane. The composition consists of microparticles and microcapsules with diameters ranging from 1 to 1000 μm. The customization of BMs involves the integration of microspheres with bioadhesive characteristics. This connection improves the drug's capacity to be absorbed by the body and its specificity at the site of absorption. The polymers included in this category consist of biodegradable, non-biodegradable, insoluble, and soluble species. They are used to regulate the medication's release and provide targeted drug administration to precise anatomical locations inside the body [27].

11.3.3.2 CHITOSAN-BASED HYDROGELS

Hydrogels are polymer networks that undergo swelling and cross-linking, enabling them to effectively absorb substantial quantities of water. Hydrogels have distinct characteristics such as the capacity for swelling, mechanical robustness comparable to that of host tissues, and the ability to undergo biodegradation. Hydrogels consist of either naturally occurring or artificially produced polymers. Biopolymers, such as chitosan, have mostly been used in the fabrication of hydrogels due to their inherent ability to undergo structural modifications. Chitosan has hydrophilic characteristics and may be biocompatible and biodegradable. Hydrogels have the capability to transport minute medication molecules, mitigate their adverse effects, and augment their concentration at the targeted site of exertion. The primary use of chitosan-based hydrogels is in the regulated administration of medicinal constituents. The mucoadhesive properties of chitosan enhance its ability to adhere to tissues, hence enabling targeted medication administration [28].

11.3.3.3 PULSATILE SYSTEM

These are designed to provide medications in a consistent manner, ensuring a seamless and uninterrupted release. Nevertheless, some circumstances require sporadic administration of medication, namely a delay in time. The pulsatile drug delivery system (PDDS) is used to accomplish such delivery. The PDDS system closely replicates the physiological process by which the body releases insulin in a regulated manner as required. PDDS has the ability to efficiently provide the medication in the most optimal quantity, location, and timing. The aforementioned technique has shown efficacy in the treatment of hypercholesterolemia, asthma, hypertension, arthritis, and peptic ulcers. Pulsatile delivery systems use several mechanisms such as time-dependent systems and pH-dependent systems, which utilize polymers that exhibit sensitivity to temperature, pH fluctuations, and light. PDDS has several benefits compared to traditional drug delivery systems, such as maintaining a consistent quantity of medicine at the intended location, reducing the required dosage, eliminating variations in drug levels, managing adverse effects, and enhancing patient adherence. Therefore, the use of pulsatile medication administration, which is synchronized with biological cycles and therapeutic requirements, offers the patient minimal adverse effects and optimal health advantages [29].

11.3.3.4 SELF-EMULSIFYING DRUG DELIVERY SYSTEMS (SEDDS)

The use of self-emulsifying drug delivery has significant potential for herbal medicine formulations characterized by limited water solubility and lipophilic natural active compounds. A self-emulsifying drug delivery system (SEDDS) is a compound consisting of a drug, oil, surfactant, and cosurfactant that is thermodynamically stable. Upon mixing the solution with water and subjecting it to gentle stirring, an oil-in-water micro/nano emulsion is promptly formed. These are capable of generating oil droplets within the wavelength range of 100–250 nm, whereas self-nanoemulsifying drug delivery systems (SNEDDS) have a wider range of 50–100 nm.

SEDDS has successfully improved the bioavailability of plant metabolites with low absorption, such as patchouli alcohol and mangiferin. SEDDS is favored over other drug delivery modalities due to its straightforward and convenient characteristics, as well as its ability to be kept in both liquid and solid states. Therefore, SEDDS may be effectively used to enhance the bioavailability and solubility of herbal medications [30].

11.3.3.5 LIPOSOMES

Liposomes are drug delivery vehicles that are non-toxic and biodegradable, capable of accommodating both hydrophobic and hydrophilic molecules. Spherical structures are characterized by the presence of one or more concentric membranes and a solvent that facilitates their unrestricted diffusion. Liposomes have the potential to enhance several aspects of drug delivery, including solubility, stability, bioavailability, intracellular absorption, and biodistribution. Drug delivery systems are used to enhance and sustain the therapeutic properties and concentration of medications over an extended period of time. Liposomes have been used as carriers for physiologically active chemicals, including proteins, tiny medicinal molecules, viruses, nucleotides, and other bioactive. A novel approach has been used to transport plant-derived bioactive compounds with anti-cancer capabilities using nano liposomal vesicles containing herbal remedies [31].

11.3.3.6 PHYTOSOMES

The bioavailability of bioactive substances is often lower as a result of their oral administration. Biomembranes that are rich in lipids impede the movement of water-soluble phytoconstituents. Therefore, it is possible to dissolve herbal extracts that exhibit insolubility in lipids in phospholipids at a precise ratio, resulting in the formation of lipid-compatible molecular complexes that possess therapeutic capabilities. The technological process described herein is founded upon the phospholipid complex methodology, whereby a chemical interaction occurs between polyphenolic plant compounds and phospholipids that include phosphatidylcholine, often referred to as phytosomes. The approach further generates cellular vesicles that serve as protective barriers for water-soluble phytocomponents, such as flavonoids, terpenoids, and phenolics, against degradation caused by gut bacteria and gastric secretions. This methodology improves the therapeutic index of the active chemicals found in the plants. It guarantees superior quality and effective delivery of active plant components to the intended recipients. This technological advancement has facilitated enhanced chemical bonding of the pharmaceutical compound, hence expediting its transdermal permeation at lower dosage levels. Therefore, the use of the phytophospholipid complex approach has facilitated a sophisticated and comprehensive assimilation of plant extracts. These phytophospholipid complexes exhibit potential as viable options for enhanced drug dosage treatment, particularly in the context of anti-inflammatory, cardiovascular, anticancer, and hepatoprotective applications [32].

11.4 FUTURE PROSPECTS IN HERBAL DRUG DEVELOPMENT

11.4.1 REGULATORY ASPECTS

From a global perspective, herbal medicine has been widely recognized as a significant alternative to contemporary allopathic treatment. While herbal remedies have widespread popularity in society, only a limited number of medicinal plants have undergone scientific evaluation to assess their potential in medical therapy. In the majority of nations, the regulation of herbal pharmaceuticals is inadequate, with a notable absence of registration and oversight by health authorities. The safety of herbal medications continues to be a significant area of concern. According to estimates provided by the Food and Drug Administration (FDA) in the United States, botanical and other dietary supplements are responsible for more than 50,000 adverse occurrences. Furthermore, the effectiveness of most herbal treatments has not been shown, and their purity is not guaranteed. The main goal of the WHO Traditional Medicine Strategy 2014–2023 is to improve the safety, effectiveness, and quality of TM by advancing knowledge and offering guidance on regulatory and quality assurance standards. As of 2012, herbal medicines were regulated by 119 member nations of the WHO [33].

Herbal medicine products include a range of botanical substances, including herbs, herbal materials, herbal preparations, and completed herbal products. These compositions consist of active compounds derived from plant parts, other plant materials, or a combination thereof. The category of herbs includes many forms of plant material, such as leaves, flowers, fruit, seeds, and stems. Finished herbal goods are derived from herbal preparations, which include comminuted or powdered herbal ingredients, as well as extracts, tinctures, and fatty oils derived from herbal sources. Finished herbal products are herbs that have been prepared using one or more herbs.

The regulatory framework pertaining to herbal remedies differs among nations [34]. Various regulatory techniques are now popular worldwide, including:

- The regulatory criteria for all items are uniform, except for herbal treatments, which do not need certain sorts of proof.
- Natural medicines are exempt from all regulatory requirements.
- Natural medicines are exempt from all regulatory requirements regarding registration or marketing authorization.
- Natural medicines are subject to all regulatory requirements.
- Natural medicines are subject to regulatory requirements regarding registration or marketing authorization.

In the European market, herbal remedies undergo classification into three distinct groups for the purpose of marketing clearance:

- The recognition of traditional medical use provisions, commonly referred to as "traditional use," relies on substantial safety evidence and credible efficacy. This acknowledgment is based on the proven effectiveness and a satisfactory level of safety, leading to the appropriate classification of the product.
- The safety and effectiveness data of the company can be acquired either through independent research and development or through a combination of their own studies and bibliographic data, termed as a "mixed application" [35].

The guidance provided by the FDA on the development of botanical pharmaceuticals outlines the recommended development plans for submission in new drug applications (NDAs), as well as specific recommendations for the submission of INDs. Botanical refers to items that include plant components, algae, macroscopic fungi, and their mixtures. According to FDA advice, the Investigational New Drug (IND) must include enough evidence to prove that the drug is safe for human testing and that the clinical procedure is well-structured for its intended goals. In addition to the overarching regulatory prerequisites for a NDA, which include nonclinical pharmacology/toxicology investigations, botanical medications are subject to specific standards aimed at safeguarding their safety and quality [36]. These criteria pertain specifically to clinical proof of effectiveness and safety:

- Description of product and documentation of prior human experience
  - Description of botanical raw materials used and known active constituents or chemical constituents
  - Prior human experience
- Quality control
  - Botanical raw materials
  - Botanical drug substance and drug product
- Overview of the product's identity, chemical composition, production methods, biological analysis, specifications, stability, current manufacturing standards, and environmental evaluation.
- Evidence to ensure therapeutic consistency
  - Botanical raw material control
  - Quality control by chemical test(s) and manufacturing control
  - Biological assay
  - Clinical data: Dose-response data and multiple batch clinical data

The primary category of Ayurveda, Siddha, or Unani (ASU) medications included under Indian legislation are:

a. The classical medications of the ASU system, as documented in the authoritative books, are produced and labelled based on the formulae outlined in the authoritative texts. The issuance of a license to manufacture in this particular category is contingent upon citation in authoritative books and published literature, unless the medication is intended for a novel indication, in which case evidence of its efficacy is necessary.
b. Patented or proprietary medicine utilizes components mentioned in authoritative literature, but incorporates intellectual intervention, creativity, or invention to produce medicines that exhibit distinct characteristics from classical medicine. In order to get a license to

manufacture for this category, it is necessary to provide evidence of efficacy, which should be based on a pilot study conducted in accordance with the applicable methodology for ASU medicines.

The Department of AYUSH implemented Rule 158(B) in 2010, which mandated the submission of evidence demonstrating the efficacy of a patent or proprietary Ayurvedic Substance Use (ASU) drug in order to obtain a license. Subsequently, the GCP guidelines were made available for researchers who express interest in conducting clinical studies with ASU medicine on a voluntary basis.

ASU medications in India are under the jurisdiction of the Department of AYUSH. Conversely, the CDSCO is responsible for overseeing the regulatory standards for phytopharmaceuticals as of 2015. This gazette announcement outlines the regulatory regulations for phytopharmaceuticals and the procedures for submitting scientific evidence on quality, safety, and effectiveness. The purpose is to assess and approve the marketing of herbal drugs in a manner comparable to synthetic chemical compounds.

A PPD denotes a refined and standardized fraction comprising no fewer than four bioactive or phytochemical compounds. These compounds undergo both qualitative and quantitative assessment to guarantee their effectiveness and consistency. This drug is derived from an extract of a medicinal plant or its components. It is intended for internal or external use by humans or animals for the purpose of diagnosing, treating, alleviating, or preventing any disease or disorder. However, it is important to note that parenteral administration is not included in this definition.

The inclusion of Appendix I B in Schedule Y delineates the requisite data that must be provided in conjunction with the application for the execution of a clinical trial or the importation or production of a phytopharmaceutical medicine within the nation. The regulatory prerequisites for the NDA of the PPD encompass established criteria pertaining to the safety and pharmacological information of the new medicine, as well as the inclusion of human research and confirmatory clinical trials. PPDs are subject to significant emphasis on:

- The provided information encompasses details regarding the plant, formulation, route of administration, dosages, therapeutic class, claims made for the phytopharmaceutical, as well as evidence from published literature pertaining to safety, efficacy, and human or clinical pharmacology.

- Data generated on:
  - The plant used for extraction and fractionation will be identified, authenticated, and its source will be determined.
  - The technique for extraction, fractionation, and purification will be described. The formulation details of the phytopharmaceutical medicine will be provided.
  - The manufacturing process of the formulation will be described.
  - Stability data will be collected.

The recently implemented rule on phytopharmaceuticals allows for the advancement of drug research via the use of sophisticated methodologies such as solvent extraction, fractionation, potentiating stages, and current formulation creation, among others. The recently implemented rule pertaining to phytopharmaceuticals aligns with the regulatory frameworks seen in the United States, China, and other nations, which emphasize scientific assessment and data gathering. The implementation of this novel legislation is anticipated to facilitate advancements and progress in the scientific exploration of novel pharmaceuticals derived from botanical sources. Moreover, it is anticipated to contribute to the widespread use of herbal items within the contemporary medical field. The promotion of phytopharmaceutical medication development would serve as a catalyst for academic, scientific, and industrial endeavors.

11.5 OCCURRENCE, ISOLATION AND CHARACTERISTIC FEATURES (CHEMICAL NATURE, USES IN PHARMACY, MEDICINAL AND HEALTH BENEFITS) OF PHYTOCHEMICALS

11.5.1 CAROTENOIDS

11.5.1.1 ALPHA-CAROTENE

The nutritional supplement known as alpha-carotene has several health advantages. The substance in question is a nutritional supplement derived from carotene, a plant pigment often presents in many fruits and vegetables. It has strong antioxidant properties that aid in safeguarding cells from harm inflicted by free radicals. Additionally, it has the potential to enhance the immune system and mitigate the likelihood of certain forms of cancer. It is used to enhance ocular well-being, improve the immune system, and safeguard against some forms of cancer. Additionally, it is used to reduce the likelihood of cardiovascular disease (CVD) and stroke. Numerous fruits and vegetables, such as carrots, sweet potatoes, spinach, kale, and cantaloupe, contain alpha-carotene [37].

In the food sector, alpha-carotene is used as a natural food colorant. The purpose of this substance is to provide a yellow or orange coloration to many food items, including margarine, cheese, and processed grains and vegetables. Additionally, it serves as an antioxidant, aiding in the preservation of food products' freshness. Alpha-carotene is further used as a dietary supplement to promote optimal visual acuity, skin health, and immune system function. Additionally, it has the potential to reduce the likelihood of certain forms of cancer, cardiovascular ailments, and age-related macular degeneration (AMD). Moreover, it has the potential to enhance the immune system, improve visual acuity, and mitigate inflammation. Although alpha-carotene is usually regarded as safe, there are some possible dangers that may be associated with its use. These factors include a heightened susceptibility to lung cancer in individuals who smoke, an elevated susceptibility to prostate cancer in males, and an increased susceptibility to heart disease in those with elevated cholesterol levels. Moreover, it is worth noting that alpha-carotene has the potential to interact with some drugs, including anticoagulants, hence potentially inducing adverse effects such as nausea, vomiting, and diarrhea [38].

The regulation of alpha-carotene varies throughout various regions globally. The Food and Drug Administration in the United States regulates dietary supplements under the Dietary Supplement Health and Education Act (DSHEA). The Therapeutic Goods Administration (TGA) regulates dietary supplements in Australia. The Food Safety and Standards Authority of India (FSSAI) regulates dietary supplements in India [39].

11.5.1.2 BETA-CAROTENE

Beta-carotene is a phytochemical compound that imparts vivid hues to red, orange, and yellow foods. The compound in question is classified as a provitamin A carotenoid, indicating its capacity for conversion into vitamin A (retinol) inside the human body. Moreover, beta-carotene has potent antioxidant effects. The term "carrot" originates from the Latin word meaning carrot. The physicist Heinrich Wilhelm Ferdinand Wackenroder discovered beta-carotene by crystallizing it from carrots in 1831. Beta-carotene not only serves as a dietary source of provitamin A but also exhibits antioxidant properties. Antioxidants, such as beta-carotene, play a crucial role in mitigating or averting oxidative stress inside the human body. Numerous study sources indicate that diets rich in antioxidants have the potential to enhance overall health. Antioxidants have the potential to mitigate oxidative stress inside the human body, hence offering potential protection against several ailments, including certain types of cancer, cardiovascular problems, and cognitive impairments such as Alzheimer's disease. Several studies have shown that beta-carotene may enhance cognitive performance as a result of its antioxidant properties. The findings of a Cochrane review conducted in 2018, which included eight studies examining antioxidants, including beta-carotene, revealed modest advantages linked to the administration of beta-carotene supplements in relation to cognitive function and memory. It is important to note that the cognitive advantages linked to beta-carotene were exclusively associated with extended periods of supplementation, with an average duration of 18 years. However, the researchers did not see a statistically significant impact in the immediate term, leading them to the conclusion that more investigation is needed. Further investigation is required to explore the possible advantages of beta-carotene supplementation in relation to cognitive health. Nevertheless, there is compelling data indicating that consuming fruits and vegetables, particularly those rich in beta-carotene, might effectively reduce the likelihood of cognitive decline and illnesses such as dementia [40].

Beta-carotene has the potential to enhance the overall health of the skin. Once again, this may be attributed to its antioxidant properties. According to a 2012 analysis, consuming enough amounts of antioxidant micronutrients, such as beta-carotene, may enhance the skin's ability to protect against UV radiation and promote the overall health and appearance of the skin. However, it should be noted by the researchers that the sun protection offered by dietary beta-carotene is much inferior to that provided by the use of a topical sunscreen. Studies on the impact of beta-carotene on lung health provide inconclusive results. Vitamin A, synthesized by the human body from beta-carotene, plays a crucial role in maintaining optimal lung function. Moreover, those who consume a substantial quantity of food rich in beta-carotene may have a reduced susceptibility to certain types of cancer, such as lung cancer. Research conducted in 2017, including over 2500 individuals, indicated that consuming fruits and vegetables abundant in carotenoids, such as beta-carotene, had a safeguarding impact against lung cancer. However, research has not shown that supplements provide the same outcome as consuming fresh vegetables. Indeed, the use of beta-carotene supplements may potentially elevate the susceptibility to lung cancer among those who engage in smoking [41].

Diets that are abundant in carotenoids, such as beta-carotene, have the potential to enhance ocular well-being and provide defense against ocular ailments, including AMD, a condition characterized by visual impairment. Studies have shown that elevated blood concentrations of carotenoids, such as beta-carotene, might potentially decrease the likelihood of developing severe AMD by up to 35%. Studies indicate that consuming diets abundant in antioxidant-rich foods, such as beta-carotene, may provide a safeguard against the onset of several types of cancer, including premenopausal breast cancer, lung cancer, and pancreatic cancer. Typically, health professionals advise consuming a diet abundant in fruits and vegetables, since they include a multitude of vitamins, minerals, and plant chemicals that synergistically promote well-being, rather than relying on beta-carotene supplementation [42].

Fruits and vegetables that have a red, orange, or yellow color have a high concentration of beta carotene. Several studies have shown that cooked carrots have a higher concentration of carotenoids compared to raw carrots. The incorporation of olive oil has the potential to enhance the bioavailability of carotenoids. Beta carotene is classified as a fat-soluble molecule, hence enhancing its absorption when consumed in conjunction with a fat source. Green vegetables, namely spinach, sweet potatoes, carrots, broccoli, butternut squash, cantaloupe, red and yellow peppers, apricots, peas, romaine, and lettuce are the foods that have the greatest levels of beta carotene. Herbs and spices such as paprika, cayenne, chili, parsley, cilantro, marjoram, sage, and coriander also contain beta carotene [43].

According to the findings of the National Center for Complementary and Integrative Health (NCCIH), there is no significant association between beta carotene supplements and adverse effects, even when administered at high levels ranging from 20 to 30 mg per day. There is no evidence to suggest that prolonged consumption of a carotenoid-rich diet is linked to toxicity. Prolonged use of excessive quantities of beta carotene may lead to the development of a benign disease known as carotenodermia, characterized by the skin exhibiting a yellow-orange hue. Nevertheless, it is recommended that those who smoke refrain from using beta carotene pills. It is advisable for those who smoke, as well as those who have a history of smoking, to refrain from using beta carotene supplements and multivitamins that exceed the recommended daily intake of vitamin A, either via preformed retinol or beta carotene. Numerous investigations have shown a correlation between elevated supplement dosages of these essential nutrients and an increased susceptibility to lung cancer among individuals who smoke. It is crucial to consider that excessive amounts of any antioxidant in a supplementary form might disrupt the absorption of other vital nutrients and have a detrimental impact on the body's innate defense mechanism. Health professionals often advise consuming a diet abundant in fruits and vegetables, since they contain many antioxidants and other vital nutrients, rather than relying on beta carotene supplementation [44].

11.5.1.3 XANTHOPHYLL (LUTEIN)

Xanthophylls, first known as phylloxanthins, are a class of yellow pigments that are abundantly found in the natural environment. They constitute one of the primary categories within the carotenoid group. The remaining portion is composed of carotene. The term "*Xanthos*" originates from the Greek words "*Xanthos*" (v), which signifies "yellow," and "*Phyllon*" (v), which signifies "leaf." This etymology is based on the observation of a yellow hue in the first chromatography of leaf pigments. The phenomenon may be traced back to the emergence of bands. Xanthophylls and carotenes exhibit structural similarities since they both belong to the class of carotenoids. However, it is important to note that xanthophylls contain oxygen atoms, whereas carotenes are hydrocarbons devoid of oxygen. Xanthophylls possess a higher degree of polarity in their molecular structure compared to carotenes due to the presence of oxygen. Consequently, several chromatography techniques are used to separate xanthophylls from carotenes. Carotenes often exhibit a more vibrant orange color compared to xanthophylls. Xanthophylls serve as a bridge to generate an epoxide by presenting oxygen as a hydroxyl group and/or as a hydrogen atom that replaces an oxygen atom [45].

Xanthophylls, similar to other carotenoids, are mostly found in the leaves of green plants. They play a role in regulating light energy and are likely non-photochemical substances that interact with triplet chlorophyll, which is the higher energy form of chlorophyll. It functions as a suppressor and is generated excessively under intense light conditions during photosynthesis. Xanthophylls, which are present in the bodies of animals, including humans, as well as in animal-derived meals, ultimately derive from plant sources within the dietary context. The yellow hue seen in chicken egg yolks, fat, and skin may be attributed to the consumption of xanthophylls, particularly lutein, which is intentionally included in chicken feed for this specific function. These compounds provide ocular protection by effectively absorbing ionizing light, namely blue light and UV light. Nevertheless, xanthophylls are incapable of undergoing conversion into retinal (also known as retinaldehyde or vitamin A aldehyde), rendering them ineffective in the visual process [46].

One of the chemicals within the xanthophyll group includes lutein, zeaxanthin, neoxanthin, violaxanthin, flavoxanthin, as well as α- and β-cryptoxanthin, among others. The molecule in question is the only xanthophyll that has been identified as possessing a beta-ionone ring. Consequently, β-cryptoxanthin stands as the sole xanthophyll that has been seen to have provitamin A action in mammals. Indeed, this vitamin is only present in plant-eating animals that possess an enzyme capable of synthesizing retinal pigments from carotenoids, such as beta-ionone (although certain carnivores lack this enzyme). Certain xanthophylls in non-mammalian animals have the ability to undergo conversion into hydroxylated retinal analogues, which play a direct role in visual function. As an example, except for certain flies, the majority of insects use the R isomer of xanthophyll-derived 3-hydroxyretinal for their visual functions. This implies that β-cryptoxanthin and other xanthophylls, including lutein and zeaxanthin, have the potential to function as a kind of visual stimulus [47].

The xanthophyll cycle encompasses the enzymatic elimination of epoxy groups from xanthophylls, such as violaxanthin, antheraxanthin, diazinoxanthin, and others, resulting in the formation of de-epoxidized xanthophylls, including diatoxanthin and zeaxanthin. The enzyme cycles have been identified as significant contributors to the promotion of energy dissipation in light-harvesting antenna proteins via non-photochemical quenching. One of the primary methods to safeguard against photoinhibition is through non-photochemical quenching. Higher plants possess three carotenoid pigments, namely violaxanthin, antheraxanthin, and zeaxanthin, which play a crucial role in the xanthophyll cycle.

Under conditions of mild stress, the conversion of violaxanthin to zeaxanthin occurs via the intermediate antheraxanthin. Antheraxanthin functions as a lipid-protective antioxidant and induces non-photochemical quenching in light-harvesting proteins, thus directly contributing to its photoprotective properties. The enzyme violaxanthin deepoxidase catalyzes the conversion of violaxanthin to zeaxanthin, whereas zeaxanthin epoxidase catalyzes the opposite process, namely oxidation. A xanthophyll cycle is seen in diatoms and dinoflagellates. The pigment diazinoxanthin is present in it and undergoes conversion to diatoxanthin (found in diatoms) or dinoxanthin (found in dinoflagellates) when exposed to strong light conditions. The study reveals that the observed rise in zeaxanthin levels in spinach surpasses the decline in violaxanthin levels. The researchers suggest that this disparity may be attributed to the process of synthesizing zeaxanthin from beta-carotene [48].

All young and yellowed leaves contain xanthophylls (Figure 11.3). Additional sources that are abundant in lutein diesters include papaya, peaches, prunes, and pumpkin. Kale has a lutein and zeaxanthin content of around 18 mg per 100 g, spinach approximately 11 mg per 100 g, parsley approximately 6 mg per 100 g, peas approximately 3 mg per 110 g, pumpkin approximately 3 mg per 100 g, and pistachio approximately 1 mg per 100 g [49].

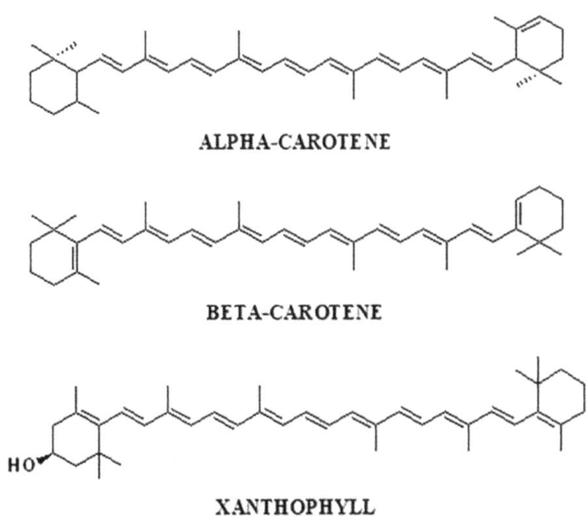

FIGURE 11.3 Structure of carotenoids.

11.5.2 LIMONOIDS

11.5.2.1 D-LIMONENE

The chemical compound known as limonene is present in the outer layer of citrus fruits, including lemons, limes, and oranges. The essential oils found in orange peels are very abundant, accounting for around 97% of the total composition of this rind. The primary chemical form of this compound is often known as D-limonene. Limonene is classified as a terpene, a class of chemicals that possess strong scents that serve to safeguard plants by repelling predators. Limonene, a prevalent terpene in nature, has the potential to provide several health advantages. Research has shown that it has anti-inflammatory, antioxidant, anti-stress, and perhaps disease-preventive characteristics. Limonene is a widely used ingredient in many consumer goods such as food items, cosmetics, cleaning agents, and natural bug deterrents. For instance, it is used in culinary products such as carbonated beverages and confections to impart a lemon-like taste. Limonene is obtained by the hydrodistillation method, wherein fruit peels are immersed in water and subjected to heat until the volatile compounds are liberated via steam, then condensed, and subsequently isolated. Limonene is used as a plant pesticide due to its powerful fragrance. It serves as a primary component in several pesticide products, including environmentally friendly insect repellents. Furthermore, limonene may be obtained as concentrated supplements in the form of capsules and liquids. These products are often promoted based on their purported health advantages. The aforementioned citrus component is further used as an aromatic oil due to its tranquilizing and medicinal qualities [50].

Several studies have shown the anti-inflammatory properties of limonene. Although short-term inflammation is a typical physiological reaction to stress and may have positive effects, persistent inflammation can have detrimental effects on the body and is a significant contributor to illness. It is crucial to minimize or eliminate this kind of inflammation to the greatest extent feasible. The efficacy of limonene in mitigating inflammatory indicators associated with osteoarthritis, a chronic inflammatory disorder, has been shown. A study conducted on human cartilage cells using test tubes observed that limonene decreased the generation of nitric oxide (NO). NO serves as a key signaling molecule in inflammatory processes. In a study conducted on rats afflicted with ulcerative colitis, a condition characterized by inflammation, the administration of limonene resulted in a significant reduction in inflammation, colon damage, and the levels of commonly seen inflammatory markers. Accumulation of free radicals may result in oxidative stress, which has the potential to initiate inflammation and illness. A study conducted in a test tube showed that limonene has the ability to suppress free radicals in leukemia cells, indicating a reduction in inflammation and cellular damage that often leads to the development of the illness [51].

Limonene has potential anticancer properties. According to a population study, those who ingested citrus fruit peel, which is the primary dietary source of limonene, had a decreased likelihood of acquiring skin cancer compared to those who only consumed citrus fruits or their juices. A further investigation conducted on a cohort of 43 women who were newly diagnosed with breast cancer revealed a noteworthy decrease of 22% in the expression of breast tumor cells following the daily consumption of 2 grams of limonene for a duration of 2–6 weeks. Furthermore, a study conducted on mice revealed that the administration of limonene as a supplement effectively suppressed the proliferation of skin tumors through its ability to mitigate inflammation and oxidative stress. Additional rat studies suggest that limonene has the potential to combat other forms of cancer, such as breast cancer. Additionally, when administered to rats in conjunction with the anticancer agent doxorubicin, limonene showed efficacy in mitigating other prevalent adverse effects associated with the medication, such as oxidative stress, inflammation, and renal impairment [59].

11.5.2.2 ALPHA-TERPINEOL

A terpene alcohol known as α-terpineol (α-T) (Figure 11.4) is present in several natural oils, including pine oil and petitgrain oil derived from the bitter orange tree. The aforementioned structural isomer is the most prevalent among the four isomers, namely β-, γ-, and 4-terpineol. Terpinol, the hydrate of terpin, a terpene diol, should not be mistaken for it. A racemic combination of (R)-(+)- and (S)-(–)-enantiomers is known as α-Terpineol. Both substances are naturally occurring, however, the commercially available product, often derived from α-pinene, is referred to as the racemate. The (+)-stereoisomer was obtained from petitgrain by German scientists H. Waldbaum and O. Hüthig in the year 1903. After a span of four years, J. E. Teeple, a researcher from New York City, successfully isolated the enantiomer of long-leaf pine oil [51].

In addition to their optically active forms, α- and β-Terpineol are also found as racemates. Both α-T and T-4-ol are the primary commercially significant compounds and are present in a wide range of essential oils. In contrast, the occurrence of β-, γ-, and ι-terpineols in natural environments is rather infrequent. Terpineols, particularly the well-known molecules such as α-T and T-4-ol, have diverse biological effects on people, animals, and plants. Not only are they widely used as aroma components in perfumes, cosmetics, and home cleaning products, but they are also employed for the purpose of flavoring various food and beverage items. Additionally, they exhibit a multitude of significant biological and therapeutic qualities [52].

The primary constituent of essential oils derived from many aromatic plant species, including *Origanum vulgare* L. and *Ocimum canum* Sims, is α-T, a volatile monoterpenoid alcohol. These oils are extensively used for medical applications. In addition to cajeput oil, pine oil, and petitgrain oil, α-T may also be obtained from many sources. It is a transparent, crystalline substance with a lilac scent. It is an optically active monoterpenoid that naturally exists in the (+)-, (-)-, and ([3]) forms. Geranium oils and Morio-Muscat-wine fragrance were found to have natural racemic mixtures of α-T. The separation of α-T enantiomers, which are present in the Myrtaceae family, was achieved by the use of a two-column linked system and a combination of two chiral phases, specific to citrus and lavender oil. α-T is extensively used in the production of cosmetics, soaps, perfumes, and antibacterial agents, and is regarded as one of the most often employed fragrance compounds due to its pleasant scent reminiscent of lilac. Acetate and other basic esters of α-T are often used in the production of perfumes and aromatic fragrances. Hence, the esterification of terpinyl acetate has significant importance in the fragrance business, specifically in terms of its acetylation. Furthermore, α-T demonstrates a diverse array of biological uses due to its ability to reduce hypertension and prevent the growth of human erythroleukemic cells. Additionally, it displays anti-inflammatory capabilities by effectively inhibiting the formation of superoxide. Numerous investigations have shown the evident anticancer properties of α-T [53].

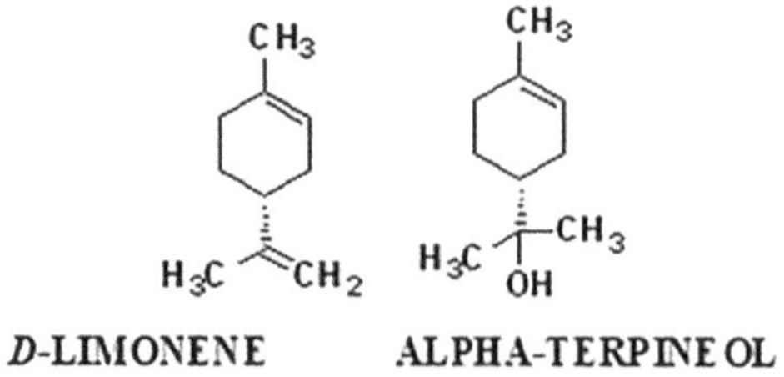

FIGURE 11.4 Structure of limonoids.

11.5.3 SAPONINS

11.5.3.1 SHATAVARINS

Shatavari, the root of *Asparagus racemosus* (AR), is extensively used due to its steroidal saponins known as shatavarins (Figure 11.5). Antiretroviral (AR) compounds have garnered therapeutic attention owing to their diverse range of properties, including immunomodulatory, galactagogue, adaptogen, antitussive, anticarcinogenic, antioxidant, antidiarrheal, and general tonic effects. The plant is at risk of extinction due to several seasonal and developmental limitations in the traditional methods used for its reproduction. The standard way of propagating AR involves the use of seeds, which exhibit poor efficacy. Consequently, there is a need to explore alternate approaches for propagating AR. In the 1980s, many techniques for cultivating AR tissue were experimented with. However, our research team has recently developed a methodology for creating callus and suspension cultures (SCs) of AR. These cultures may be readily maintained in laboratory settings to ensure efficiency. These cultures consistently exhibit elevated quantities of saponins, both inside their cells and outside of them. The effectiveness of using a tissue culture methodology as a means of supporting conservation efforts will be contingent upon the caliber and abundance of shatavarins generated via *in vitro* methods. The root extract of the wild type AR (WRE) is well recognized as an immunomodulator. WRE has been shown to have immunomodulatory effects in many investigations. According to reports, it has the ability to replenish lymphocyte and neutrophil levels. It regulates the activation of macrophages and slows down the growth of tumors in animals used in experiments. The study also reports the immunomodulatory effects of crude WRE extracts on the release of tumor necrosis factor-alpha and phagocytosis. Additionally, it functions as an immunotherapeutic agent in animals and has a significant influence on systemic Th1/Th2 immunity. Steroidal saponins, together with minor steroids and their glucosides, alkaloids, flavonoids, and triterpenoids, have been identified as a prominent class of compounds found in the plant AR. The roots were found to contain significant amounts of steroidal glucosides, namely shatavarin I to X (shatavarins). The immunopharmacological action of cancer treatment is shown by the entire extract, polar and non-polar extracts, and their formulations. The plant extracts have been shown to have inhibitory effects on breast carcinogenesis produced by 7, 12-dimethylbenz[a]anthracene (DMBA) in rats [54].

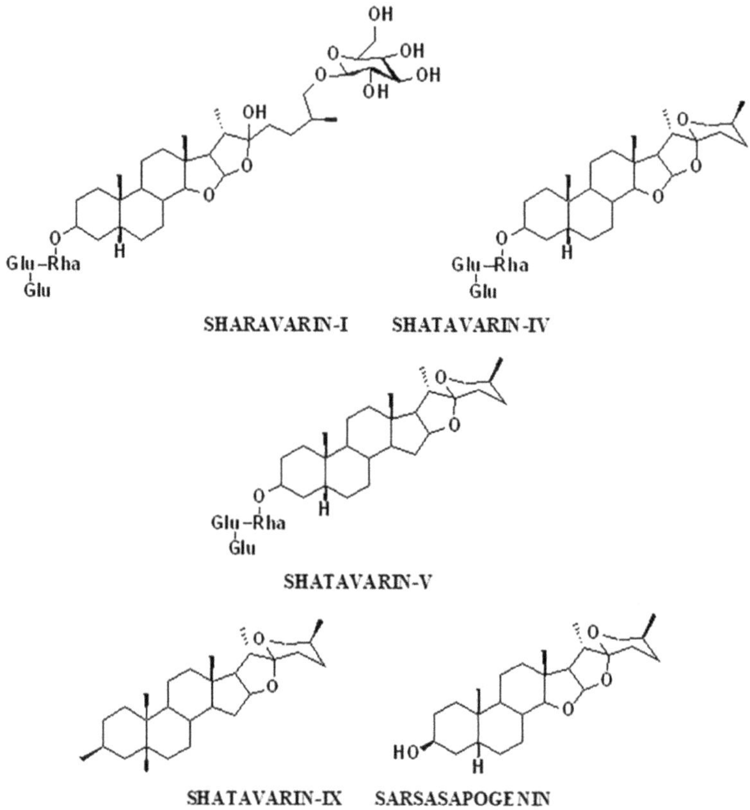

FIGURE 11.5 Structure of shatavarins.

11.5.4 FLAVONOIDS

11.5.4.1 RESVERATROL

A polyphenolic phytoalexin known as resveratrol (3,5,4'-trihydroxystilbene) is present. The compound in question is a stilbenoid, which is a derivative of stilbene. It is synthesized in plants by the enzymatic activity of stilbene synthase. The compound is present in both cis-(Z) and trans-(E) isomers. When subjected to heat or UV irradiation, the trans form may undergo isomerization to the cis form. Dr. Sinclair from Harvard University said in a 2004 publication of science that safeguarding resveratrol against oxidation is a challenging task. There have been assertions made about its susceptibility to degradation when exposed to light, heat, and oxygen.

Nevertheless, research indicates that trans-resveratrol experiences little oxidation under typical atmospheric conditions at ambient temperature.

Resveratrol, a phytoalexin, has been seen to hinder the reproduction of both herpes virus types 1 and 2 in a way that depends on the dosage and may be reversed. However, it is important to note that this is only one of the several pharmacological characteristics of resveratrol. There is a correlation between increased red wine intake and a decreased prevalence of heart disease in some nations. Resveratrol has other advantages, such as its anti-inflammatory and antioxidant properties. Resveratrol has shown promising anticancer effects in preclinical investigations. Resveratrol inhibits the activation of NF-kappaB in cells infected with HSV. Reports suggest that HSV triggers the activation of NF-kappaB during productive infection, which may play a crucial role in its reproduction mechanism [55].

11.5.4.2 RUTIN

Rutin is a bioflavonoid found in certain vegetables and fruits and is classified as a plant pigment. Apples contain tons of rutin. Rutin is present in buckwheat, most citrus fruits, figs, and both black and green tea. The compound rutin has strong antioxidant effects. It also aids in the production of collagen and the utilization of vitamin C by the body. Historically, rutin has been used for its circulatory-enhancing properties. There is a prevailing belief that rutin has the potential to enhance the strength and flexibility of blood vessels, including arteries and capillaries. Enhanced vascular integrity has the potential to improve one's overall well-being. This intervention has the potential to alleviate associated ailments, such as bruising, venous congestion, and varicose veins. Additionally, there is data suggesting that rutin may assist in the treatment of hemorrhoids, which are a result of enlarged veins, as well as in the recovery process after surgery to remove hemorrhoids [56].

Studies indicate that rutin has the ability to inhibit the development of blood clots in some animal species. These findings suggest that rutin may have a potential anticoagulant effect. Implementing measures to prevent blood clots may significantly reduce the likelihood of developing severe medical disorders such as myocardial infarctions, cerebrovascular accidents, pulmonary embolisms, and deep vein thrombosis. There is ample data supporting the efficacy of rutin in reducing LDL cholesterol levels. In a particular study, individuals diagnosed with diabetes and a prior medical history of hypertension were given a daily dosage of 500 milligrams (mg) of rutin. A reduction in the plasma LDL cholesterol levels of the subjects was observed by the researchers. The study posits that this phenomenon might be attributed to the antioxidant capabilities of rutin. Rutin is often used to alleviate arthritic discomfort. Research revealed that it facilitated the reduction of oxidative stress in individuals suffering from arthritis. This might be attributed to the potent anti-inflammatory and antioxidant characteristics of rutin. Additionally, there is research suggesting that rutin enhances knee functionality in individuals with arthritis.

Consuming fruits and vegetables that are high in rutin is generally considered safe. Nevertheless, the use of rutin supplements is associated with some adverse effects. These often occur due to the use of it in larger and more concentrated quantities. Several common adverse effects associated with the use of rutin supplements include visual impairment, gastrointestinal disturbances, headaches, erythema, dermatitis, anxiety, cardiac arrhythmia, edema in the knees, muscle rigidity, elevated leukocyte count, and so on. It is contraindicated for pregnant or lactating women to use rutin supplements. Insufficient data exists to establish the safety of the subject matter. Nevertheless, the use of natural sources of this bioflavonoid does not pose any risk [57].

11.5.4.3 HESPERIDIN

Hesperidin, a flavanone glycoside belonging to the flavonoid class, was extracted from the mesocarp, the gelatinous inner peel of oranges. Citrus fruits such as oranges, lemons, clementines, mandarins, and grapefruits contain a significant amount of hesperidin (Hsd). Hesperidin is named from the term "hesperidium," which refers to a fruit with a fleshy, divided inside and a tough outer layer that contains fragrant oils. The aglycone version of the compound, which lacks a glycosyl group, is referred to as hesperetin.

Experiments investigating the anti-inflammatory effects of hesperidin have shown inconclusive findings. According to a meta-analysis, the consumption of hesperidin, whether via citrus juice or oral supplements, resulted in a non-dose-dependent reduction in pro-inflammatory markers such as C-reactive protein (CRP), interleukin-6 (IL-6), and interleukin-4 (IL-4). Nevertheless, a subsequent meta-analysis failed to reproduce similar results pertaining to CRP and IL-6. However, it did see a noteworthy reduction in the concentrations of the inflammatory biomarker known as vascular cell adhesion molecule-1 (VCAM-1). The divergent results seen may be ascribed to variations in the quality of studies, methodologies used, and characteristics of participants, hence highlighting the need for more research to substantiate the anti-inflammatory effects of hesperidin.

Furthermore, a meta-analysis has shown that the administration of hesperidin resulted in a noteworthy decrease in several risk variables associated with CVD. These advantages included reduced levels of triglycerides (TG), total cholesterol (TC), low-density lipoprotein (LDL), TNF-α, and systolic blood pressure (SBP). It is worth mentioning that the aforementioned results were mostly noticed when hesperidin dosages exceeded 500 mg per day. Furthermore, these effects were significantly impacted by several variables, including the length of hesperidin therapy (which tends to be more effective when it exceeds 6 weeks) as well as the participants' BMI, age, and general health condition [58].

Hesperidin has been shown to enhance blood circulation, as demonstrated by a randomized controlled trial (RCT) that included individuals with metabolic syndrome who were given a daily dose of 500 mg of hesperidin for a duration of 3 weeks. Hesperidin demonstrated a 2.5% increase in blood flow, as evaluated using flow-mediated dilation (FMD). A further investigation observed a notable enhancement in microcirculation, namely the blood flow inside the tiny capillaries, six hours after the administration of either hesperidin capsules or standardized orange juice to overweight men who were in a state of full stomach. This intervention was administered over a period of four weeks. Notwithstanding the encouraging nature of these findings, there is ambiguity about the durability of these effects and their potential influence on blood pressure [59].

In addition, a RCT was conducted to assess the effects of hesperidin methyl chalcone (HMC), a synthetic derivative of hesperidin, on muscle damage and discomfort related to delayed onset muscle soreness (DOMS) resulting from a rigorous anaerobic exercise regimen. The administration of HMC supplements enhanced muscular recuperation, athletic performance, and postural equilibrium. The experimental group administered HMC exhibited enhanced physical performance, as indicated by the duration of repetitions until failure, and showed reduced muscle soreness during passive quadriceps palpation. However, these improvements were not seen during activities such as ascending and descending stairs. No negative effects related to hesperidin supplementation have been identified in studies. Nevertheless, it is crucial to acknowledge that the lack of side effects in studies does not unequivocally exclude them, and more examination is necessary. According to research, the administration of a 500 mg dosage of HMC did not have any significant impact on indicators of renal and hepatic function. A meta-analysis revealed a correlation between hesperidin administration and weight gain, which may be worrisome for those who are obese or overweight. Nevertheless, this phenomenon has not been consistently shown in other research, and it might be impacted by several variables other than the administration of hesperidin [60].

The exact method by which hesperidin exerts its effects remains elusive. Nevertheless, other research, mostly focused on animals, has emphasized various mechanisms by which hesperidin may exert its effects. Hesperidin has the ability to enhance lipid metabolism via many mechanisms. Hesperidin has been shown to potentially block the enzymes.

Moreover, clinical research on G-hesperidin indicates that it improves the breakdown of very low-density lipoprotein (VLDL), resulting in decreased levels of TG and LDL. G-hesperidin has been shown to exert its effects via the activation of lipoprotein lipase (LPL), an enzyme that plays a crucial role in the hydrolysis of TG. Additionally, *in vitro* investigations have shown that G-hesperidin has the potential to inhibit the excessive production of LDL in the liver by reducing the release of apolipoprotein B, a crucial component of LDL. In terms of its anti-inflammatory effects, hesperidin has been discovered to potentially alleviate inflammation by inhibiting key inflammatory enzymes like inducible nitric oxide synthase (iNOS) and cyclooxygenase-2 (COX-2), as well as inflammatory markers such as TNF-κ and IL-6. This mechanism is believed to result in a reduction of prostaglandin levels. These findings are supported by both *in vitro* and *in vivo* research [61].

Furthermore, a theory posits that the blood pressure-lowering action of hesperidin may be attributed to its ability to enhance the generation of NO. This, in turn, triggers vasodilation by inducing relaxation of the smooth muscles in blood vessels, ultimately resulting in a decrease in blood pressure. Another plausible mechanism is the reduction of vasoconstrictor angiotensin-2 levels by hesperidin via the inhibition of the angiotensin-converting enzyme. It is important to acknowledge that these pathways are still theoretical and need clinical validation. Hesperidin and hesperetin have been observed to exhibit a moderate effect on blood flow. This effect can be attributed to two mechanisms: firstly, by promoting the generation of intracellular hydrogen peroxide, which subsequently activates the Src family kinase enzymes responsible for regulating NO production in blood vessels; and secondly, by modulating estrogen signaling, which is also implicated in the production of NO [62].

11.5.4.4 NARINGIN

Naringin, a flavonoid compound, is mostly found in grapefruits and other citrus fruits. It is a glycoside composed of the disaccharide neohesperidose and the flavone naringenin, as described in chemical terms. Naringin is composed of a flavonoid backbone, two phenolic rings, and a heterocyclic pyran ring in its chemical structure. The compound has a molecular weight of 580.54 g and is represented by the chemical formula $C_{27}H_{32}O_{14}$. Naringin has garnered significant attention in the field of pharmaceutical and nutraceutical research due to its distinctive bitter taste and diverse range of biological attributes, including antioxidant, anti-inflammatory, anticancer, and cardioprotective activities. Multiple scientific studies have shown that the concurrent administration of naringin has been found to modify the blood concentrations of some drugs by disrupting the functioning of enzyme proteins and transporters inside the gastrointestinal tract. The compound known as naringin has potent inhibitory effects on many transporter proteins, including the multidrug resistance protein (MDR), organic anion transporting polypeptide (OATP) isoforms, and sulfotransferase (SULT). Naringin has inhibitory effects on several cytochrome isoenzymes (CYP). Research has shown that the anticancer medicine naringin decreases the expression of P-glycoprotein, a drug efflux pump located on the cell membrane. Increased production of P-glycoprotein leads to resistance to doxorubicin, an anticancer therapy. Naringin, a flavanone, inhibits the generation of carcinogens by preventing CYP isoenzymes, suggesting its possible function in cancer mitigation. Naringinase, a particular enzyme, may eliminate the bitter taste caused by naringin in the production of commercial grapefruit juice. The aglycon component of naringenin is linked to two rhamnose units at the 7-carbon position. Naringin and naringenin have potent antioxidant properties.

The potency of naringin is comparatively lower than that of naringenin due to the presence of a sugar moiety in the former, which leads to steric inhibition of the scavenging group. Naringin exhibits modest solubility in water. Within the intestine, gut microflora breaks down naringin into its aglycon form, naringenin, which is subsequently absorbed. The enzyme naringinase, present in the gastric environment of humans, facilitates the conversion of naringin into aglycone naringenin [63].

In 1928, the chemical structure and molecular formula of naringin were found and characterized by Asahina and Inubuse. An alpha-L-rhamnopyranosyl group is added to position 7 of the disaccharide derivative naringin via a glycosidic link, replacing a 2-O-(alpha-L-rhamnopyranosyl)-beta-D-glucopyranosyl moiety. Naringin has a melting point of 83C, with a solubility of 1 mg/mL at a temperature of 40C. Additionally, the molecular weight of naringin is determined to be 580.5 g/mol. As the temperature increases, the solubility of naringin and its aglycon counterpart, naringenin, is enhanced in different solvents. Naringin exhibited solubility in six solvents, namely methanol, ethyl acetate, n-butanol, isopropanol, petroleum ether, and hexane. The solubility of naringin complexes in water at a temperature of 37 ± 0.1°C is 15 times greater than that of free naringin. The degradation process begins at temperatures over 100°C or in the presence of light. The broad and intense absorption of –OH ranging from 3300 cm^{-1} to 2500 cm^{-1} indicates the existence of a carboxylic group. The strong and broad hydrogen-bonded O-H stretching bands, centered at 3300 cm^{-1} and 3400 cm^{-1}, reflect alcohols and phenols. The $C = C$ stretching bands associated with aromatic rings are often seen beyond the conventional area of $C = C$ emergence observed in alkenes (1650 cm^{-1}), spanning from 1600 to 1450 cm^{-1}. The occurrence of these peaks is exclusive to naringin. The investigation of flavonoid-cyclodextrin inclusion complexes revealed the absence of the distinctive peaks associated with aromatic rings and phenols in naringin at 1519 cm^{-1} and 1361 cm^{-1}. A correlation coefficient (r) of 0.97 IBU was observed between the measured quantity of naringin and the perceived bitterness [64].

11.5.4.5 QUERCETIN

Quercetin is a plant, fruit, and vegetable pigment. Quercetin has strong antioxidant capabilities and perhaps confers resistance against certain health ailments, such as CVD. Plants, fruits, herbs, vegetables, and nuts contain phytochemical substances known as flavonoids. The human body lacks the ability to synthesize quercetin; nevertheless, several fruits, vegetables, and beverages are rich sources of this compound. Quercetin may be found in several foods and beverages such as broccoli, onions, peppers, buckwheat, capers, Brassica vegetables, apples, grapes, berries, tea, wine, nuts, and seeds. The typical individual ingests around 10–100 mg of it on a daily basis from diverse dietary sources. Additionally, it is accessible in the form of powder and capsules as a dietary supplement.

Research indicates that quercetin has the potential to mitigate inflammation. Quercetin decreased the levels of inflammatory markers in human cells, such as TNF-α and IL-6. In an 8-week trial involving a sample of 50 women diagnosed with rheumatoid arthritis, it was discovered that the administration of 500 mg of quercetin resulted in a notable decrease in early morning stiffness, morning discomfort, and post-activity pain among the participants. In addition, they exhibited decreased levels of inflammatory markers, such as TNF-α, in comparison to those who were administered a placebo. Further human study is required to fully comprehend the compound's potential anti-inflammatory capabilities, despite the encouraging nature of these results.

The existing body of research indicates that the antioxidant properties of quercetin may have potential protective effects against degenerative brain illnesses, including Alzheimer's disease and dementia. A study was conducted where mice diagnosed with Alzheimer's disease were given quercetin injections every 2 days for a duration of 3 months. At the conclusion of the trial, the injections effectively reversed many indicators of Alzheimer's disease, and the mice exhibited much improved performance on cognitive assessments. In a separate investigation, a meal abundant in quercetin was shown to decrease indicators of Alzheimer's disease and enhance cognitive abilities in rats during the first intermediate phase of the disorder. Nevertheless, the impact of the diet on animals exhibiting middle-late-stage Alzheimer's was minimal or negligible. Coffee, a widely enjoyed beverage, has been linked to a reduced risk of developing Alzheimer's disease. Research suggests that quercetin, not caffeine, is the primary compound in coffee responsible for its potential protective effects against this condition [65].

Moreover, studies indicate that quercetin may help lower blood pressure levels. In laboratory experiments, quercetin demonstrated a vasodilatory effect on blood vessels. Administered daily for 5 weeks, quercetin led to a decrease in systolic and diastolic blood pressure values in hypertensive mice, with an average reduction of 18% and 23%, respectively.

Likewise, a thorough examination of nine human trials comprising 580 individuals revealed that consuming quercetin supplements daily at doses exceeding 500 mg resulted in an average reduction of 5.8 mm Hg in SBP and 2.6 mm Hg in diastolic blood pressure. Quercetin's potential in fighting cancer may be attributed to its antioxidant capabilities. Quercetin (Figure 11.6) was seen to inhibit cell proliferation and trigger apoptosis in prostate cancer cells, as evidenced by an analysis of test-tube and animal experiments. Additional experiments conducted on test tubes and animals revealed that the substance had comparable effects on cancer cells in the liver, lung, breast, bladder, blood, colon, ovarian, lymphoid, and adrenal glands [66].

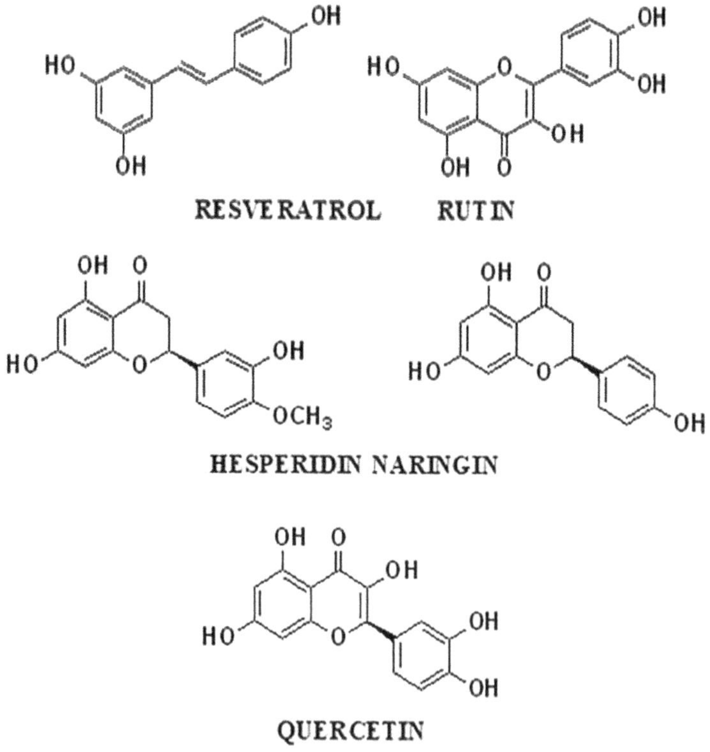

FIGURE 11.6 Structure of flavonoids.

11.5.5 PHENOLIC ACIDS

11.5.5.1 ELLAGIC ACID (EA)

EA was first identified in 1831 by Henri Braconnot, a French chemist and pharmacist. He dubbed it "acide ellagique" based on the word "Galle" when read backwards. Nevertheless, the comprehensive comprehension of the existence of this compound in botanical specimens remained elusive until the commencement of the 20th century. During this period, it was synthesized from diverse botanical origins, including oak bark, valonea, pomegranate (*Punica granatum* L.), divi-divi (*Caesalpinia coriaria* (Jacq.) Willd.), myrobalan (*Terminalia catappa* L.), and algarrobilla (*Prosopis humilis* Hook.). Currently, EA is recognized as a naturally extracted bioactive and pharmacologically active polyphenolic chemical that is prevalent in several taxonomically varied plant groupings, particularly within the eudicotyledonous classification. EA is a dilactone of hexahydroxydiphenic acid (HHDP), which is a dimeric derivative of gallic acid. Ethanol (EA) is primarily synthesized in plants by the process of hydrolyzing ellagitannins, which are a diverse set of secondary metabolites found in plants. In addition to free ellagitannins, plants that have the ability to produce ellagitannins also have a variety of ellagitannin derivatives with different levels of structural complexity. These derivatives are formed by processes such as methylation, methoxylation, glycosylation, and glucuronidation of the ellagitannin molecule. The hydrolysable derivatives of ellagic acid (EA), known as ellagitannins, have the ability to release EA in a free form inside the human gastrointestinal system subsequent to the consumption of plant-based diets [67].

In recent years, there has been a significant increase in the interest surrounding EA, mostly owing to its notable antioxidant, anti-inflammatory, antimutagenic, and antiproliferative characteristics, as well as its potential therapeutic applications in the management of many human ailments. Multiple studies have provided evidence indicating that EA potentially has a role in the regulation of many cellular signaling pathways, hence potentially preventing, mitigating, or decelerating the advancement of chronic conditions such as cardiovascular and neurodegenerative illnesses, diabetes, and cancer. This chemical has shown neuroprotective, hepatoprotective, nephroprotective, cardioprotective, antifibrotic, antiatherosclerotic, antiallergic, antinociceptive, antiestrogenic, skin-protecting, wound-healing, osteogenic, antibacterial, antiviral, and antiparasitic properties. Furthermore, EA has shown a safeguarding impact against the harmful effects of metals and metalloids, organic xenobiotics, and natural poisons. Additionally, there is evidence supporting the beneficial therapeutic impact of combining EA with other antioxidants, such as selenium (in the form of selenomethionine), which is recognized for its diverse biological activity and potential for treatment [68].

Electrolyte (EA) is a thermostable compound characterized by a melting point of 350°C, a molecular weight of 302.19 g/mol, and limited solubility in water and alcohol. EA may be classified as 2,3,7,8-tetrahydroxy-chromeno [5,4,3-cde]chromene-5,10-dione from a chemical perspective. EA has the characteristics of an amphiphilic molecule. It is composed of a planar biphenyl lipophilic moiety connected by two lactone rings. Additionally, it contains four hydroxyl groups, which, when combined with lactone groups, provide a hydrophilic moiety. The presence of hydrogen bonding acceptor (lactone) and donor (–OH) sites in the hydrophilic portion of the EA molecule is crucial for its biological action. These sites consist of phenolic hydroxyl groups that may dissociate under physiological circumstances, resulting in the formation of negatively charged phenolate ions. Within the cellular structure of plants, ethylene (EA) exists in two distinct forms: free EA and covalently bound EA glycosides and ellagitannins. These forms exhibit varying chemical reactivity, solubility, and bioavailability. From diverse plant species, a wide range of ellagitannins and EA glycosides have been extracted and examined so far. Glycosides of the EA family consist of sugar residues, including glucose, arabinose, xylose, and rhamnose. Both ellagitannins and EA glycosides are biodegradable chemicals that have the ability to release EA via hydrolysis. This phenomenon may occur in plants as well as in the gastrointestinal system of humans and herbivore animals [69].

Edible plants that contain ellagic acid (EA) and its hydrolysable derivatives, particularly ellagitannins, are considered a good source of EA for humans. These plants are classified as functional foods that have the potential to boost health and perhaps lower the risk of illness. Numerous botanical species used in traditional medical practices across various regions, such as Traditional Chinese Medicine and Ayurveda, have been identified as possessing endocrine-acting (EA) and ellagitannins. The use of EA is now prevalent within the pharmaceutical and cosmetics sectors. As a result, researchers are now investigating different plant species to determine their ethylene glycol (EA) content. This research aims to identify new sources of EA for human nutrition, as well as potential raw materials for the development of functional nutritional supplements and nutraceuticals [70].

While ellagitannins and EA derivatives are abundant in plants, only a few plant species have been shown to have very high amounts of these phytochemicals. As a result, these plant species serve as abundant natural sources of EA in human diet. Specifically, fruits (particularly berries), nut kernels, and sometimes other plant components contain significant amounts of both ellagitannins and EA. Considering the level of conversion of ellagitannins to EA, the highest concentrations of EA are found in fruits of plants of the genus Rubus (raspberry, cloudberry, arctic bramble, blackberry, and boysenberry), strawberry (*Fragaria* × *ananassa* (Duchesne ex Weston) Duchesne ex Rozier), pomegranate, muscadine grape (*Vitis rotundifolia* Michx.), and tropical fruits such as camu-camu (*Myrciaria dubia* (Kunth) McVaugh); walnuts (*Juglans* spp.) and pecan (*Carya illinoinensis* (Wangenh.) K.Koch) have also relatively high EA content. The aforementioned plants serve as the primary sources of dietary EA in humans. Additional sources of ellagitannin (EA) in human nutrition include the juices, jams, and other processed goods derived from plants that contain ellagitannin, which are often found in the food business. Pomegranate juice (PJ) may have a total ellagic acid (EA) concentration of 811 mg/L or more, mostly because of the abundant ellagitannins found in P. granatum fruits. It is important to acknowledge that although initial research did not demonstrate the existence of EA in plants belonging to the Fabaceae family, recent findings indicate the presence of comparatively elevated concentrations of this phytochemical in various sprouted legumes, including sprouted adzuki bean (Vigna angularis), certain bean varieties (*Phaseolus vulgaris* L.), cowpea (*Vigna unguiculata* (L.) Walp.), pea (*Pisum sativum* L.), and soybean (*Glycine max* (L.) Merr.). The EA content of sprouted soybeans has been shown to be much greater compared to other sprouted legumes, with values ranging from 45.6 to 48.9 mg/100 g dry weight and 8.96 to 18.3 mg/100 g dry weight, respectively [71].

The distribution of free and bound forms of ethylene acetate (EA) in plant tissues exhibits significant variation among different plant species. Nevertheless, the fraction of unbound EA may also be influenced by the specific technique used for its detection. Some writers argue that free EA constitutes a very modest fraction of the overall EA pool in plants, whilst others propose that its proportion might potentially approach and surpass 50% of the entire content. It is noteworthy that among the fruits of *Terminalia ferdinandiana* Exell, a native Australian plant often referred to as the Kakadu plum, the predominant form of EA was seen to be free form, accounting for a significant proportion of 70.6% in the overall EA pool. In comparison, the research reveals that strawberries contain 7.4% of their total composition in the form of free EA [72].

Research has shown that the storage and freezing of fruits, together with their processing for the purpose of producing drinks and jams, might potentially provide varying impacts on the concentration of essential amino acids (EA). The concentration of EA in juices is notably elevated as a result of industrial processing of pomegranates for juice production. Conversely, juice derived from frozen fruits exhibits a twofold decrease in this chemical compared to juice derived from fresh fruits. The processing of raspberries for jam manufacturing and the preservation of raspberry jam resulted in significant increases in the content of EA, with a range of 2-3 times. The processing of strawberries for the purpose of jam making has been shown to result in a 20% reduction in the overall EA content. Certain tree species, such as Quercus spp., Eucalyptus spp., and Castanea spp., have a notably elevated EA content in both their wood and bark. Therefore, the by-products derived from the forestry and wood-processing sectors, together with the by-products generated from juice production such pomegranate husk, provide a promising avenue for industrial production in the field of EA [73].

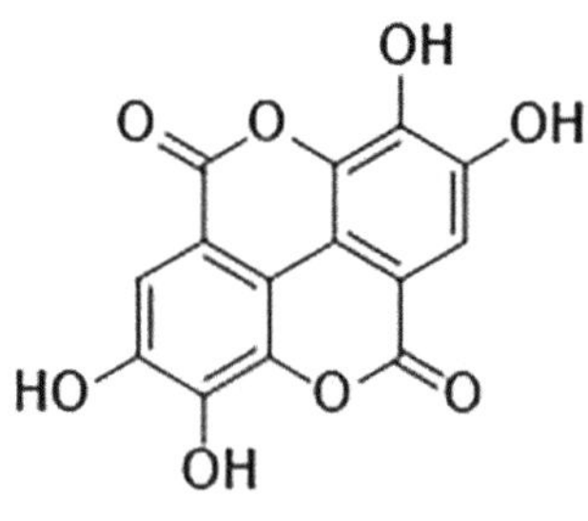

11.5.6 VITAMINS

Vitamins (Figure 11.7) are essential chemical substances that the body needs in minimal quantities. The inclusion of these nutrients in the diet is necessary since their synthesis inside the body is not feasible. Vitamins are needed for a multitude of bodily functions and for preserving the integrity of the skin, bones, nerves, eyes, brain, blood, and mucous membranes. They might be either soluble in water or soluble in fat. Vitamins A, D, E, and K exhibit solubility in fat, but vitamin C, along with the B-complex vitamins including thiamin (B1), riboflavin (B2), niacin (B3), pantothenic acid (B5), pyridoxine (B6), biotin (B7), folic acid (B9), and cyanocobalamin (B12), demonstrates solubility in water. Beta-carotene, a pro-vitamin, undergoes conversion into vitamin A inside the body. The body has the ability to retain fat-soluble vitamins, but water-soluble vitamins are not stored and are readily eliminated in urine. The B-complex vitamins and vitamin C exhibit heat lability, rendering them susceptible to degradation when exposed to heat, air, or subjected to drying, cooking, and food processing. Nutritional deficiencies manifest when an individual's consumption of essential nutrients continuously fails to meet the required threshold.

Nutritional deficiencies have the potential to give rise to a range of health problems; however, their occurrence may be mitigated through the adoption of a well-balanced diet or the consumption of a nutrient-dense diet that aligns with the body's requirements [74].

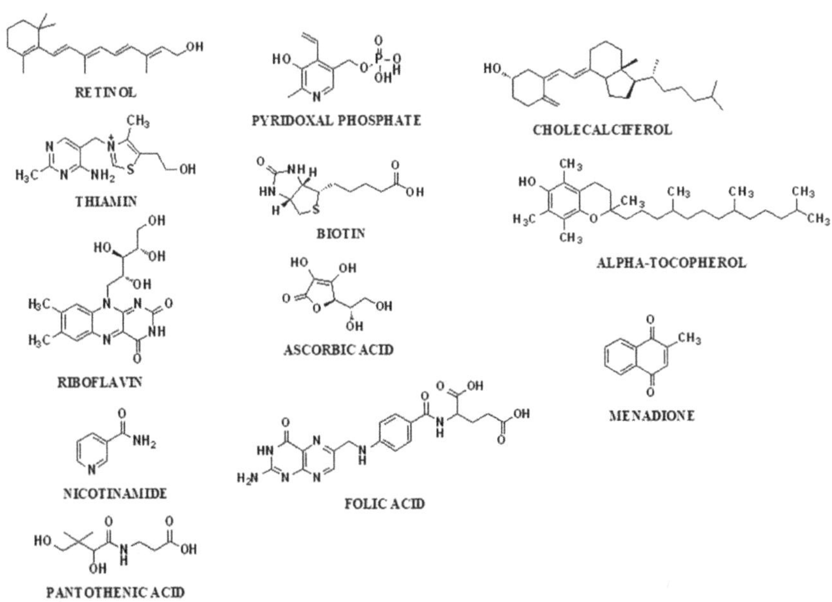

FIGURE 11.7 Structure of some important vitamins.

11.5.7 MISCELLANEOUS BIOACTIVE COMPOUNDS

11.5.7.1 ANDROGRAPHOLIDE

The diterpene lactone chemical known as Andrographolide is derived from the plant species *Andrographis paniculata* (Burm. F) Nees. *Andrographis paniculata* is often referred to by several names such as lanhelian, yijianxi, zhanshecao, kucao, kudancao, and others. Due to its origin in India, this product is sometimes referred to as Indian grass. The dry ground component of the *A. paniculata* plant, scientifically known as Conus, is believed to have its origins in South Asia. The cultivation of this crop is prevalent in several regions of China, including Fujian, Guangdong, Hainan, Guangxi, and Yunnan. Additionally, it has been brought to Australia and has also been introduced in Jiangsu and Shaanxi [75].

The use of *Andrographis paniculata* is prevalent within the realm of traditional Chinese medicine. The "Lingnan herbal medicine records" documented its efficacy in alleviating symptoms of "snake venom and internal injuries cough." According to "Quanzhou Materia Medica," the substance is characterized as possessing heat-clearing and detoxifying properties, as well as anti-inflammatory, detumescent, and inhibitory effects on throat irritation, diarrhea, and high fever. *A. paniculata*'s aboveground portion includes compounds such as andrographolide, neo-andrographolide, and 14-deoxygenated andrographolide, while its root mostly contains flavonoids. The crystalline material from *Andrographis paniculata* was first isolated by Gorter in 1911. Gorter subsequently characterized this substance as a diterpene lactone chemical and assigned it the name andrographolide. The structure of andrographolide is intricate and poses challenges in its artificial synthesis, hence necessitating its extraction from the plant. Andrographolide extraction encompasses several techniques, including water extraction, alcohol extraction, and other approaches. However, these procedures are plagued by challenges such as time-consuming and difficult operations, as well as the loss of active components. Therefore, modifications are necessary to address these concerns. In recent years, the extraction of andrographolide has seen the use of novel technological procedures, including enzymatic pretreatment, microwave-assisted extraction, and ultrasonic-assisted extraction. These advancements have yielded notable reductions in extraction time and enhancements in extraction efficiency [76].

The water solubility of andrographolide is limited, resulting in low bioavailability. Despite its wide pharmacological effects, these effects are rather modest, necessitating tight preparation conditions. Hence, since the 1970s, extensive efforts have been made by researchers in the field of drugs and organic chemistry to modify and transform andrographolide. These efforts primarily focus on various techniques such as Michael addition, redox reactions, selective esterification of hydroxyl groups, oxidation and substitution reactions, intramolecular cyclization, and replacement of lactone rings. A variety of novel derivatives were acquired. Pharmacological research primarily investigates the anticancer, antiviral, and other biological actions of andrographolide derivatives, and has achieved notable advancements in this area. The research on Andrographis has expanded to include both oral preparations of andrographolide and injectables of andrographolide derivative compounds, such as potassium dehydroandrographolide succinate and potassium sodium dehydroandrographolide succinate. These compounds have gained popularity and are now widely used drugs. For more information, refer to potassium dehydroandrographolide succinate and potassium sodium dehydroandrographolide succinate [77].

To date, there have been over 600 different procedures used for the creation of andrographis. The SFDA has authorized a total of 14 different types of andrographolide preparations, including 14 tablets, 2 capsules, and sodium nitrite andrographolide, 5 soft capsules, and one tablet. Recent pharmacological research has shown that andrographolide has anti-inflammatory, antibacterial, antiviral, anticancer, and immune-modulating properties. Consequently, it holds potential for therapeutic applications in the management of cardiovascular-cerebrovascular disorders, as well as the safeguarding of the liver and gallbladder. The antipyretic action of andrographolide in treating fever produced by pneumococcus and hemolytic Streptococcus mutans is mostly attributed to its inhibition of hypothalamic PGE2 and cAMP content. However, it is worth noting that the fundamental mechanism behind its anti-inflammatory activity may include the reduction of chemotaxis (fMLP) CD+11b and CD+18. *In vitro* studies have shown the antagonistic properties of andrographolide against Hong Kong virus (HKV), Ebola virus (EBOV), and respiratory syncytial virus (RSV). Additionally, it has been observed to have inhibitory effects on HIV, SARS, and viral myocarditis ST2 [78].

Furthermore, andrographolide has the potential to improve myocardial ischemia and provide protection against ischemia-reperfusion damage. Additionally, it has protective properties for vascular endothelial cells, regulates lipid disorders, reduces blood pressure, and exhibits anti-atherosclerosis effects. Additionally, it has the potential to inhibit angiogenesis during restenosis and enhance blood rheology. The primary mechanisms of action of this substance are attributed to its ability to scavenge free radicals and inhibit platelet aggregation. Andrographolide has been seen to enhance bile flow, bile salt levels, bile acid production, and deoxycholic acid levels in experimental rats and guinea pigs. Additionally, it has been found to counteract the decrease in bile and cholic acid secretions induced by paracetamol, hence promoting liver function improvement [79].

It is often used in therapeutic settings for the treatment of dysentery, leptospirosis, meningitis, pneumonia, upper respiratory tract infection, and the improvement of adrenal cortical function. Given the need for immediate treatment of clinical viral infections, it is crucial to incorporate the hydrophilic group into various lactone structures, increase its water solubility, and boost its effectiveness. Various types of andrographolide injections exist, such as the potassium dehydroandrograpolide succinate needle and the potassium sodium dehydroandrographolide succinate needle. Lianbizhi serves as the exemplar of this category of pharmaceuticals in contemporary therapeutic practice. Administering andrographolide orally might cause the occurrence of bitter vomiting. The ingestion of this product and other preparations in high quantities by oral administration may result in epigastric distress and a decrease in appetite. Instances of drug eruption, upper abdominal discomfort, and anaphylactic shock resulting from intramuscular injection have been documented. The patient had a pronounced symptomatic reaction, including chest tightness, dyspnea, pallor, lip bruising, cold sweats, weak pulse, and reduced blood pressure, among others. Common symptoms of light responses include stomach discomfort, vomiting, asthma, urticaria, acne, dizziness, cranial edema, sneezing, and chest pain, among others. The response occurs instantaneously and occurs within 5–20 minutes after injection. It progressively improves between 5–45 minutes after rescue, and the person recovers within 24 hours. Additionally, there have been documented instances of acute amniotic fluid obstruction resulting from the interchange of weaning lotion. Furthermore, considering the detrimental impact of andrographolide on reproduction, it is advisable for infertile couples and pregnant women to exercise caution while using it [80].

11.5.7.2 GLYCOLIPIDS

Glycolipids are a class of lipids characterized by the presence of a carbohydrate and a glycosidic (covalent) link. The primary function of these entities is to maintain the structural integrity of the cellular membrane and to promote the process of cellular recognition, which plays a pivotal role in the immune response and the establishment of intercellular connections that enable tissue formation. Glycolipids are ubiquitously present on the cellular membranes of all eukaryotic organisms, spanning from the phospholipid bilayer to the extracellular milieu. A glycolipid is characterized by the inclusion of a monosaccharide or oligosaccharide that is attached to a lipid molecule. Glycerolipids and sphingolipids are the predominant lipids found in cellular membranes, characterized by the presence of glycerol or sphingosine backbones, respectively. The fatty acids are linked to this structural framework, resulting in a lipid with a polar head and a non-polar tail. The cell membrane is composed of a lipid bilayer, which is divided into two layers of lipids. The inner and outer surfaces of the membrane are composed of polar head groups, while the interior half of the membrane is composed of non-polar fatty acid tails.

The ligand components of glycolipids are the saccharides connected to the polar head groups on the exterior of the cell. These saccharides are also polar, which enables them to dissolve in the aqueous environment surrounding the cell. A glycoconjugate is formed between the lipid and the saccharide via a glycosidic link, which is a kind of covalent bond. A free hydroxyl group on the lipid backbone is bound by the anomeric carbon of the sugar. The configuration of these saccharides varies depending on the configuration of the molecules to which they are attached [81].

Glycolipids primarily operate as recognition sites for intercellular interactions throughout the body. The glycolipid's saccharide has the ability to form a complex with either a complementary carbohydrate or a lectin, which is a protein that binds to carbohydrates, in a nearby cell. The identification of cell surface markers serves as the foundation for cell interactions, triggering cellular responses that play a role in several processes including regulation, proliferation, and death. One instance illustrating the role of glycolipids in physiological processes is the interplay between leukocytes and endothelial cells in the context of inflammation. The immune response is initiated by selectins, which are a kind of lectins that are present on the surface of leukocytes and endothelial cells.

These selectins bind to the carbohydrates that are connected to glycolipids. This interaction induces the migration of leukocytes from the bloodstream and their accumulation in close proximity to the site of inflammation. This is the first process of binding, which is then followed by the activation of integrins that establish more robust connections and enable leukocytes to move towards the location of inflammation. Additionally, glycolipids have a role in several reactions, including in the identification of host cells by viruses. Glycolipids on cell membranes facilitate cell interactions with the surrounding environment, as shown by blood types. The classification of human blood types into four primary categories (A, B, AB, O) is based on the presence of an oligosaccharide that is linked to a certain glycolipid on the outer layer of red blood cells, serving as an antigen. The H antigen, which remains unaltered, serves as the distinguishing feature of type O and is found on erythrocytes across all blood types. The key defining structure of blood type A is N-acetylgalactosamine, whereas type B contains galactose. Type AB has all three of these antigens. The absence of antigens in an individual's bloodstream triggers the production of antibodies, which subsequently attach to the alien glycolipids. Due to this rationale, individuals with blood type AB have the capacity to undergo transfusions from all blood types, often referred to as the universal acceptor. Conversely, those with blood type O may serve as donors for all blood types, also known as the universal donor [82].

11.5.7.3 GUGULIPIDS

The gum resin known as guggul is derived from a diverse range of plant species indigenous to India, Bangladesh, and Pakistan. Several notable species may be identified, including *Commiphora wightii*, *Commiphora gileadensis*, *Commiphora mukul*, *Boswellia serrata*, and *Boswellia sacra*. Every species belongs to the *Burseraceae* family, which is often referred to as the incense family. The extraction of guggul sap, known by several names such as guggul, gum guggul, guggula, or gugulipid, is conducted in a manner similar to the extraction of maple syrup from maple trees. For ages, guggul has been used in Ayurvedic medicine, a comprehensive medicinal system developed from plants, to address a range of health ailments, including obesity, arthritis, and inflammation. Guggul is composed of a diverse array of botanical constituents, including steroids, essential oils, lignans, flavonoids, carbohydrates, and amino acids. These constituents all contribute to the many health benefits associated with guggul. Alleged to possess anti-inflammatory and antioxidant characteristics, this substance has been used in traditional medicinal practices to safeguard against a diverse range of ailments [83].

The anti-inflammatory qualities of guggul have garnered recognition. Initial investigations indicate that it might potentially aid in the treatment of certain anti-inflammatory ailments, including acne, eczema, psoriasis, and arthritis. Additionally, it has been used for the purpose of facilitating weight reduction, addressing hypothyroidism, and regulating cholesterol and blood glucose levels. Guggul has undergone research to assess its efficacy in treating acne. Research has shown the efficacy of this therapy in both complementary and alternative therapies for nodulocystic acne, a very severe manifestation of acne that mostly affects the facial, chest, and back regions. A study conducted on a sample of 21 individuals revealed that the oral administration of 25 mg of guggulsterone had comparable efficacy to tetracycline, a frequently used antibiotic for the treatment of acne. In addition, those with conspicuously oily skin had a considerably more favorable response to guggulsterone compared to the tetracycline therapy. A previous study showed that oral administration of guggul for a duration of 6 weeks effectively alleviated acne symptoms without inducing significant negative consequences [84].

Eczema and psoriasis are noncommunicable dermatological disorders mostly resulting from skin inflammation. The majority of studies on the efficacy of guggul in treating various skin irritations have focused on the impact of guggul derived from the *Boswellia serrata* plant. Studies have shown that lotions containing guggul can effectively alleviate symptoms of itching, redness, skin pigmentation, and inflammation in those suffering from psoriasis and eczema. Additionally, a recent study revealed that a cream containing guggul effectively addressed skin responses that arose as a consequence of radiation treatments for breast cancer. The study revealed that the cream containing guggul showed enhancements in skin symptoms, including redness, inflammation, soreness, and discomfort. Additionally, it decreased the need for topical steroid creams in the therapy process. Thyroid diseases are prevalent, particularly among females [85].

Hypothyroidism is a medical disorder characterized by insufficient production of thyroid hormones by the thyroid gland, resulting in impaired bodily functioning. Animal studies, including those that are outdated, indicate that guggul extracts enhance hypothyroidism by augmenting iodine absorption and enhancing the functionality of thyroid gland enzymes. A human study was conducted to examine the efficacy of *Triphladya Guggulu* tablets and a *Punarnavadi Kashayam* decoction in the treatment of hypothyroidism. The findings demonstrated that this intervention had a substantial positive impact on the manifestations and indications linked to hypothyroidism, including debility, exhaustion, and myalgia.

Guggul is often said to aid in the treatment of obesity by facilitating fat reduction and inhibiting appetite. Nevertheless, there is a scarcity of reliable data to substantiate its use for this objective. A test-tube study indicates that guggul may facilitate weight reduction by stimulating the catabolism of fat, hence decreasing the quantity of adipose tissue. A further study conducted on rats revealed that guggul had beneficial effects on the hormones responsible for controlling hunger, namely ghrelin and leptin. Nevertheless, the applicability of these effects to human beings remains uncertain. A previous study conducted on a sample of 58 individuals with obesity observed that the administration of guggul resulted in an average weight reduction of 5 pounds (2.25 kg) compared to the group that did not receive any treatment. Further research has shown that the use of herbal supplements with guggul extract may potentially contribute to the management of obesity via the facilitation of weight reduction and the mitigation of skinfold thickness and body circumference. While the findings of these studies are encouraging, they do not directly investigate the impact of guggul on weight reduction. Guggul is well recognized as a prevalent natural remedy for hyperlipidemia, a medical condition characterized by elevated levels of cholesterol and TG. Animal studies suggest that guggul may have a beneficial effect in lowering triglyceride, TC, and LDL cholesterol levels. Nevertheless, the impact of guggul on concentrations of cholesterol and TG in the human population remains uncertain. While several studies have shown that guggul has cholesterol-lowering properties, other research indicates a lack of substantial advantages. Indeed, guggul has the potential to elevate LDL cholesterol levels in individuals diagnosed with hypercholesterolemia; however, the substantiating data remains outdated [86].

Preliminary investigations indicate that guggul has the potential to mitigate symptoms often linked with osteoarthritis. A previous study involving 30 individuals with knee osteoarthritis who received guggul treatment demonstrated enhancements in knee pain and knee swelling, along with heightened knee flexion. In addition, those who received guggul treatment had an increase in their walking distance.

11.5.7.4 WITHANOLIDES

Withanolides, scientifically known as *Withania somnifera* (L.) Dunal or Ashwagandha, belongs to the Solanaceae family and is a prominent therapeutic plant in Ayurveda, the comprehensive system of Indian medicine. C-28 steroidal lactones are the primary bioactive constituents, which are a collection of secondary metabolites known as withanolides. Withaferin A, a steroidal lactone, was originally extracted from *W. somnifera* (winter cherry) in 1965, making it the first ever withanolide to be identified. Withanolides are a group of tiny compounds that are often present in the Solanaceae family. The Solanaceae plant has been historically used for the treatment of several health conditions, including asthma, parasite illnesses, constipation, edema, glaucoma, headache, hepatopathy, anti-inflammatory effects, postpartum discomfort, and skin problems. Over the course of the previous decade, there has been a significant acceleration in the research pace of compounds within the solanaceae family due to the rapid advancement and utilization of diverse separation techniques and spectral analysis methods, particularly nuclear magnetic resonance spectroscopy. Consequently, substantial progress has been made in the field of structural research pertaining to these compounds. To far, a total of over 900 distinct varieties of withanolides have been identified globally. Numerous studies have shown the anti-inflammatory and cytotoxic properties of withanolides in recent times. This compound primarily targets the NF-κB and STAT3 signaling pathways in its pharmacological actions. Numerous physiological processes, including as cellular proliferation, development, differentiation, immunity, apoptosis, inflammation, and metabolism, are regulated by NF-κB. The dysregulation of growth and survival, promotion of angiogenesis, migration, and invasion of tumor cells, and induction of tumorimmune tolerance are seen as a result of abnormal STAT3 activation. The crucial function in regulating the communication between cancer cells and inflammatory cells is attributed to the activation and interaction between STAT3 and NF-κB. Furthermore, the synergistic effects of TNF-α in conjunction with withanolides have been shown to augment its anti-cancer properties. Given that the etiology of cancer and psoriasis has similarities in terms of cell proliferation, inflammation, angiogenesis, and associated signaling pathways, it is plausible to explore the potential of withanolides in the treatment of psoriasis, arthritis, cancer, and other autoimmune illnesses [87].

It has a significant amount of pharmaceutically active triterpenoids called withanolides, which are steroidal lactones. It has a broad global distribution and mostly thrives in xeric and arid locations within tropical and subtropical areas. These regions include a wide range, including the Canary Islands, the Mediterranean region, Northern Africa, and Southwest Asia. In the distant past, the Solanaceae plant Flos Datura, together with Buddhism, was brought from India to China and subsequently spread extensively over the southern and northern regions of the nation. Li Shizhen, a prominent Chinese medical expert during the Ming Dynasty, meticulously documented the effectiveness and properties of the Flos Datura in the Compendium of Materia Medica. Additionally, he conducted personal experiments to evaluate the medicinal properties of this plant. A group of Chinese scholars identified a total of nine novel withanolides with anti-inflammatory properties in the leaves of Flos Daturae. Although several anticancer medications have been developed, the worldwide prevalence of different types of malignancies, as well as their associated death rates, continues to increase. It is estimated that the number of fatalities caused by cancer will grow by a factor of two in the next 50 years. Various types of solanol lactones exhibit variations in their anticancer action and target, although their shared pharmacological property is their ability to combat cancer. NF-κB is a typical signaling pathway involved in the development of tumors. The control of cell survival mediated by mitochondrial fission was shown to entail an interaction between the TP53 and NF-κB pathways. Due to recent advancements in the field of molecular biology, researchers have started the process of elucidating crucial oncogenic pathways involved in the development of cancer. This has paved the way for a new age of chemotherapy, whereby it becomes feasible to propose targeted therapies for cancer. Multiple studies have consistently shown that many types of cancer exhibit abnormal or increased levels of intermediate filaments, including keratin (type I or II), nestin (type VI), and vimentin (type III). The cytoskeletal components known as type III Intermediate Filaments (IFs) play a crucial function in mechanosignal transmission and are of utmost importance in the process of tissue healing.

While there is currently no known antineoplastic medication that directly targets abnormal amounts of keratin or nestin in cancerous cells, withanolides have shown potential as a powerful inhibitor of type III intermediate filaments [88].

Withaferin A has shown strong inhibitory effects on several proteins, including vimentin and other type III intermediate filaments. Furthermore, withaferin A has shown a consistent ability to impede angiogenesis by suppressing the NF-κB signaling pathway, in addition to its affinity for intermediate filaments. In addition to its ability to suppress estrogen receptor-α expression in human breast cancer cells, withaferin A has been reported to inhibit the STAT3 signaling pathway. Furthermore, in the treatment of ovariectomized osteoporosis models, withaferin A has been found to promote bone formation by inhibiting the NF-κB pathway. These findings suggest a potential role for both withaferin A and estrogen in this context. By directly reducing neoplastic development, Withaferin A exhibits antineoplastic efficacy in a wide range of cancer cell lines, such as head and neck carcinomas, ovaries, thyroid carcinomas, glioblastoma multiforme, and melanoma [89].

Due to its strong ability to prevent blood vessels from forming new blood vessels, withaferin A has shown significant combined effects with the multikinase inhibitor sorafenib. This suggests that withaferin A could be a useful addition to treatment for renal cell carcinomas and other cancers that are particularly affected by the prevention of new blood vessel formation. It is important to acknowledge that other closely related congeners, such as withaferin A and withalongolide A (a 19-hydroxy derivative of withaferin A), have the potential to impact signaling pathways mediated by the PI3K/AKT/mTOR pathway. These congeners inhibit the phosphorylation of RET and Akt, as well as the expression of proteins. They also limit the activity of mTOR, the translational activity of 4EBP1, and protein synthesis facilitated by p70S6 kinase activation in neoplastic cells, including patient-derived medullary thyroid carcinoma cells and human and murine glioblastoma cells in laboratory settings. The findings presented suggest the existence of a possible synergistic association between withanolides and mTOR inhibitors that are being used in clinical practice. Consequently, more preclinical research is justified. According to traditional Chinese medicine, Physalin A, a bioactive withanolide obtained from *Physalis alkekengi*, has anti-tumor properties in non-small cell lung cancer cell lines via the inhibition of JAK/STAT3 signaling.

According to reports, withaferin A has the ability to directly disrupt the two-dimer structure of NF-κB, hence impeding the DNA-binding activity. Additionally, it inhibits the development of the NEMO/IKKβ association complex and directly targets the catalytic kinase activity of IKKβ. The findings indicate that the extract derived from *Withania somnifera* leaves has the ability to hinder the activation and migration of microglia. This implies that it might be a promising therapeutic option for mitigating neuroinflammation in the management of neurodegenerative disorders. An extract of *W. somnifera* was evaluated and shown to have the ability to decrease the activity of NF-κB P65–luciferase reporter in microglial cultured BV2 cells in a dose-dependent manner. The aqueous extract of *W. somnifera* decreases the activity of NF-κB generated by LPS in DI TNC1 astrocytes. Withaferin A exhibits potential as a viable therapeutic option for addressing neuroinflammatory and stress-related disorders that are distinguished by a significant astrocytic contribution. The first function of withanolides may include the inhibition of mitochondrial oxidative stress [90].

11.5.7.5 VASICINE

It is mostly derived from the plant *Adhatoda vasica* (AV) (zeylanica)/ *Justicia adhatoda* (Acanthaceae) and is classified as a quinazoline alkaloid. Several key chemical elements of this plant include vasicine (Figure 11.8), which is formed from leaves, 2'-hydroxy-4-glucosyloxychalcone, vasicol, vasicinone, vasicinol, and deoxyvasicinone, which are found in the leaves, stem, and roots, respectively. Sen and Ghose first isolated it in 1924. Various morphotypes of this particular plant species may be seen in natural environments. These species are categorized into several categories and may be identified using fingerprint profiles and vasicine content. The geographical distribution of *Adhatoda vasica* includes tropical areas in Southeast Asia, notably India. The plant's pharmacological effects have been recognized since ancient times. Vasicine is widely recognized as the primary and most significant active compound found in this medicinal plant. The majority of its properties, including antioxidant, anti-inflammatory, and bronchodilatory activity, are attributed to it. In its native state, this molecule exhibits optical activity; however, upon extraction, it undergoes racemization. Despite its long-standing recognition and widespread usage in herbal formulations for respiratory disorders and female reproductive system-related ailments, there is a scarcity of evidence on its molecular mode of action.

Researchers have conducted research on the pollination biology of the plant, recognizing its therapeutic significance. Numerous investigations have been conducted to elucidate various techniques used in the extraction of vasicine from the plant AV. The establishment of HPLC determination of vasicine using a photodiode (PD) detector is currently lacking. A C18 column with a pH of 3.9 and a buffer consisting of acetonitrile, phosphate, and acetic acid in a ratio of 15:85:1, v/v/v, may be used for the separation of vasicinone and vasicine. Investigators conducted a comparative analysis of several techniques for extracting vasicine. These techniques included the traditional approach, where crushed leaves are heated using moist heat and then squeezed to get the extract. Another modernized method included exposing the leaves to steam at a pressure of 15 pounds. The alkaloid content exhibited a range of 0.3 mg/ml to 5.93 mg/ml, whereas the vasicine concentration ranged from 0.2 mg/ml to 5.64 mg/ml across several methodologies. Global Application: In 2003, a technique for the synthesis of vasicine was released under the Patent Cooperation Treaty (PCT) [91].

While AV serves as the primary means of acquiring vasicine, several botanical species have also been investigated with the purpose of isolating this particular compound. Scientists successfully isolated vasicine from *Sida cordifolia*, a distinct plant species. The isolation of vasicine from two species of *Afrogalega*, namely *Galega battiscombei* (Bak.f) Gillett and *Galega lindblomi* (Harms) Gillett, was conducted. In a study, investigators documented the separation of vasicine from *A. beddomei* and conducted a comparative analysis of its content with that of *Adhatoda zeylanica/vasica.* According to their findings, *Adhatoda zeylanica/vasica* exhibited significant seasonal fluctuations throughout the course of the year. The variability of vasicine was shown to range from 1.22% to 2.57% on a biannual basis. Researchers extracted peganine/vasicine hydrochloride from dehydrated *Peganum harmala* seeds.

In their study, the safety of vasicine was investigated in 24 human volunteers. They administered a dose of 0.5–16 mg of vasicine intravenously in 500 mL of saline over a period of 3 hours. The aim was to assess acute human toxicity, tolerance, pharmacological effects, adverse effects, and establish a safe dosage range. According to clinical observations, hematological and biochemical investigations, as well as kidney and liver function tests conducted before, during, and after vasicine treatment, a maximum dose of 16 mg of vasicine was administered to hospital inpatients between the 2nd and 8th day of normal puerperium. The results indicated that vasicine was well tolerated and did not exhibit any adverse effects. Nevertheless, the uterus exhibited firmness and contraction after vasicine administration, demonstrating its efficacy as an oxytocic agent, as previously mentioned, and its abortifacient properties. The chronic toxicity research of AV was undertaken in rats (at doses of 2.5 mg/kg, 5 mg/kg, and 10 mg/kg, representing low doses with 2x ED50, and medium doses with 4x ED50 and 8x ED50, respectively) and monkeys (at doses of 5, 10, and 20 mg/kg, as per the aforementioned criteria) over a period of 6 months. According to their study, there has been no change in the death rate and body weight. No abnormalities were detected during the autopsy and histological evaluation of the main organs.

Only a limited number of precise chemical pathways underlying the function of the vasicine molecule have been documented so far. The primary attribute attributed to the physiological benefits of the plant AV and its constituents is believed to be their antioxidant nature. It was proposed that vasicine exerts its bronchodilatory effects by targeting both respiratory sensors and peripheral receptors. If a cardio-depressant impact occurs, it is recommended to widen the blood vessels in the local area in order to lower blood pressure. Two primary mechanisms have been proposed for its anti-diabetic properties: firstly, it inhibits glucosidase activity, and secondly, it affects glycoprotein metabolism and release in blood plasma and urine, hence regulating blood sugar levels [92].

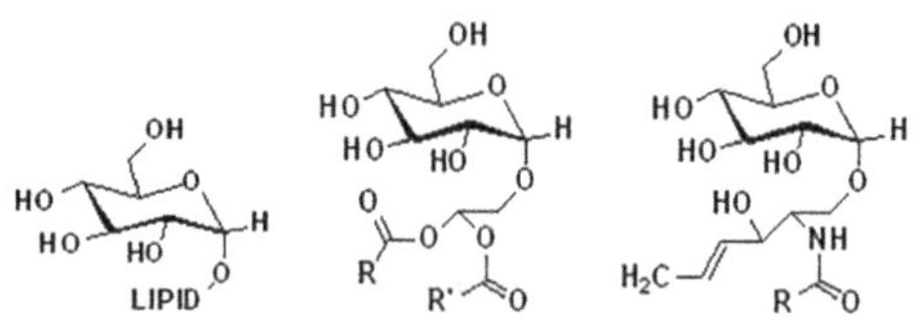

GLYCOLIPIDGLYCERO-GLYCOLIPID SPHINGO-GLYCOLIPID

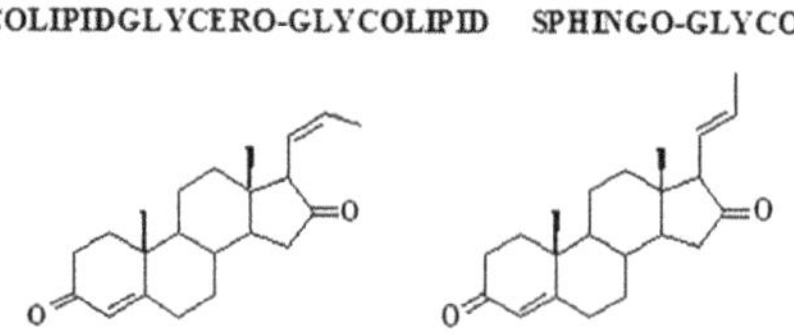

Z-GUGGULSTERONE *E*-GUGGULSTERONE

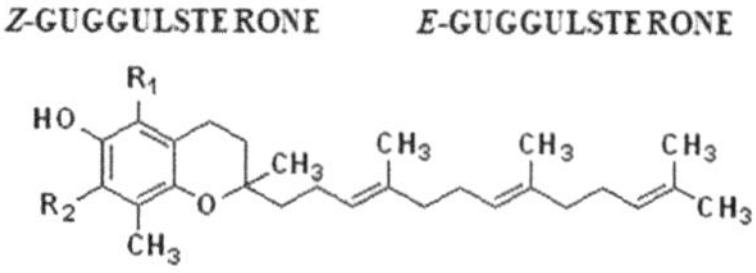

TOCOTRIENOLS

$\alpha = R_1 = CH_3, R_2 = CH_3; \beta = R_1 = CH_3, R_2 = H; \gamma = R_1 = H, R_2 = CH_3; \delta = R_1 = H, R_2 = H$

(Continued)

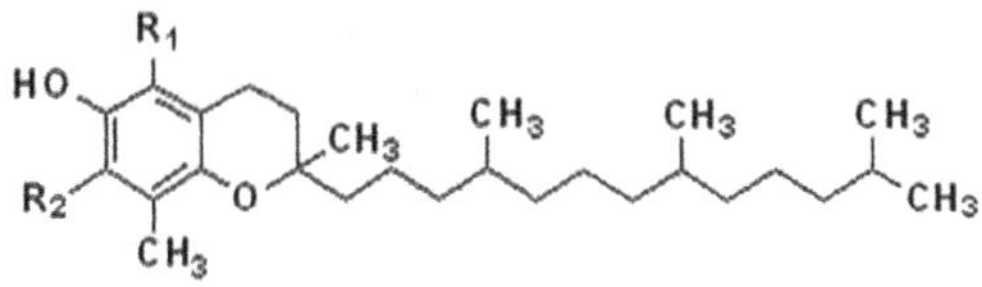

TOCOPHEROLS

$\alpha = R_1 = CH_3, R_2 = CH_3; \beta = R_1 = CH_3, R_2 = H; \gamma = R_1 = H, R_2 = CH_3; \delta = R_1 = H, R_2 = H$

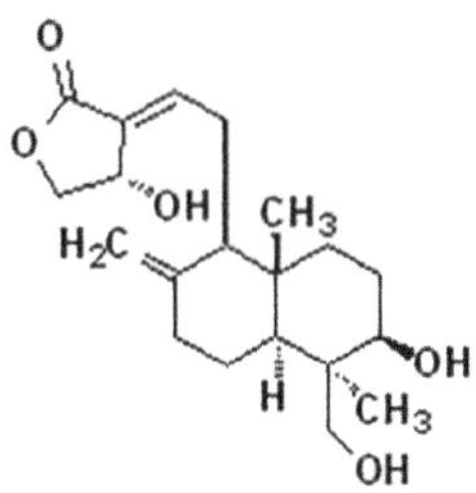

ANDROGRAPHOLIDE

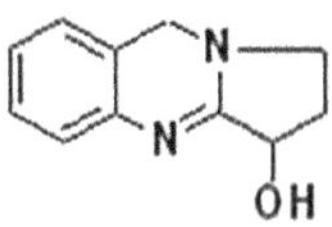

VASICINE

FIGURE 11.8 Structure of bioactive compounds.

11.6 CONCLUSION

Throughout history, natural remedies have been employed by nearly all documented human societies as efficacious treatments for a wide range of health ailments, including but not limited to eczema, wounds, skin infections, swelling, aging, mental disorders, cancer, asthma, diabetes, jaundice, scabies, venereal diseases, snakebite, gastric ulcers, and various other conditions. This is mostly due to the prevailing notion that herbal medications are devoid of any adverse effects, inexpensive, and readily accessible in the local area. Due to the growing demand, policymakers, health experts, and the general public are becoming more concerned about the safety, standardization, effectiveness, quality, availability, and marketing of herbal products. Herbal medications, similar to conventional pharmacological treatment, are subject to less stringent regulation in several nations, including the United States. Moreover, the phenomenon of globalization has significantly enhanced the availability of herbal medications to consumers worldwide, regardless of their geographical location. It is evident that there exists a pressing need for collaborative endeavors aimed at conducting the requisite clinical studies to investigate the effectiveness and safety of herbal medications. Numerous scholars are now examining herbal medicines in relation to their therapeutic applications as recorded in ancient texts from Ayurveda, Unani, TCM, and other traditions. The assessment and validation of herbal medicinal usage in accordance with contemporary drug standards have been facilitated by the recent use of advanced analytical methods and research approaches.

KEYWORDS

- **drugs**
- **future trends**
- **herbal**
- **natural products**
- **phytochemicals**
- **phytoconstituents**

REFERENCES

1. Prakash, O., Usmani, S., Singh, R., Mahapatra, D. K., & Gupta, A. (2019). Cancer chemotherapy by novel bio-active natural products: Looking towards the future. *Current Cancer Therapy Reviews, 15*(1), 37-49.
2. Mahapatra, D. K., Bharti, S. K., & Asati, V. (2015). Anti-cancer chalcones: Structural and molecular target perspectives. *European Journal of Medicinal Chemistry, 98*, 69–114.
3. Hardeland, R. (2016). Melatonin in plants – Diversity of levels and multiplicity of functions. *Frontiers in Plant Science, 7*, 1–14.
4. Meng, X., Li, Y., Li, S., et al. (2017). Dietary sources and bioactivities of melatonin. *Nutrients, 9*(4), 1–64.
5. Chuffa, L. G. A., Reiter, R. J., & Lupi, L. A. (2017). Melatonin as a promising agent to treat ovarian cancer: Molecular mechanisms. *Carcinogenesis, 38*, 945–952.
6. Chuffa, L. G. A., Alves, M. S., Martinez, M., et al. (2016). Apoptosis is triggered by melatonin in an *in-vivo* model of ovarian carcinoma. *Endocrine-Related Cancer, 23*, 65–76.
7. Colombo, J., Jardim, P. B. V., Ferreira, J. P. S., et al. (2018). Melatonin differentially modulates NF-KB expression in breast and liver cancer cells. *Anticancer Agents in*

Medicinal Chemistry, 18(12), 1688–1694. https://doi.org/10.2174/1871520618666180131112304.

8. Torre, L. A., Bray, F., Siegel, R. L., et al. (2015). Global cancer statistics, 2012. *CA: A Cancer Journal for Clinicians, 65*, 87–108.
9. Prakash, O., Amit, K., Pawan, K., et al. (2013). Anticancer potential of plants and natural products: A review. *American Journal of Pharmaceutical Sciences, 1*(6), 104–115.
10. Asati, V., Mahapatra, D. K., & Bharti, S. K. (2016). PI3K/Akt/mTOR and Ras/Raf/MEK/ERK signaling pathways inhibitors as anticancer agents: Structural and pharmacological perspectives. *European Journal of Medicinal Chemistry, 109*, 314–341.
11. Donaldron, M. S. (2004). Nutrition and cancer – A review of the evidence for an anticancer diet. *Nutrition Journal, 3*, 1–21.
12. Riboli, E., & Norat, T. (2003). Epidemiological evidence of the protective effect of fruit and vegetables on cancer risk. *American Journal of Clinical Nutrition, 78*(3), 559–569.
13. Nichenametla, S. N., Taruscio, T. G., Barney, D. L., et al. (2006). A review of the effects and mechanisms of polyphenolics in cancer. *Critical Reviews in Food Science and Nutrition, 46*, 161–183.
14. Nirmala, M. J., Samundeeswari, A., & Sankar, P. D. (2011). Natural plant resources in anti-cancer therapy – A review. *Research in Plant Biology, 1*(3), 1–14.
15. Paller, C. J., Samuel, R., et al. (2016). Challenges of conducting clinical trials of natural products to combat cancer. *Clinical Advances in Hematology & Oncology, 14*(6), 447–455.
16. Newman, D. J., & Cragg, G. M. (2012). Natural products as sources of new drugs over the 30 years from 1981 to 2010. *Journal of Natural Products, 75*(3), 311–335.
17. Amin, A. R., Kucuk, O., Khuri, F. R., et al. (2009). Perspectives for cancer prevention with natural compounds. *Journal of Clinical Oncology, 27*, 2712–2725.
18. Ishikawa, H., Saeki, T., Otani, T., et al. (2006). Aged garlic extract prevents a decline of NK cell number and activity in patients with advanced cancer. *Journal of Nutrition, 136*, 816S–820S.
19. Tanaka, S., Haruma, K., Yoshihara, M., et al. (2006). Aged garlic extract has potential suppressive effects on colorectal adenomas in humans. *Journal of Nutrition, 136*, 821S–826S.
20. Natelson, E. A., Giovanella, B. C., Verschraegen, C. F., et al. (1996). Phase I clinical and pharmacological studies of 20-(S)-camptothecin and 20-(S)-9-nitrocamptothecin as anticancer agents. *Annals of the New York Academy of Sciences, 803*, 224–230.
21. Verschraegen, C. F., Gilbert, B. E., Loyer, E., et al. (2004). Clinical evaluation of the delivery and safety of aerosolized liposomal 9-nitro-20(S)-camptothecin in patients with advanced pulmonary malignancies. *Clinical Cancer Research, 10*, 2319–2326.
22. Shimada, Y., Yoshino, M., Wakui, A., et al. (1993). Phase II study of CPT-11, a new camptothecin derivative, in metastatic colorectal cancer CPT-11 gastrointestinal cancer study group. *Journal of Clinical Oncology, 11*, 909–913.
23. Cheng, A. L., Hsu, C. H., Lin, J. K., et al. (2001). Phase I clinical trial of curcumin, a chemo-preventive agent, in patients with high-risk or pre-malignant lesions. *Anticancer Research, 21*, 2895–2900.

24. Dhillon, N., Aggarwal, B. B., Newman, R. A., et al. (2008). Phase II trial of curcumin in patients with advanced pancreatic cancer. *Clinical Cancer Research, 14*, 4491–4499.
25. Bettuzzi, S., Brausi, M., Rizzi, F., et al. (2006). Chemoprevention of human prostate cancer by oral administration of green tea catechins in volunteers with high-grade prostate intraepithelial neoplasia: A preliminary report from a one-year proof-of-principle study. *Cancer Research, 66*, 1234–1240.
26. Jian, L., Xie, L. P., Lee, A. H., et al. (2004). Protective effect of green tea against prostate cancer: A case-control study in Southeast China. *International Journal of Cancer, 108*, 130–135.
27. Gao, Y. T., McLaughlin, J. K., Blot, W. J., et al. (1994). Reduced risk of esophageal cancer associated with green tea consumption. *Journal of the National Cancer Institute, 86*, 855–858.
28. Ji, B. T., Chow, W. H., & Hsing, A. W. (1997). Green tea consumption and the risk of pancreatic and colorectal cancers. *International Journal of Cancer, 27*, 255–258.
29. Choan, E., Segal, R., Jonker, D., et al. (2005). A prospective clinical trial of green tea for hormone refractory prostate cancer: An evaluation of the complementary/alternative therapy approach. *Urologic Oncology, 23*, 108–113.
30. Kim, J. H., & Park, C. Y. (2006). Effects of Sun Ginseng on subjective quality of life in cancer patients: A double-blind, placebo-controlled pilot trial. *Journal of Clinical Pharmacy and Therapeutics, 31*, 331–334.
31. Suh, S. O., Kroh, M., Kim, N. R., et al. (2002). Effects of red ginseng upon postoperative immunity and survival in patients with stage III gastric cancer. *American Journal of Chinese Medicine, 30*, 483–494.
32. Cragg, G. M., & Newman, D. J. (2005). Plants as a source of anti-cancer agents. *Journal of Ethnopharmacology, 100*, 72–79.
33. Okouneva, T., Hill, B. T., Wilson, L., et al. (2003). The effects of vinflunine, vinorelbine, and vinblastine on centromere dynamics. *Molecular Cancer Therapeutics, 2*, 427–436.
34. Simoens, C., Lardon, F., Pauwels, B., et al. (2008). Comparative study of the radiosensitising and cell cycle effects of vinflunine and vinorelbine *in vitro*. *BMC Cancer, 8*(65), 1–12.
35. Shoeb, M., MacManus, S. M., Jaspars, M., et al. (2006). Montamine, a unique dimeric indole alkaloid from the seeds of *Centaurea montana* (Asteraceae), and its *in vitro* cytotoxic activity against the $CaCo_2$ colon cancer cells. *Tetrahedron, 62*, 11172–11177.
36. Lee, K. H., & Xiao, Z. (2005). Podophyllotoxins and analogs. In G. M. Cragg, D. G. I. Kingston, & D. J. Newman (Eds.), *Anticancer Agents from Natural Products* (p. 71). Boca Raton, FL: Taylor & Francis Group.
37. Kingston, D. G. I. (2007). The shape of things to come: Structural and synthetic studies of Taxol and related compounds. *Phytochemistry, 68*(14), 1844–1854.
38. Hait, W. N., Rubin, E., Alli, E., et al. (2007). Tubulin targeting agents. *Update on Cancer Therapeutics, 2*, 1–18.
39. Srivastava, V., Negi, A. S., Kumar, J. K., et al. (2005). Plant-based anticancer molecules: A chemical and biological profile of some important leads. *Bioorganic & Medicinal Chemistry, 13*, 5892–5898.

40. Creemers, G. J., Bolis, G., Gore, M., et al. (1996). Topotecan, an active drug in the second-line treatment of epithelial ovarian cancer: Results of a large European phase II study. *Journal of Clinical Oncology, 14*, 3056–3061.
41. Fuchs, C., Mitchell, E. P., & Hoff, P. M. (2006). Irinotecan in the treatment of colorectal cancer. *Cancer Treatment Reviews, 32*, 491–493.
42. Mineko, I., Michio, I., Ikuo, M., et al. (2000). Growth inhibitory effect of a new camptothecin analog, DX-8951f, on various drug-resistant sublines including BCRP-mediated camptothecin derivative-resistant variants derived from the human lung cancer cell line PC-6. *Anti-Cancer Drugs, 11*, 353–362.
43. Reichardt, P., Nielsen, O. S., Bauer, S., et al. (2007). Exatecan in pretreated adult patients with advanced soft tissue sarcoma: Results of a phase II study of the EORTC soft tissue and bone sarcoma group. *European Journal of Cancer, 43*, 1017–1022.
44. Zhang, J. A., Xuan, T., Parmar, M., et al. (2004). Development and characterization of a novel liposome-based formulation of SN-38. *International Journal of Pharmaceutics, 270*, 93–107.
45. Cao, Z., Kozielski, A., Liu, X., et al. (2009). Crystalline camptothecin-20(s)-opropionate hydrate: A novel anticancer agent with strong activity against 19 human tumor xenografts. *Cancer Research, 69*, 4742–4749.
46. Xie, J., Ma, T., Gu, Y., et al. (2009). Berbamine derivatives: A novel class of compounds for anti-leukemia activity. *European Journal of Medicinal Chemistry, 44*, 3293–3298.
47. Xu, R., Dong, Q., Yu, Y., et al. (2006). Berbamine: A novel inhibitor of bcr/abl fusion gene with potent anti-leukemia activity. *Leukemia Research, 30*, 17–23.
48. Wang, F., Gao, Y., Gao, L., et al. (2011). Study on the electrochemical behavior of the anticancer herbal drug berberine and its analytical application. *Journal of the Chinese Chemical Society, 58*(4), 450–456.
49. Patil, J. B., Kim, J., & Jayaprakasha, G. K. (2010). Berberine induces apoptosis in breast cancer cells (MCF-7) through mitochondrial-dependent pathway. *European Journal of Pharmacology, 645*, 70–78.
50. Li, Y., Li, C. J., Yu, D., et al. (2000). Potent induction of apoptosis by β-lapachone in human multiple myeloma cell lines and patient cells. *Molecular Medicine, 6*, 1008–1015.
51. De Almeida, E. R. (2009). Preclinical and clinical studies of lapachol and beta-lapachone. *The Open Natural Products Journal, 2*, 42–47.
52. Jeong, S. Y., Park, S. J., Yoon, S. M., et al. (2009). Systemic delivery and preclinical evaluation of Au nanoparticle containing β-lapachone for radiosensitization. *Journal of Controlled Release, 139*, 239–245.
53. Fulda, S. (2008). Betulinic acid for cancer treatment and prevention. *International Journal of Molecular Sciences, 9*, 1096–1107.
54. Liao, L. L., Kupchan, S. M., & Horwitz, S. B. (1976). Mode of action of the antitumor compound bruceantin, an inhibitor of protein synthesis. *Molecular Pharmacology, 12*, 167–176.
55. Dubey, K. K., Ray, A. R., & Behera, B. K. (2008). Production of demethylated colchicines through microbial transformation and scale-up process development. *Process Biochemistry, 43*, 251–257.

56. Thomson, P., Naylor, M. A., Everett, S. A., et al. (2006). Synthesis and biological properties of bioreductively targeted nitrothienyl pro-drugs of combretastatin A-4. *Molecular Cancer Therapeutics, 5*, 2886–2894.
57. Ley, C. D., Horsman, M. R., & Kristjansen, P. E. G. (2007). Early effects of combretastatin-A4 disodium phosphate on tumor perfusion and interstitial fluid pressure. *Neoplasia, 9*, 108–112.
58. Molavi, O., Ma, Z., Mahmud, A., & Alshamsan, A. (2008). Polymeric micelles for the solubilization and delivery of STAT3 inhibitor cucurbitacins in solid tumors. *International Journal of Pharmaceutics, 347*, 118–127.
59. Bernard, S. A., & Olayinka, O. A. (2010). Search for a novel antioxidant, anti-inflammatory/analgesic, or antiproliferative drug: Cucurbitacins hold the ace. *Journal of Medicinal Plants Research, 4*, 2821–2826.
60. Sa, G., Das, T., Banerjee, S., et al. (2010). Curcumin: From exotic spice to modern anticancer drug. *Al Ameen Journal of Medical Sciences, 3*, 21–27.
61. Goel, A., Kunnumakkara, A. B., & Aggarwal, B. B. (2008). Curcumin as "Curecumin": From kitchen to clinic. *Biochemical Pharmacology, 75*, 787–789.
62. Surh, Y. J., & Chun, K. S. (2007). Cancer chemopreventive effects of curcumin. In B. B. Aggarwal, Y. J. Surh, & S. Shishodia (Eds.), *The Molecular Targets and Therapeutic Uses of Curcumin in Health and Disease* (pp. 149–172). Springer.
63. Kim, S., Hwang, B. Y., Su, B. N., et al. (2007). Silvestrol, a potential anticancer rocaglate derivative from *Aglaia foveolata*, induces apoptosis in LNCaP cells through the mitochondrial/apoptosome pathway without activation of executioner caspase-3 or -7. *Anticancer Research, 27*, 2175–2183.
64. Lu, C. L., Li, Y. M., Fu, G. Q., et al. (2011). Extraction optimization of daphnoretin from root bark of *Wikstroemia indica* (L.) C. A. and its antitumor activity tests. *Food Chemistry, 124*, 1500–1506.
65. Diogo, C. V., Felix, L., Vilela, S., et al. (2009). Mitochondrial toxicity of the phytochemicals daphnetoxin and daphnoretin—Relevance for possible anti-cancer application. *Toxicology in vitro, 23*, 772–779.
66. Kaufman, P. B., Duke, J. A., Brielmann, H., et al. (1997). A comparative survey of leguminous plants as sources of the isoflavones, genistein and daidzein: Implications for human nutrition and health. *Journal of Alternative & Complementary Medicine, 3*, 7–12.
67. Moon, Y. J., Wang, X., & Morris, M. E. (2006). Dietary flavonoids: Effects on xenobiotic and carcinogen metabolism. *Toxicology in Vitro, 20*, 187–210.
68. Dixon, R. A., & Ferreira, D. (2002). Molecules of interest: Genistein. *Phytochemistry, 60*, 205–211.
69. Kuo, Y. C., Kuo, P. L., Hsu, Y. L., et al. (2006). Ellipticine induces apoptosis through the p53-dependent pathway in human hepatocellular carcinoma HepG2 cells. *Life Sciences, 78*, 2550–2557.
70. Huang, Z., Chen, G., & Shi, P. (2009). Effects of emodin on the gene expression profiling of human breast carcinoma cells. *Cancer Detection and Prevention, 32*, 286–291.
71. Mans, D. R. A., Da Rocha, A. B., & Schwartsmann, G. (2000). Anti-cancer drug discovery and development in Brazil: Targeted plant collection as a rational strategy to acquire candidate anti-cancer compounds. *The Oncologist, 5*, 185–198.

72. Smith, M. E., Cimica, V., Chinni, S., et al. (2008). Rhabdoid tumor growth is inhibited by flavopiridol. *Clinical Cancer Research, 14*, 523–532.
73. Efferth, T., Li, P. C. H., Konkimalla, V. S. B., et al. (2007). From traditional Chinese medicine to rational cancer therapy. *Trends in Molecular Medicine, 13*, 353–361.
74. Nam, S., Buettner, R., Turkson, J., et al. (2005). Indirubin derivatives inhibit Stat3 signaling and induce apoptosis in human cancer cells. *Proceedings of the National Academy of Sciences, 102*, 5998–6003.
75. Liu, X. M., Wung, L. G., Li, H. Y., et al. (1996). Induction of differentiation and downregulation of c-myb gene expression in ML4 human myeloblastic leukemia cells by the clinically effective leukemia agent meisoindigo. *Biochemical Pharmacology, 51*, 1545–1551.
76. Hampson, P., Wang, K., & Lord, J. M. (2005). Treatment of actinic keratoses, acute myeloid leukemia therapy, treatment of basal cell carcinoma, protein kinase C activator. *Drugs of the Future, 30*, 1003.
77. Hazra, B., Sarma, M. D., & Sanyal, U. (2004). Separation methods of quinonoid constituents of plants used in oriental traditional medicines. *Journal of Chromatography B, 812*, 259–275.
78. Herst, P. M., Davis, J. E., Neeson, P., et al. (2009). The anticancer drug, phenoxodiol, kills primary myeloid and lymphoid leukemic blasts and rapidly proliferating T cells. *Hematologica, 94*, 928–934.
79. Pan, L., Chai, H., & Kinghorn, A. D. (2010). The continuing search for antitumor agents from higher plants. *Phytochemistry Letters, 3*, 1–8.
80. Bardona, S., Foussard, V., Fournel, S., et al. (2002). Monoterpenes inhibit proliferation of human colon cancer cells by modulating cell cycle-related protein expression. *Cancer Letters, 181*, 187–194.
81. Yeruva, L., Pierre, K. J., Elegbede, A., et al. (2007). Perillyl alcohol and perillic acid induced cell cycle arrest and apoptosis in non-small cell lung cancer cells. *Cancer Letters, 257*, 216–226.
82. Mi, Q., Cui, B., Silva, G. L., et al. (2001). Pervilleines A: A novel tropane alkaloid that reverses the multidrug resistance phenotype. *Cancer Research, 61*, 4030–4037.
83. Mi, Q., Cui, B., Silva, G. L., et al. (2002). Pervilleines B and C: New tropane alkaloid aromatic esters that reverse multidrug resistance in the hollow fiber assay. *Cancer Letters, 184*, 13–20.
84. Mi, Q., Cui, B., Lantvit, D., et al. (2003). Pervilleine F: A new tropane alkaloid aromatic ester that reverses multidrug resistance. *Anticancer Research, 23*, 3607–3615.
85. Deng, F., Lu, J. J., Liu, H. Y., et al. (2011). Synthesis and antitumor activity of novel salvicine analogues. *Chinese Chemical Letters, 22*, 25–28.
86. Shoeb, M., Celik, S., Jaspars, M., et al. (2005). Isolation, structure elucidation, and bioactivity of schischkiniin, a unique indole alkaloid from the seeds of *Centaurea schischkinii*. *Tetrahedron, 61*, 9001–9006.
87. Kinghorn, D., de Blanco, E. J. C., Chai, H. B., et al. (2009). Discovery of anticancer agents of diverse natural origin. *Pure and Applied Chemistry, 81*, 1051–1063.
88. Kim, J. H., Xu, C., Keum, Y. S., et al. (2006). Inhibition of EGFR signaling in human prostate cancer PC-3 cells by combination treatment with β-phenylethyl isothiocyanate and curcumin. *Carcinogenesis, 27*, 475–482.

89. Liu, Q. (2011). Triptolide and its expanding multiple pharmacological functions. *International Immunopharmacology, 11*, 377–383.
90. Ancuceanu, R. V., & Istudor, V. (2004). Pharmacologically active natural compounds for lung cancer. *Alternative Medicine Review, 9*, 402–419.
91. Helong, L., Liangxing, T., Yongxin, Z., et al. (2017). Improved bioavailability and antitumor effect of docetaxel by TPGS-modified proniosomes: *In vitro* and *in vivo* evaluations. *Scientific Reports, 7*, 43372.
92. Abir, K. P., Dwaipayan, C., Irene, S., et al. (2017). New insights into therapeutic activity and anticancer properties of curcumin. *Journal of Experimental Pharmacology, 9*, 31–45.

Index

D

E

Q

T

W

X

Y

Z

For Product Safety Concerns and Information please contact our EU representative GPSR@taylorandfrancis.com
Taylor & Francis Verlag GmbH, Kaufingerstraße 24, 80331 München, Germany

www.ingramcontent.com/pod-product-compliance
Lightning Source LLC
LaVergne TN
LVHW020627300926
849161LV00004B/635
* 9 7 8 1 9 9 8 5 1 1 7 6 1 *